VITAL YOGA

A SOURCEBOOK FOR STUDENTS AND TEACHERS

META CHAYA HIRSCHL

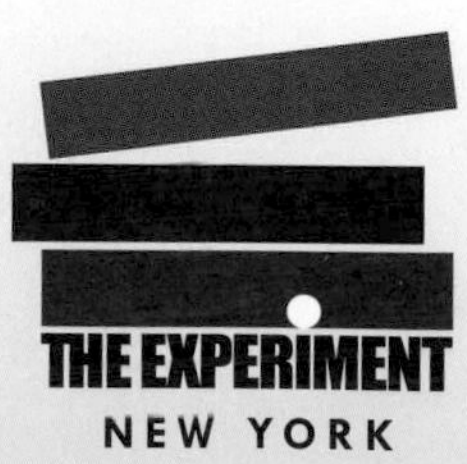
THE EXPERIMENT
NEW YORK

VITAL YOGA: *A Sourcebook for Students and Teachers*

The Experiment, LLC
260 Fifth Avenue
New York, NY 10001–6408
www.theexperimentpublishing.com

The Experiment's books are available at special discounts when purchased in bulk for premiums and sales promotions as well as for fundraising or educational use. For details, contact us at info@theexperimentpublishing.com.

The contents of this book are for educational purposes only and are not intended as a replacement for diagnosis or treatment of any medical or psychiatric ailment. Individuals with such an ailment should first see their physician or psychiatrist for treatment and make use of yoga therapy only as an adjunct to such treatment.

Library of Congress Cataloging-in-Publication Data:

Hirschl, Meta Chaya.
Vital yoga : a sourcebook for students and teachers / Meta Chaya Hirschl.
p. cm.
Originally published: Albuquerque, NM : Prajna Pub. Co., 2010.
Summary: "A resource on yoga practices, including mantras, poses, breath work, meditation, yoga therapy, a historical overview of yoga and yogic texts, and wisdom of both historic and contemporary yogis"— Provided by publisher.
Includes bibliographical references and index.
ISBN 978-1-61519-040-9 (pbk.)—ISBN 978-1-61519-144-4 (ebook) 1. Yoga—Study and teaching. 2. Hatha yoga—Study and teaching. 3. Meditation. 4. Breathing exercises. 5. Yoga—Therapeutic use. I. Title.
RA781.7.H57716 2011
613.7'046076—dc23
2011032905

ISBN 978-1-61519-040-9
Ebook ISBN 978-1-61519-144-4

Cover design by Alison Forner
Front cover illustrations by Jodi Call-Swedberg
Back cover illustration by Angela Werneke
Back cover photographs by Tina Larkin

Interior book design by Pauline Neuwirth of Neuwirth & Associates, Inc., based on an original design by Angela Werneke
Photography by Tina Larkin

Manufactured in the United States of America
Distributed by Workman Publishing Company, Inc.
Distributed simultaneously in Canada by Thomas Allen & Son Ltd.

First published by The Experiment in November 2011
10 9 8 7 6 5 4 3 2 1

Praise for *Vital Yoga*

"[Meta Chaya Hirschl] offers an excellent overview of yoga styles, as well as sections on classical asana, advice on selecting teachers and classes, tips on becoming part of a community, and her take on applying yogic precepts to daily life via 'stealth' yoga. For instructors, Hirschl offers sample yoga sequences and advice about the initial steps of opening a studio. As reference and inspiration, Hirschl's beautifully illustrated compendium will best serve novice students and teachers, as well as those aspiring to change careers."

—*Publishers Weekly*

"Meta Chaya Hirschl's contemporary journey through the wonder of yoga gently nudges superficial fads into perspective and shares refreshingly relevant insights. *Vital Yoga*'s illustrations, poetic imagery, and key texts enrich the inner life of both the teacher and student of yoga: students will inhabit poses with feeling and energy, while teachers will gain pragmatic advice on teaching. This is an aesthetically beautiful book, but above all it is a book permeated with explorative joy!"

—Liz Lark,
yoga teacher based in London, author, retreat leader, and artist

"A book with plenty of heart and lots of information."

—Nicolai Bachman,
author of *The Language of Yoga*

"Meta Chaya Hirschl's enthusiasm and love for yoga shine throughout these pages. Modern and accessible, bridging to the ancient truths, she reaches out to those of us who are yogis and yet don't realize it, those of us who want to grow yet may have been put off by modern-day stereotypes about this ancient science. . . . [The book] also includes a therapeutic view of yoga, which may expand our view of health care for future generations."

—Amadea Morningstar, MA, RPP,
author of *The Ayurvedic Cookbook* and founder of
Ayurveda Polarity and Yoga Therapy Institute in Santa Fe, New Mexico

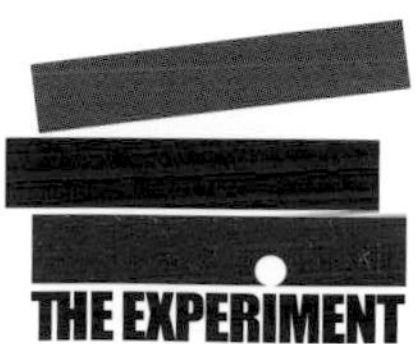

BECAUSE EVERY BOOK IS A TEST OF NEW IDEAS

"The yoga of self-mastery through the breathless state, as practiced for eons in the East, particularly before the Dark Ages, is a very difficult science to investigate. For those looking for a more approachable and less intimidating introduction to the yogas adopted in the West, *Vital Yoga* provides numerous welcoming doors to a bevy of paths and practices."

—Sankara Saranam,
founder of The Pranayama Institute
and author of *God Without Religion*

"*Vital Yoga* supports yoga students on their search for inner freedom. Meta Chaya Hirschl blends her life experiences with the lightness that only wisdom can give. She takes the reader by the hand along the many paths of yoga tradition."

—Rossella Baroncini,
yoga teacher based in Florence, Italy
and longtime student of Vanda Scaravelli

"Having been a student of yoga for fifty years and teaching for twenty, and buying countless books on yoga, I finally stopped buying them, since it seemed there was nothing new to be said. When *Vital Yoga* fell into my hands, I read it cover to cover in one sitting. It is a gem! If a person could have only one book on yoga, Meta's would be the one! It is an invaluable resource for both students and teachers (no matter how many trainings they may have attended)."

—Barbara Luboff,
yoga teacher based in Santa Fe, New Mexico

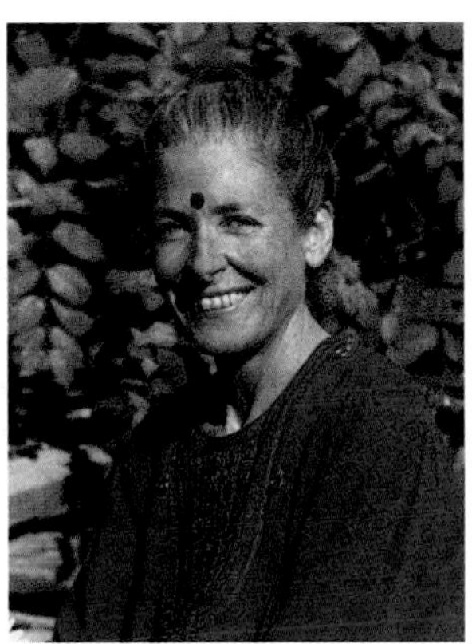

This book is dedicated to Betheyla, my teacher,
who became my colleague and cherished friend.
Betheyla embodied yoga, and I am profoundly grateful
to have been in her presence.

Whenever I visited her in the hospital as she lay dying in the fall of 2007, after the usual discussion on the progress of her illness she wanted to know about my life—what my daughters were doing, how my yoga was going, what was happening in my love life, and how the current astrological array was affecting it all. She was as completely present, engaging, and interested as she'd ever been. And when I looked into her eyes as we compared stories and ideas, I'd stop seeing her shriveled body and instead see only her brilliance, which lit the way of many.

May her memory be a blessing.

Contents

PART III. INTO THE WORLD

Preface

If you'd told me as I was walking the catwalk high in the night sky checking the release valves of the two-story fermenters as a twenty-three-year-old manufacturing supervisor for Miller Brewing Company in Milwaukee, Wisconsin, that later in life I would not only be practicing yoga but teaching it, I would have had a great belly laugh over a few beers with my buddies after work.

If you'd suggested to me at age thirty-three, when I was teaching the use of computers in business to undergraduates at Purdue University and writing software books, that in a later decade I'd be teaching students how to teach yoga, I would have thought you had me confused with someone who actually regarded yoga as more than part of the annoying babble of New Age pomposity.

If you'd said to me while I was sitting in a room with fifty other systems consultants and terminals with cable strung like Christmas lights as we wrote software in the business programming language COBOL for the international management firm Arthur Andersen & Co. that later, to celebrate my fiftieth birthday, I would prefer to sit in a ten-day silent meditation retreat rather than attend an extravagant party, I would have been sure you didn't know me.

Many well-known yoga teachers find yoga at a young age and spend most of their lives in the world of gurus, ashrams, and yoga poses. But I've come to yoga from a different cosmology. I grew up vowing that my work would be about making it in the world, unconstrained by the traditional limitations of women's work: restrictions on job choices, lower pay, often harder work, and usually not self-supporting in a way that allows real freedom. The women I grew up around—my mother, grandmothers, great-grandmother, and neighborhood mothers—almost without exception stayed at home while their husbands worked as professors, doctors, lawyers, or businessmen. And it was always clear to me that the women were at least as smart as the men and often resented the division of labor, and that the men had the better deal in terms of recognition, success, and ease of life. I also listened to Gloria Steinem at Wabash College and Kate Millett at Purdue University and read about all the changes for women happening in the 1970s. So when it came time to choose a major in college, I was motivated by the availability and pay rates of jobs.

This strategy was successful. I did find interesting and challenging jobs in industry, business, and academia. And I was remunerated well enough to support my family and have choices. But something was missing. My options seemed to vary between a burger from McDonald's or Wendy's; veggie burgers or fresh steamed vegetables weren't even on the menus. Whether the job was in a brewery, a corporation, or a university, lifestyle choices didn't seem that different. And, tellingly, I could never make the commitment to stay with any of the jobs more than about five years.

When a partner at Arthur Andersen & Co. made a strong case for me to stick around and move from manager to partner, I looked at him and thought, Why would I want your life? I could see the money and status he had, but ultimately it seemed like such a life just meant long hours, tedious business lunches, and evenings that could be described as glamorous, but only if you didn't mind being told whose trust to cultivate so you could build more business.

When a professor at Purdue University took me aside and with touching sincerity told me I would have a fabulous future as a PhD candidate since I had so much business experience, I looked at him and thought, And then what—I'd be part of your club? The academic life seemed so narrow.

I looked like I knew what I wanted: I appeared strong and confident at work, and was also a wife of twenty years and the mother of two daughters. I was focused about what I thought I should be doing. But once in a while I'd get an inkling that some inner awareness was missing. I remember attending a women's group therapy session in my early thirties and talking about my latest embarrassing exchange while working as the only female manufacturing supervisor in a Pepsi-Cola Bottling Plant in East Canarsie, Brooklyn. I'd insisted to workers that the pornography on the factory equipment be removed, and I was ridiculed, even though I was eventually obeyed. At that point, I said I hated the way I was treated in my workplace. My therapist asked me why I stayed then. I thought for a moment and replied that the job was how I was supporting my husband and myself. Then she asked me what kind of work I'd enjoy. Suddenly I realized that although my dissatisfaction with my job circumstances was obvious I had no idea what I actually wanted. And even though I eventually quit my job and went to graduate school at New York University, it would be years before I could begin cultivating inner awareness and happiness.

It was yoga that helped me forge a connection to my inner self. I took my first yoga class in 1978, while working at an extremely stressful job as a manufacturing supervisor in a graham cracker pie shell plant. I signed up for the yoga class because I was overwhelmed in this first job out of undergraduate school and thought yoga might help. Unfortunately, the yoga teacher discouraged me from continuing after I fell asleep at the end of class, telling me that if I couldn't stay awake I couldn't be a yogi.

Decades later yoga helped me acquire strength and renewed health following an illness. While working as a systems consultant for Consolidated Edison of New York, I had developed a disease described as a triad: asthma, nasal polyps severe enough to eliminate my sense of smell, and continual sinus infections. All the doctors I consulted said the condition was genetic so I would have it for the rest of my life. They recommended taking drugs indefinitely, which were expensive and caused jitteriness, headaches, bloating, and other side effects. Unable to accept this grim prognosis and limited treatment, I explored alternative ways to regain my health. Yoga was the major support for my recovery, in addition to other holistic and surgical solutions. Although yoga didn't eradicate the disease, since it is genetic, as a result of yoga my perspective was transformed. I could see painful truths about my work, my marriage, and my physical well-being, and glimpses into what creates inner happiness in life. Soon, with the help of yoga and other lifestyle changes (finding new work, divorcing, and embarking on a healthy diet without alcohol), I was able to stop taking the drugs.

Finally understanding why I could no longer tolerate work that didn't feed my soul, I began searching for another path. I was determined not to make computers and software my focal points, but I wasn't sure what else I should do. On a yoga retreat in Mexico, I meditated on the question, then asked for divine guidance in my dreams. One morning I woke from a dream in which I was living in Manhattan wearing a 1980s suit that didn't fit and looking for my car. I met a man who told me to stop looking, and then I woke up.

Minutes later I walked to the beach and sat to meditate. I was watching my breath and my mind when I heard a voice instruct me, in a firm yet loving tone: "You didn't get better just for yourself. You must teach yoga and help others feel better, too." A sense of calm melted over me, and I smiled, knowing that was exactly what I had to do. I realized that yoga would require everything I'd learned in life, and I also understood a puzzling episode from my past. Many years before, a friend named Radha had gone home to India to visit her family and returned with an odd gift for me—a large sculpture of Shiva as cosmic dancer—telling me her instinct was that I should have it. I later learned that Shiva as cosmic dancer symbolizes yoga, and I realized just how prescient Radha's gift had been.

Once I knew that my path was teaching yoga, I began to take teacher training courses in earnest. I earned a Registered Yoga Teacher/Therapist 500-hour status, the highest level of training, from Gabriella Hansen; studied with John Friend and his teachers of Anusara yoga; learned from Irene Beer and her translations of Vanda Scaravelli's teachings; trained with Iyengar-inspired teachers, as well as those of more eclectic persuasions; and took college courses in anatomy and physiology.

Initially, I taught yoga from my home, then at various rented spaces and local health clubs. Finally, another teacher advised me that to make a living as a yoga teacher I would have to open a yoga studio so I would have a permanent location for students. Although it was a leap of faith, I wrote a business plan and created the name YogaNow. I liked its sound, its sense of the moment, and the way it mimicked the ancient text of the Yoga Sutras, written in approximately the second century BCE by Patanjali, which begins, "Now, the instruction of yoga."[1]

In March 2001, I opened YogaNow, presided over by the sculpture of Shiva as cosmic dancer announcing that yoga is practiced here (see figure 0.1). Since then I have enjoyed not only teaching yoga but also running retreats and creating a community of individuals who appreciate the benefits of yoga. After teaching yoga for ten years, I am still inspired by the process. When I teach, I feel as if a force much greater and wiser than myself is at work. In fact, when I teach students they also teach me and one another as we explore together the many possibilities for transformation that yoga provides. I have witnessed incredible growth in the students and seen in their eyes such energy and happiness that I know teaching yoga is my mission.

After the studio was opened a few years, students began urging me to also instruct others to teach yoga. I realized, despite the wealth of books on yoga, there was no comprehensive guidebook available on how to teach it. And even though teachers with training and certificates come to teach at YogaNow, although they might know the intricacies of teaching yoga poses they don't always know how to delve into the heart of yoga for their own and their students' liberation. Contrary to widespread belief, yoga is not simply a series of postures to promote flexibility, balance, and strength. Although it does these things, to see it only in such terms is to miss its real potential, for yoga is ultimately about personal transformation. Therefore, teaching yoga does not simply involve instructing students in a series of poses with preferred alignment details. It also guides students to connect to their inner selves through breath awareness, quiet the mind to witness thought, and posture alignment. It encourages students to embrace who they are in the moment and show compassion for others. In addition, teaching yoga requires an understanding of aspects of anatomy, as well as the ability to read bodies energetically to assist students with specific challenges. With this perspective, I developed and then taught a teacher training program, in which I witnessed the incredible blossoming of teachers and students.

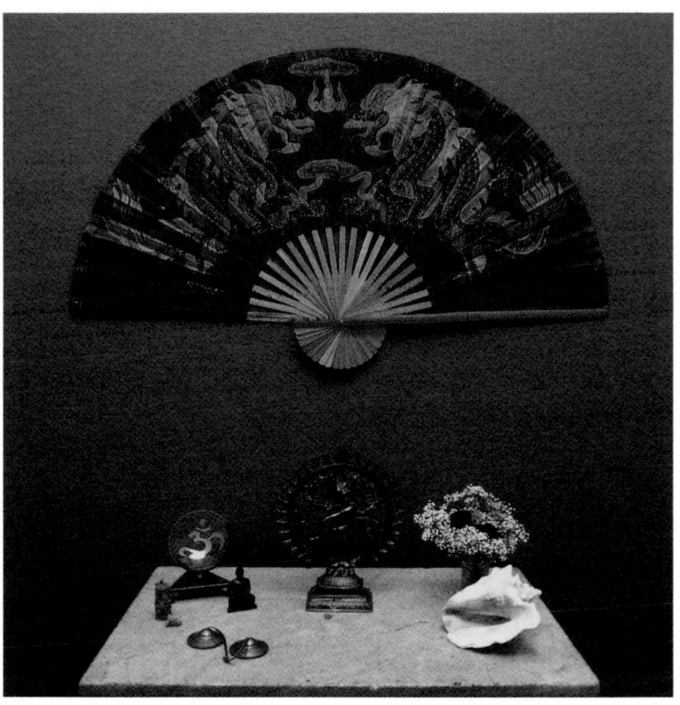

Figure 0.1. Nataraj Shiva on altar at YogaNow studio

Vital Yoga, an outgrowth of those efforts, provides a way to teach yoga first to yourself and then to others, tapping into your unique inner gifts and offering them to the world. As such, the book is a guide for liberation in the fullest sense—freedom from fear of living and dying, freedom from pain and emotional turmoil, and freedom from attachment to the daily stresses and difficulties of life. To reinforce this mission, I've designed the book with multiple learning styles in mind: along with the text there are diagrams; photographs; illustrations; reading, writing, and living assignments; and recipes and other creative projects to aid readers in working with the material in their own manner, in their own time. While some may remember the illustrations more than the words, others may benefit more from journaling, doing assignments, or chanting mantras. The book is also designed to support the reader's gradual transformation, both as a student and, if applicable, while teaching students.

It is intended to enrich any chosen style of practice—such as Ashtanga, Bikram, Iyengar, Anusara, Kripalu, integral, flow, hot, or yin yogas—and doesn't require following anyone other than an inner guru. The book is not, however, a substitute for taking a teacher training course with a professional yoga teacher or for reading the literature of the ancient sages, but is meant to supplement both endeavors.

Finally, it is as much for people who are simply interested in learning more about yoga as for those intent on becoming yoga teachers or for yoga teachers wishing to refresh their perspectives.

Today, we are living in a time of great change and global concern about the welfare of the planet and its inhabitants. I reject the notion that we are doomed. I believe that change begins within, that as we alter ourselves we also alter the world.

Mahatma Gandhi said, "Be the change you wish to see in the world."[2] May you find in this book a way to be the change and then bring it to the world.

Introduction

Yoga is a universal tool for exploring the deeper aspects of body, mind, and spirit. An ancient expression in Sanskrit, *neti neti*, meaning not this, not that, was used to help understand who we are by observing what we are not. With this principle in mind, perhaps we can better comprehend what yoga is by determining what it is not. For example:

Yoga isn't a New Age invention.

It isn't a fad invented by New Age enthusiasts or the marketing geniuses of corporate America. The word *yoga* is first mentioned in the Sanskrit classic the *Rig Veda* in approximately 4000 BCE.[1] Having evolved over at least a few millennia, yoga has had many adherents who have found it useful as a path to liberation and happiness. Since yoga also has benefits for life in the modern world, its popularity has grown along with the interest in many other spiritual disciplines.

Yoga isn't a religion.

While yoga guides us to examine our spiritual aspects and form a deep connection to self, it doesn't impose a belief system on us. And even though many people who practice yoga in India are Hindu, yoga isn't a religion. In fact, it was rejected by Hinduism because yoga does not mandate the existence of God.[2] One of the great yogi sages, Swami Sivananda Saraswati, who helped bring yoga to America by establishing yoga training centers worldwide beginning in the late 1950s, said, "Yoga is not a religion but an aid to the practice of the basic spiritual truths in all religions. Yoga is for all and is universal."[3] Yoga enhances whatever religion we believe in by helping us open to the intrinsic love at our core and then to community and all humanity. In the seminal Yoga Sutras, after discussion about how to overcome obstacles to self-knowledge, it is stated:

> *Or another way,*
> *is persistent meditation*
> *in harmony with your*
> *religious heritage.*[4]

Yoga isn't a fitness program or self-improvement plan.

Although yoga classes are sometimes taught at gyms or health clubs, yoga is not fundamentally concerned with appearance, or even fitness, so much as inner transformation. Yoga practice may in fact make your waist smaller; increase the firmness of your abdominal muscles; build strength, flexibility, and balance; improve posture; and even reduce high blood pressure. But these physical advantages are not the goal of yoga, which is ultimately enlightenment and happiness. Yoga is also unlike self-improvement plans, which imply the existence of some personal deficit and the idea of hostility toward self, to paraphrase American Buddhist nun Pema Chödrön.

Then what is yoga, if not this and not that, *neti neti*? Yoga is an ancient approach to discovering our true nature so we can cultivate our inner gifts and offer them to the world. Yoga is about how to be happy, right now, with exactly what we have. Yoga teaches, through movement and breathing, how to focus attention on our inner self to achieve enlightenment beyond our material world. Yoga offers practice in challenging techniques on the mat so we can take the resulting discipline, flexibility, and balance wherever we go and apply them to daily situations. If we can stay still in Downward Facing Dog Pose, for example, maybe we can remain unperturbed and relaxed the next time we are cut off on the freeway, narrowly escaping an accident after a long day's work. If we can balance in Headstand Pose, perhaps we can balance our needs with those of our loved ones, not accommodating others when it's not good for us. And if we can stay present, watching our breath, in Half Moon Pose, maybe in difficult moments at work or home, we can say to ourselves, "Well, I'll just keep breathing and watching, and allow the experience to happen without a lot of judgment."

Misunderstandings also abound over what is required to teach—or practice—yoga:

You don't have to be a vegetarian to teach or practice yoga.

It's true that the Yoga Sutras discuss a fundamental precept of inner nonviolence that then creates an atmosphere capable of changing the world:

By abiding
in nonviolence,
one's presence
creates an atmosphere
in which hostility ceases.[5]

But although there is widespread agreement that such nonviolence means not killing other human beings, it is not so clear whether it precludes killing to eat. In fact, according to some surveys nearly two-thirds of today's yogis are not vegetarian.[6] Additionally, there are many types of vegetarians, from people who eat no animal products (vegans) to those who eat only animal products that don't require killing, such as milk and eggs (ovo-lacto vegetarians) and individuals who shift eating patterns (flexo-tarians).

It is also true that many yoga practitioners change what they eat after becoming attuned to what feels right and nonviolent in their bodies and to the planet. As we develop strength, flexibility, and balance with focus on our breath, opening energetic channels so our bodies function more efficiently, our desire for foods that support our health increases. You may notice, for example, that even though eating a quart of ice cream may be your first inclination when you're depressed after a difficult conversation with a parent or friend, upon sensing your body's needs you may select another type of self-care, such as a restorative yoga pose, a walk in the park, or sitting quietly and meditating. A teacher-training student in her sixties recently reported that every Memorial Day during her adult life she had eaten two hamburgers with her family. This year she only wanted one, and figured that next year she'd eat something else entirely. The important thing is to choose a diet based on your experiences, not on some externally imposed mandate.

You don't have to be strong, flexible, and have good balance to teach or practice yoga.

The common concern that to teach or practice yoga you have to be strong, flexible, and have good balance is ironic since one goal of yoga postures is to create strength, flexibility, and good balance. In fact, teachers graced with extreme flexibility often have to work harder to understand the challenges faced by most yoga students, who struggle with inflexibility and tightness.

Gaining strength, flexibility, and good balance through yoga practice leads to increased physical well-being and also a decreased risk of accidents. And it improves mental and emotional clarity, suppleness, and equanimity so we are less likely to get upset when plans change or friends disappoint us.

You don't have to be in good shape or of a certain age to teach or practice yoga.

People of all ages and physical conditions, including individuals with disabilities, become students and eventually take teacher training and benefit enormously. Since the work of yoga is ultimately inner work, all individuals can focus on that aspect. Additionally, there are so many poses, as well as modifications, that everyone can practice physical yoga as well.

You don't have to travel to India to teach or practice yoga.

Many people have a perception that authentic yoga is only practiced in India. Yoga used to be practiced primarily by Indians, and the yoga practiced during Patanjali's time was for men and nonhouseholders only. Today, however, yoga is practiced worldwide by all types of people. According to a *Yoga Journal* survey, 15.8 million Americans were practicing yoga in February 2008. Bill Harper, publisher of *Yoga Journal*, said, "Yoga is no longer simply a singular pursuit but a lifestyle choice and an established part of our health and cultural landscape. People come to yoga and stick with it because they want to live healthier lives."[7]

Americans want healthier lives, less stress, a deeper connection to their inner self, and better relationships with one another—all objectives of yoga. In the United States, it is possible to practice a wide range of yoga styles, including flow yoga; hot yoga; therapeutic yoga for specific sports or ailments; and brand yogas, such as Iyengar, Ashtanga, Bikram, Anasura, Kundalini, and Svaroopa. Famous teachers from India and from the United States travel all over the country, as well as offer retreats around the world. Teacher training programs exist in most cities, and yoga classes are available in numerous yoga studios and almost all gyms and universities.

You don't have to learn Sanskrit to teach or practice yoga.

Sanskrit is the ancient language used in writings about yoga and also spoken around the world to refer to the names of yoga poses. Even so, learning Sanskrit while practicing yoga is optional. Some teachers use only the English translation of poses, while others use not only the Sanskrit names for poses but also Sanskrit words and phrases throughout their classes. Because Sanskrit is a mantric language, whose sounds vibrate with our being at all levels, including the cellular, saying pose names or other words in Sanskrit may enable students to experience the poses more deeply. For readers who wish to learn the names of key poses and more in Sanskrit, a glossary of Sanskrit terms is included at the end of the book.

Yoga is beneficial for achieving many goals. You may be searching for more meaning, joy, and peace in your life. Or perhaps you are looking for help with life's stresses and seek more balance. Or maybe you believe in the power of body, mind, and spirit and want to manifest these beliefs. Whatever attracts you to it, as you begin practicing yoga or preparing to become a yoga teacher it is helpful to remember the following. Come to yoga with an empty stomach and an open mind; other helpful qualities are enthusiasm, sincerity, perseverance, willingness to explore your inner self, and a sense of humor. It is important to give yourself time and space to explore your inner self with an attitude of curiosity and joy, as if you were a child investigating playground equipment for the first time—the swings, merry-go-round, teeter-totter. Such an attitude will facilitate progress both on the mat and off the mat in daily life.

Consider, for example, a retired couple in their sixties and seventies who began practicing yoga, enthusiastically embracing the connection to their bodies and their inner selves. After traveling to Ecuador, they reported that while much younger adventurers had had trouble with balance and anxiety, especially while taking small boats around the Galapagos Islands, they themselves had moved about spryly and confidently, both on water and when climbing steep steps to monuments. The yogis were pleased that the strength, flexibility, and balance they had acquired through yoga had allowed them to journey easily to this and other world cultures.

The way yoga can transform people mentally, emotionally, and spiritually is equally impressive. For example, one of my students told me that she'd suffered from depression for most of her life but since practicing yoga she'd not only felt better but been able to stop taking antidepressants. Another student related how yoga had first brought her relief from physical aches and pains and then opened up a connection to others in the yoga studio community and ultimately people everywhere. In short, yoga cannot solve all personal problems or eradicate all social ills, but it is a major catalyst for all aspects of physical, mental, emotional, and spiritual growth.

This book offers a way to approach yoga by reading ancient and contemporary sacred texts, doing writing and life assignments, and experimenting with various yoga poses and methods of learning the discipline. It differs from other books about yoga primarily by encouraging readers to explore other texts that support the study of yoga, as well as investigate several methods and techniques for practicing yoga to access what works best for transforming body, mind, and spirit. As Pema Chödrön says, "Live your life as an experiment."[8]

Vital Yoga is divided into three parts, or *padas* (Sanskrit for "feet"), mimicking the terminology of the Yoga Sutras. The first *pada*, "Before the Mat," details the rich history and philosophy that gave birth to yoga and how we can enrich our experience of yoga before coming to the mat.

The second *pada*, "On the Mat," describes the many options for yoga practice, including *pranayama*-based breath work, *bandhas* and mudras, and meditation. This *pada* also includes key anatomical terms, core strength practices, and broad categories of poses for both yoga teachers and practitioners.

Finally, the third *pada*, "Into the World," focuses on using yoga to change our experience of daily life and to affect the external world in a positive manner both through actions—karma yoga—and through attitude and verbal skills, using a model of relationship called Nonviolent Communication. This *pada* also addresses basic yoga therapy and ways to make yoga a profession.

Following the *padas* are a glossary of Sanskrit words and phrases and three appendixes: a table of poses, a student waiver agreement, and a listing of sample classes at various levels.

Although *Vital Yoga* follows a logical progression from personal practice to use of yoga in the world, it is possible to read some sections of the book independently to gain information for solving immediate problems.

For example, to learn what to do for a sore back, you can read the section "General Principles of Yoga Therapy"; to figure out how to talk to your boss without yelling, it might be helpful to look at "The Nonviolent Communication Model"; if you've always wondered what the ethical considerations of yoga are, you might read "The Foundational Texts of Yoga." Additional information, highlighted throughout, allows you to learn more about Sanskrit ("Sanskrit Gems") and teachers' experiences ("Sages Say") while reading the chapters, or later as your interest is drawn to a particular topic.

English spellings of Sanskrit pose names vary widely across texts, because some sounds don't exist in English and some conventions aren't easy to apply. This book uses the common spellings except in transliterations of the Sanskrit Devanagari appearing in the margins of chapter 6.

The models demonstrating poses in these chapters reflect the diversity of people drawn to yoga. The three yogis showing variations of the same poses in chapters 6 are Wyatt Heard, age eighty-three, who was a District Court judge in Houston before being bitten by the yoga bug; Cypresse Emery, age thirty-five, who has been in love with yoga since 1994, upon attending her first yoga class; and the author, Meta Chaya Hirschl, age fifty-two, who has been practicing and teaching yoga for fifteen years. Also appearing in chapter 6, as well as chapters 4, 5, and 8, is Lisa Keck who, passionate about working with overlooked groups, teaches yoga to incarcerated populations and to parent-child teams.

The models for poses in chapter 8 are Dharmashakti, Felice, and Leah. Dharmashakti is a certified hatha yoga and therapeutic yoga instructor, mediation teacher, and ordained minister, as well as an inspired kirtan leader. Felice began doing yoga in 2001 to find relief from stress and chronic back and shoulder pain. Yoga brought her not only strength but also an ability to recognize when to seek challenge, when to slow down and listen to her body and instincts, and when to release situations over which she has little or no control. For Leah, yoga is about finding balance. "Through asanas and meditation," she says, "I gain a sense of freedom and ease that helps alleviate the struggles I create for myself."

The models in chapter 9 include Irene, Jenny, and Ross, all of whom have benefited from yoga therapy. Yoga has helped Irene with flexibility and knee problems; aided Jenny, who began as a dancer, with recovery from many injuries and maintenance of her general health; and alleviated Ross's low back pain and sciatica.

Throughout your own practice of yoga, while working with the many variables that exist in this discipline, keep in mind the following verse from an ancient text, proposing that everything is already perfect as it is:

All is perfect,
So perfectly perfect!
Whatever being lives, moves
And breathes on Earth
At every level from atom
To galaxy is absolutely
Perfect in its place. . . .[9]

Whether you've been teaching for years, are contemplating becoming a teacher, or wish to delve more deeply into the world of yoga, I bow to you from the depth of my soul as we join hands on this powerful playground of life.

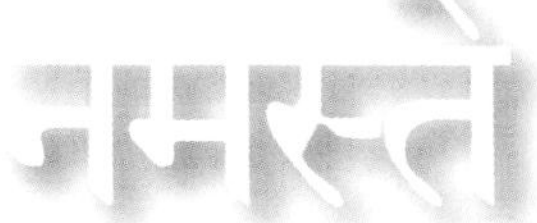

***Namaste* in Sanskrit Devanagari, meaning "I bow to you"**

PART I

BEFORE THE MAT

Yoga is so much more than the poses many people equate with it as seen on TV, at the gym, or in advertisements. Before considering the central topics of practicing poses, breathing, and meditation, we'll look at yoga from a historical perspective, including its foundational texts and the role of vibration in yoga practice.

Chapter 1, "A Panoramic View of History and Ideas," focuses on the history of yoga, first from the point of view of general themes and then from the perspective of foundational texts of yoga that exemplify these periods. Included is a discussion of how modern manifestations of yoga developed and the styles currently practiced today, which are described in many modern sources, including Web sites, video, CDs, and DVDs. Knowledge of how yoga developed up to and including its current forms provides a solid basis for determining which style would be best for you now and evaluating new yoga approaches you encounter.

Chapter 2, "The Foundational Texts of Yoga," looks at some of the pivotal ideas of yoga, beginning with the seminal book on the subject, the Yoga Sutras by Patanjali, and how its principles relate to modern life. Next, the Bhagavad Gita—a dialogue about gaining awareness between a warrior and his charioteer who is also his God—is discussed. Ways to use the ideas in your own life are included. Modern commentaries and translations are suggested to further explore the foundational texts of yoga.

Chapter 3, "Vibration As Tool," first focuses on Sanskrit, the language of yoga, the sounds of which cause vibrations in the body. We consider a few of the most commonly used Sanskrit words and how to write them in their original form. Then the topic of energetics in yoga and the chakras are discussed with suggestions for ways to experience them. Mantras, potent vibrational tools chosen for specific transformative purposes, such as healing, enlightenment, or wholeness, are introduced. Possible reasons why the number 108 is special to yogis are discussed, and finally the *koshas*, or layers of existence, are described.

CHAPTER ONE

A Panoramic View of History and Ideas

HISTORICAL OVERVIEW OF YOGA

The study of history and ideas is a good theoretical underpinning for your yoga education and also helps in understanding the divergent approaches to yoga taught today. You may have attributed the different attitudes and styles of yoga teachers to the natural differences and preferences among individuals, but differing approaches are also rooted in the philosophy and history of yoga. The following incidents highlight two distinct methods of teaching yoga and how they derive from the history of yoga.

Once while I was on holiday and taking a yoga class, as I usually do wherever I go, after class the teacher announced a special yoga workshop with a highly gifted teacher from India who'd studied with a famous yogi, B.K.S. Iyengar. The studio teacher also taught in the Iyengar tradition, which includes the use of props and detailed alignment instructions while holding poses for minutes at a time. Because I respected her, I signed up for the workshop, even though the Iyengar tradition was not my usual approach to yoga.

When I arrived at the workshop, the visiting teacher called me over and told me to turn around. I was wearing a top that read in Sanskrit Devanagari on the front, "*Yogah citta vritta nirodhah*" ("Yoga is the cessation of the fluctuations of the mind"); across the back it read, "Don't believe everything you think," which is a loose translation of a famous verse in the ancient Yoga Sutras. He shook his head and said, "No, that isn't correct." I shrugged and replied, "It's a way to make the verse more accessible." He repeated, "No, it is not correct," at which point I took my seat on my mat.

The visiting teacher was friendlier as he taught poses, until we were in a pose called Triangle, lined up along the wall. He said to move the top of our ribs down, after which I heard a loud slap. I looked up and saw that he'd hit the studio teacher to "help her ribs move down." Then he again instructed us to move our ribs down and, one by one, slapped the yogis on the ribs. As he approached me, I tried to decide what to do because I did not want to be struck. Fortunately, we changed poses before he got to me. Despite my misgivings, the studio teacher later said that she had found the slap helpful and loving, and felt her practice had progressed enormously because of it.

By contrast, another time I attended teacher training taught by an instructor who at the beginning of classes had us sit in a comfortable posture with closed eyes while he led us through a meditation. Then he asked each of us to imagine what our lives would be like if we believed we were intrinsically good, and even perfect, exactly as we existed in the moment. After that, he led the practice of poses with cues like "Open your heart" and "Radiate the light to the universe." While in the Triangle Pose, he encouraged us to "shine toward the heavens," focusing on the inner experience in addition to his external alignment instructions.

The teacher who slapped students was inspired by a classical approach, following in the tradition of his teacher, B.K.S. Iyengar. According to his approach, spirit and matter are separate, and it is advantageous to break through matter (the body) to get to spirit. Thus, hitting might be done out of a sincere desire to help students find poses to move them toward enlightenment. In contrast, the instructor of the teacher training session would find hitting a student antithetical to his concept of yoga, based on the sacredness of the body as a conduit for the Divine, as in the tantric tradition. Both teachers were trying to help their students, but they used methods originating in different philosophical foundations of yoga.

To provide a context for understanding these and other approaches to yoga, let's look at the general philosophies and periods of yoga. Figure 1.1 shows a panoramic view of the history of yoga. The main horizontal line denotes the periods: Vedic, preclassical (epic), classical, postclassical (tantric), and modern. Because the exact dates of yoga history and development are widely debated among scholars, dates are given in ranges. Below the line are principal texts of the periods and some key historical figures.

Here we'll look at a historical overview of yoga and then review the texts associated with various periods by reading short excerpts from them. Evidence of the beginnings of yoga can be seen on stone seals unearthed from the ancient Indus-Sarasvati civilization that flourished from about 2500 to 1500 BCE, beginning perhaps as early as 5000 BCE. These seals

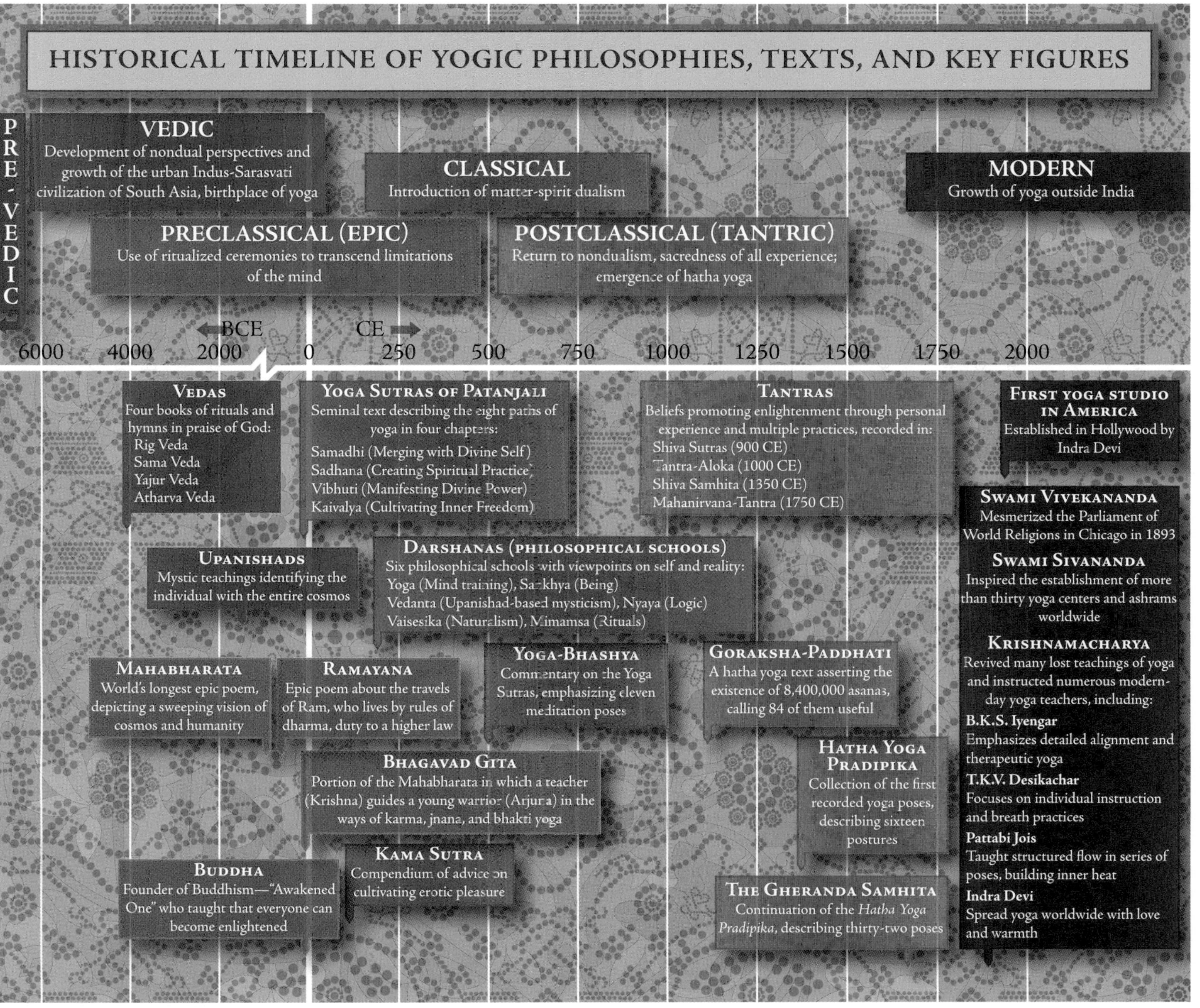

HISTORICAL TIMELINE OF YOGIC PHILOSOPHIES, TEXTS, AND KEY FIGURES
PRE-VEDIC
VEDIC
Development of nondual perspectives and growth of the urban Indus-Sarasvati civilization of South Asia, birthplace of yoga
CLASSICAL
Introduction of matter-spirit dualism
MODERN
Growth of yoga outside India
PRECLASSICAL (EPIC)
Use of ritualized ceremonies to transcend limitations of the mind
POSTCLASSICAL (TANTRIC)
Return to nondualism, sacredness of all experience; emergence of hatha yoga
BCE
CE
6000
4000
2000
0
250
500
750
1000
1250
1500
1750
2000
VEDAS
Four books of rituals and hymns in praise of God:
Rig Veda
Sama Veda
Yajur Veda
Atharva Veda
YOGA SUTRAS OF PATANJALI
Seminal text describing the eight paths of yoga in four chapters:
Samadhi (Merging with Divine Self)
Sadhana (Creating Spiritual Practice)
Vibhuti (Manifesting Divine Power)
Kaivalya (Cultivating Inner Freedom)
TANTRAS
Beliefs promoting enlightenment through personal experience and multiple practices, recorded in:
Shiva Sutras (900 CE)
Tantra-Aloka (1000 CE)
Shiva Samhita (1350 CE)
Mahanirvana-Tantra (1750 CE)
FIRST YOGA STUDIO IN AMERICA
Established in Hollywood by Indra Devi
UPANISHADS
Mystic teachings identifying the individual with the entire cosmos
DARSHANAS (PHILOSOPHICAL SCHOOLS)
Six philosophical schools with viewpoints on self and reality:
Yoga (Mind training), Sankhya (Being)
Vedanta (Upanishad-based mysticism), Nyaya (Logic)
Vaisesika (Naturalism), Mimamsa (Rituals)
SWAMI VIVEKANANDA
Mesmerized the Parliament of World Religions in Chicago in 1893
SWAMI SIVANANDA
Inspired the establishment of more than thirty yoga centers and ashrams worldwide
KRISHNAMACHARYA
Revived many lost teachings of yoga and instructed numerous modern-day yoga teachers, including:
B.K.S. Iyengar
Emphasizes detailed alignment and therapeutic yoga
T.K.V. Desikachar
Focuses on individual instruction and breath practices
Pattabi Jois
Taught structured flow in series of poses, building inner heat
Indra Devi
Spread yoga worldwide with love and warmth
MAHABHARATA
World's longest epic poem, depicting a sweeping vision of cosmos and humanity
RAMAYANA
Epic poem about the travels of Ram, who lives by rules of dharma, duty to a higher law
YOGA-BHASHYA
Commentary on the Yoga Sutras, emphasizing eleven meditation poses
GORAKSHA-PADDHATI
A hatha yoga text asserting the existence of 8,400,000 asanas, calling 84 of them useful
BHAGAVAD GITA
Portion of the Mahabharata in which a teacher (Krishna) guides a young warrior (Arjuna) in the ways of karma, jnana, and bhakti yoga
HATHA YOGA PRADIPIKA
Collection of the first recorded yoga poses, describing sixteen postures
KAMA SUTRA
Compendium of advice on cultivating erotic pleasure
BUDDHA
Founder of Buddhism—"Awakened One" who taught that everyone can become enlightened
THE GHERANDA SAMHITA
Continuation of the Hatha Yoga Pradipika, describing thirty-two poses

Figure 1.1

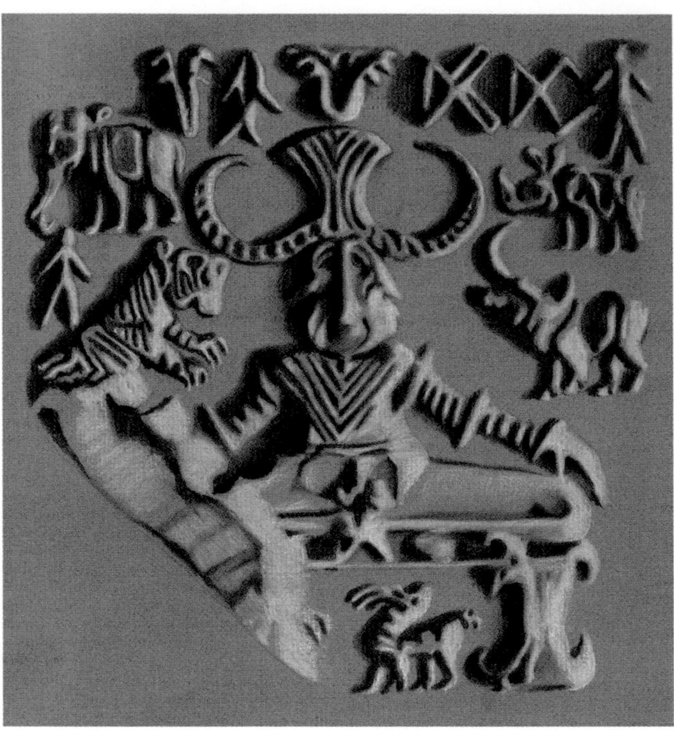

Figure 1.2. An artist's interpretation of the Pashupati seal

show yoga positions, such as the famous Pashupati seal depicting a person in a Lotus Pose, the classical position for sitting meditation (see figure 1.2). The Indus-Sarasvati civilization was a highly developed culture with multistory buildings, granaries, baths with drainage systems that led into brick-lined sewers, and many art forms as evidenced by pottery and bronze and copper objects. The Sarasvati River flowed between 5000 and 1800 BCE, when it began drying up, probably due to tectonic shifts in the Himalayas. The map in figure 1.3 shows the locations of these ancient civilizations in northwest India and today's Pakistan.

The first mention of the word *yoga* is in the Vedas, composed as early as around 4000 BCE. The term *Veda,* which comes from the root *vid,* to know, means knowledge. The Vedic period is marked by the literature of the Vedas, consisting of four books, the earliest of which is the *Rig Veda,* where the word *yoga* first appears. The other Vedas are the *Sama Veda, Yajur Veda,* and *Atharva Veda.* According to some scholars, the *Rig Veda* is the most ancient book in the world and contains sacred hymns that are considered unparalleled in global literature.[1]

Sanskrit Gem

Upanishad **is derived from the words** ***upa*** **(near),** ***ni*** **(down), and** ***s(h)ad*** **(to sit) and means sitting down near.**

The Vedas describe how to honor the Divine, including the use of prayers, hymns, mantras, and ritual specifications, all of which are sacred texts to Hindus. Many people consider the essence, or knowledge portion, of the Vedas to be the Upanishads. The word *Upanishad* means the inner or mystic teaching. In the quiet of the forest hermitages, the Upanishad thinkers would ponder questions of deep concern and communicate their knowledge to the students sitting near them eager to learn the secret doctrine. The philosophy of the Upanishads, involving the identity of the individual soul and the Supreme Soul, is sublime, profound, and soul stirring. They focus essentially on monism—that all is God or the Absolute—and reveal deep spiritual truths.

Great philosophers and writers have read these texts for inspiration. For example, the German philosopher Arthur Schopenhauer, whose book *The World As Will and Idea* was influenced by the *Chandogya Upanishad,* held that the Upanishads were the most beneficial and elevating study ever produced, stating, "It has been the solace of my life, it will be the solace of my death!"[2] Central ideas of the Upanishads are also reflected in Walt Whitman's *Song of Myself,* such as the transcendence of the ego, immanence of God, and intuitability of knowledge.

The preclassical, or epic, period (see figure 1.4) is marked by two great stories of India: the *Mahabharata* and the *Ramayana*. India's official name is Bharat; in fact, the first clause of the Constitution begins with the words "India, that is Bharat."

The *Mahabharata,* the longest epic poem in the world, telling of heroic struggles between families and complex battles, includes the Bhagavad Gita or *Song of God* (see discussion in chapter 2). The Bhagavad Gita describes the yoga of action, devotion, and wisdom. Still read today by yogis, it is now available in new, more accessible translations that capture in contemporary language the excitement and inspiration of the original text.

Dushanbe
Kabul
Islamabad
New Delhi
Kathmandu
Thimphu
Dhaka
Rangoon
Colombo

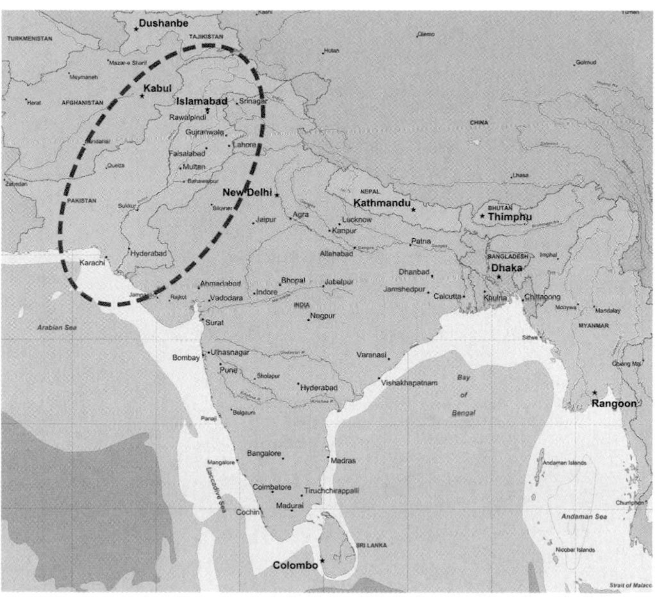

Figure 1.3. Ancient Indus-Sarasvati civilization, birthplace of yoga

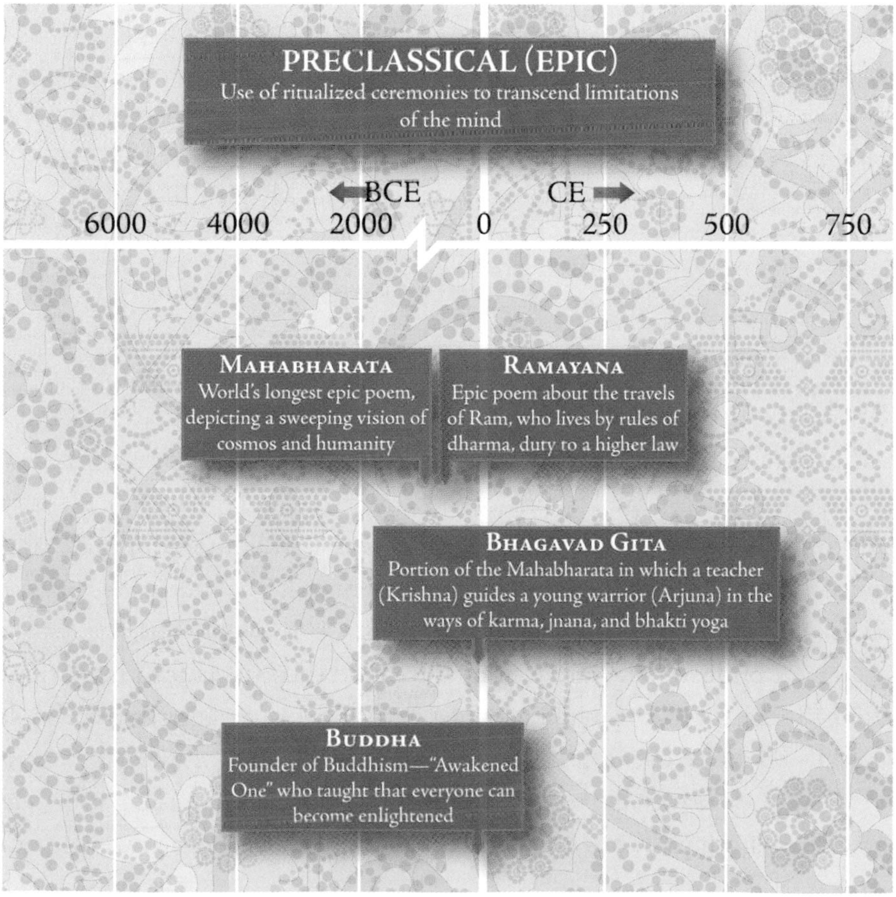

PRECLASSICAL (EPIC)
Use of ritualized ceremonies to transcend limitations of the mind
BCE
CE
6000
4000
2000
0
250
500
750
MAHABHARATA
World's longest epic poem, depicting a sweeping vision of cosmos and humanity
RAMAYANA
Epic poem about the travels of Ram, who lives by rules of dharma, duty to a higher law
BHAGAVAD GITA
Portion of the Mahabharata in which a teacher (Krishna) guides a young warrior (Arjuna) in the ways of karma, jnana, and bhakti yoga
BUDDHA
Founder of Buddhism—"Awakened One" who taught that everyone can become enlightened

Sanskrit Gem

Mahabharata is derived from the words *maha*, meaning big, great, and *bharatas*, descendants of the legendary king Bharata. The word *maha* is used often in yogic circles, as in *maharishi*, a great one with the ability to see (*rishi* means seer) and *maha mantra*, a great mantra.

Figure 1.4. Preclassical (epic) period

The *Ramayana* is usually interpreted as the travels of Rama, a mythic hero of astounding power and an incarnation of Vishnu (the preserver)—one of a triad representing the forms of the Supreme Being in Hinduism, which also includes Brahma (the creator) and Shiva (the destroyer). Three is an important number in yoga, associated with the ongoing cycle of birth, continuance, and death, or transformation. We all experience this cycle in our lives—each moment, day, or project has a beginning, middle, and end. As Sogyal Rinpoche, author of *The Tibetan Book of Living and Dying*, reminds us, we know only two things for sure: we will all die, and no one us knows when.[3] Remembering these two basic facts can motivate us to live our lives more fully.

Sanskrit Gem

Nataraj **combines the words** ***nata*****, meaning dance, and** ***raj*****, meaning royal.**

Other ways to relate to these deities is to think of them as manifestations of human characteristics and behaviors. One manifestation of Shiva, as mentioned earlier, is as cosmic dancer, *Nataraj* (see figure 1.5), demonstrating the rhythms of the universe combined with the cycles of creation and destruction. Dance helps us use the body to transcend the intellect and connect to our inner energies just as yoga does and thus represents yoga. When we practice yoga, we connect to our bodies and waves of energy, allowing us to experience not some intellectual idea of happiness but a bodily joy and feeling of universality that can forge the foundation of our spiritual life. Although such feelings may be fleeting when we begin practicing yoga, as we continue they occur more and more often.

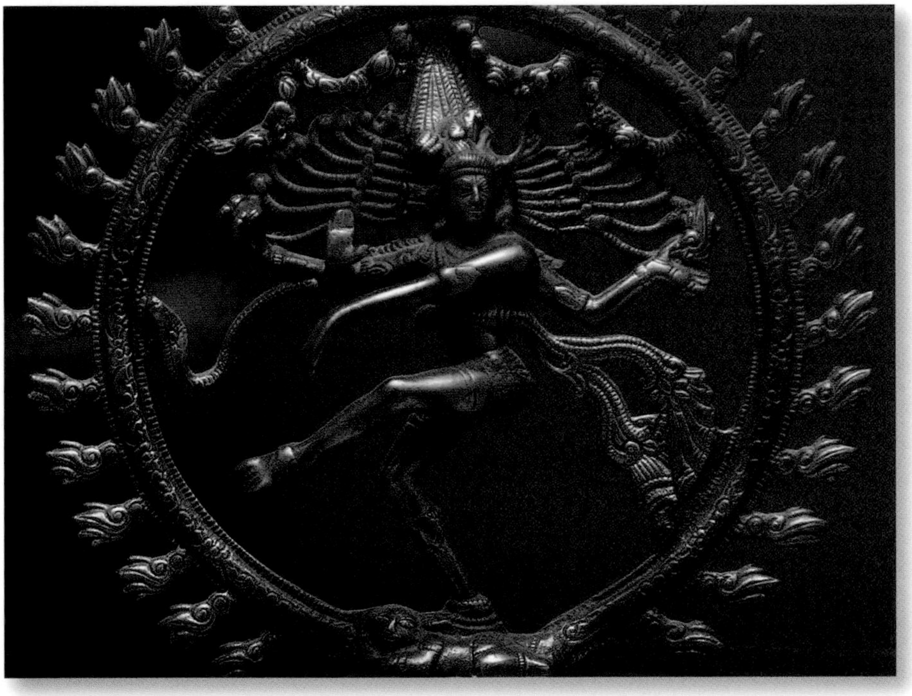

Figure 1.5. Shiva as cosmic dancer

The classical period (see figure 1.6) is defined by Patanjali's Yoga Sutras, which identify an eight-limbed path for reaching liberation, or enlightenment, through yoga (see discussion in chapter 2). The Yoga Sutras also describe a dualistic vision of the world, consisting of matter (*Prakriti*) and spirit (*Purusha*). Liberation and happiness, *kaivalya* or *moksha,* is found by overcoming the material world, including the body, to realize the spiritual realm. The path to *kaivalya* or *moksha* is to work through the body to realize the spirit in this dualistic view of the world.

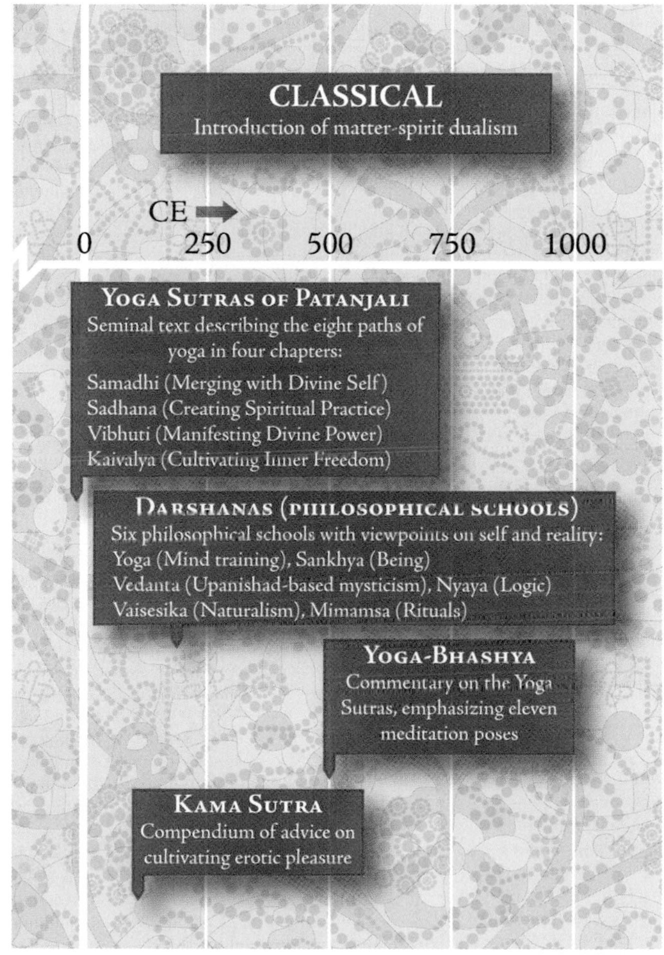

Figure 1.6. Classical period

During the period between 2 and 10 CE, six classical schools of Indian philosophy, called *darshanas,* evolved, of which yoga is one. Following is a brief summary of each school:

1. Yoga is the path of witnessing inner states to experientially find happiness within by entering the state of ecstasy, bliss, freedom, pure consciousness, and enlightenment, also known as *samadhi.*
2. *Sankhya,* meaning that which explains the whole, offers a method for dealing with all levels of manifestation—matter, consciousness, intelligence, the fundamental elements (*gunas*) of stability, activity, and lightness, the mind, cognitive and active senses, and the elements of earth, fire, water, air, and space.
3. *Vedanta,* translated as end of Vedas or the cultivation of knowledge, is a method of contemplative self-inquiry leading to the realization of one's true nature.
4. *Nyaya,* meaning that which leads the mind to a conclusion, is the study of the elements and states of matter: earth, fire, water, air, and space.
5. *Vaisesika,* originally proposed by the sage Kanada (or Kanabhuk—literally, atom-eater), postulates that all objects in the physical universe are reducible to a finite number of atoms.
6. *Mimamsa,* which is fundamental to *Vedanta* and has deeply influenced Hindu law, gives rules for the interpretation of the Vedas and provides a philosophical justification for Vedic ritual.

Sanskrit Gem

***Hatha* combines the words *ha*, meaning sun, and *tha*, meaning moon, and *hath* means to be severe. *Tantra* can mean that which expands wisdom, to weave, or book.**

The postclassical, or tantric, period (see figure 1.7) gave rise to the type of yoga most practiced today—hatha yoga, which grew out of an experimentation with Tantra, a complex philosophy with much older roots though it flourished from about the fourth to ninth century CE. Tantra was revolutionary, in part because the yoga practices it spawned for the first time included women and householders. In contrast to the classical dualistic perspective, Tantra maintains there is no division between spirit and matter; all things are sacred. Consequently, the body is not to be overcome but rather embraced as a means toward liberation. The seeds of these ideas already existed in the Upanishads thousands of years earlier, but Tantra took them further and appealed to many more groups, including Buddhists. Tantric texts include *Tantra-Aloka, Mahanirvana-Tantra, Shiva Samhita,* and *Shiva Sutras.*

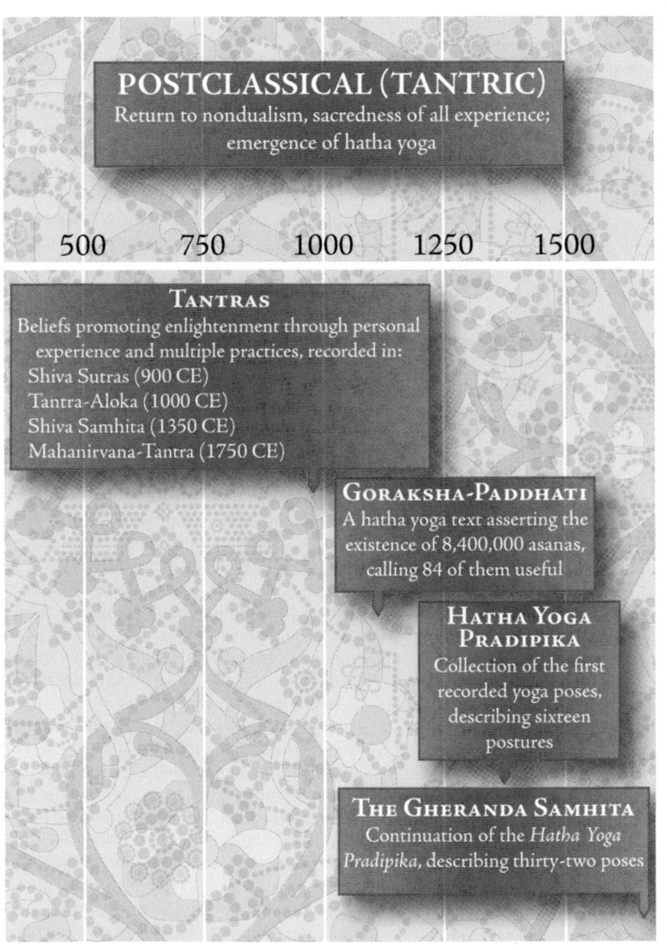

Figure 1.7. Postclassical (tantric) period

Tantra encompasses many strains, all of which focus on personal experience and experimentation. And since Tantra regards all experience as sacred, once-taboo topics like sex, death, and excretion could at last be discussed. For example, there is a "left-handed" school of Tantra that includes going into instead of avoiding sacred places like cemeteries and working ritualistically with the dead using the senses to transcend momentary reality and achieve bliss in the spiritual realm.

A central idea of Tantra is that the energy of the body, *prana,* flows like two rivers representing the masculine and feminine forces, which start at the base of the spine and spiral upward to the crown of the head (see figure 1.8), a concept known as Kundalini. Both the masculine energy (identified with Shiva) and the feminine energy (identified with Shiva's consort, Shakti) are valued. The path to liberation involves opening the thousands of energetic pathways, called *nadis,* that run throughout the body so that the flow of masculine and feminine energy can rise up the central channel, the *sushumna nadi.* The *nadis* form vortices, or wheels (chakras, in Sanskrit), along the spine, all of which must be open for the Kundalini energy to flow in both directions and extend to every part of the body. Hatha yoga developed from this tantric notion as a way to unleash the rivers of energy.

Sanskrit Gem

***Kundalini* means coiling like a snake.**

Statistics citing that 16.5 million Americans are practicing yoga refer to students of hatha yoga.[4] In hatha yoga, the body is viewed as a channel through which the Kundalini rises when the *nadis* are opened through oppositional movements—for example, pressing down with the feet and legs and lifting up with the torso and the arms. Ultimately, this opening allows the yogi to sit quietly and meditate for long periods of time so that the mind stills and the body, mind, and spirit become one.

During the modern period, specifically between 1800 and the 1900s, yoga spread to the West as yoga masters began to travel. A major turning

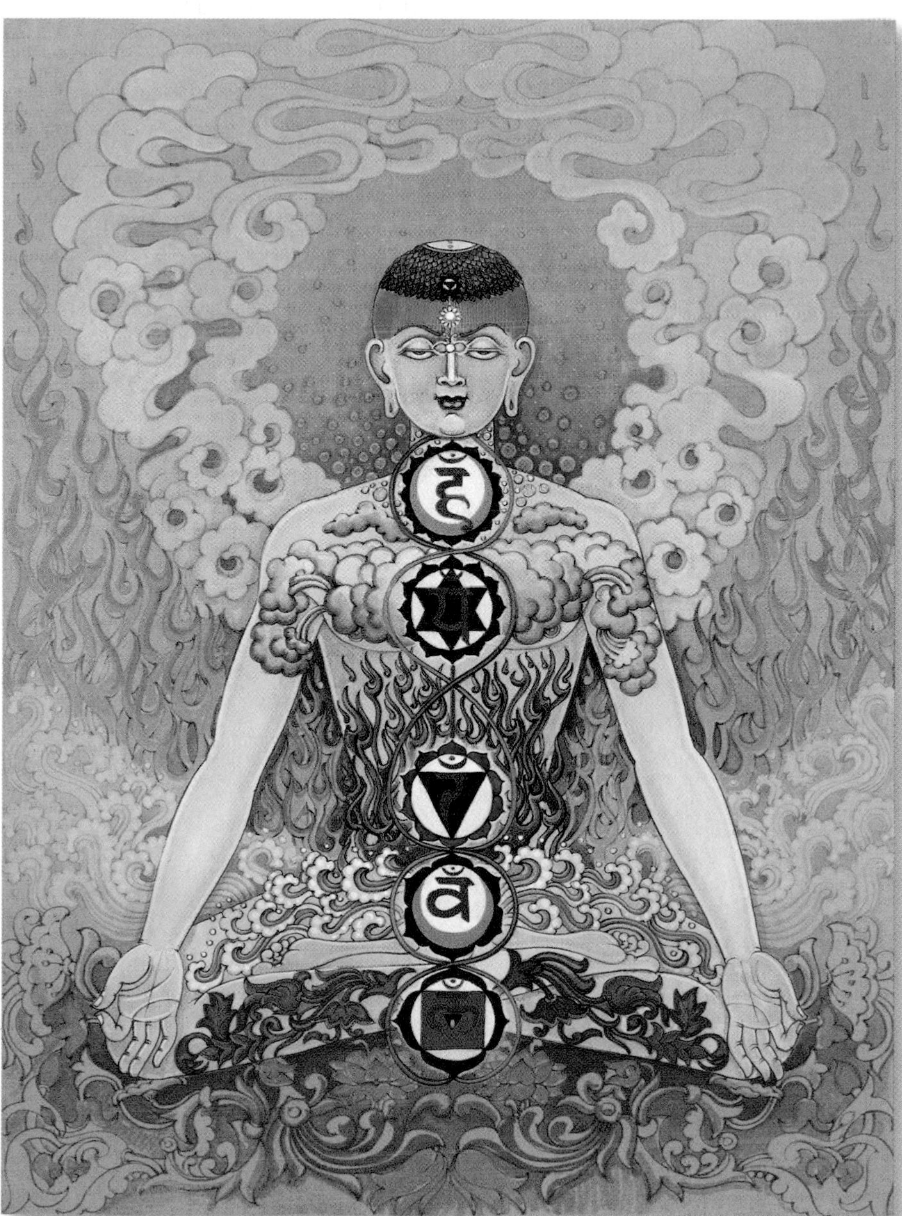

Figure 1.8. Kundalini energy channels

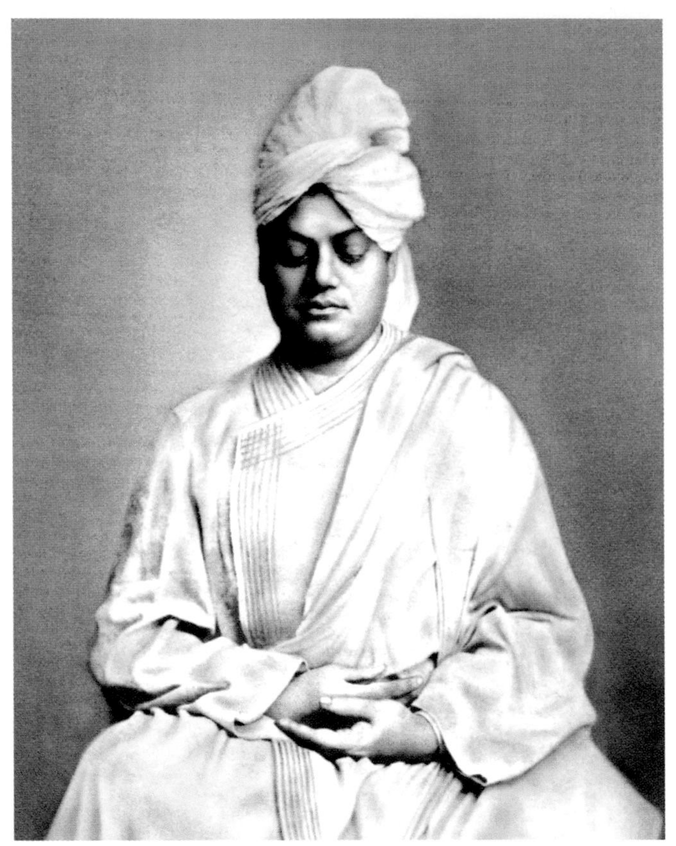

Figure 1.9. Swami Vivekananda

point for yoga in America came when Swami Vivekananda (see figure 1.9) attended the first Meeting of World Religions in Chicago, Illinois, in September 1893 and mesmerized the audience with his powerful speech. For an excerpt of his speech, see "Sages Say."

By the end of the nineteenth century, the practice of yoga had diminished in India. Fortunately, two yogis were born who revitalized it—Swami Sivananda and Krishnamacharya. Swami Sivananda wrote over two hundred books on yoga and philosophy and in his name yoga centers the world over provide instruction to yoga teachers. His main teaching is summarized in six words: serve, love, give, purify, meditate, realize.

Krishnamacharya (see figure 1.10) had encyclopedic knowledge, degrees from the best universities in India, and was known for his healing abilities. Making it his mission to bring yoga back to India and ultimately the rest of the world, he opened a yoga school in Mysore. Several of his students, including his son, T.K.V. Desikachar, his brother-in-law, B.K.S. Iyengar, Pattabi Jois, and Indra Devi, became some of the most influential modern yoga teachers, with distinctive styles.

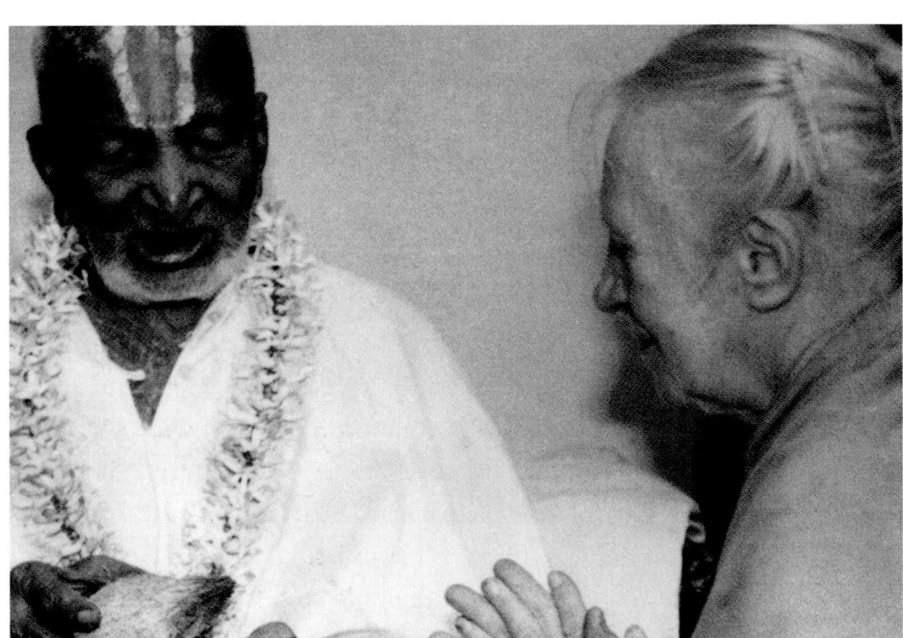

Figure 1.10. Krishnamacharya with his student Indra Devi

Sages Say

Sisters and Brothers of America—

I am proud to belong to a religion which has taught the world both tolerance and universal acceptance. We believe not only in universal toleration, but we accept all religions as true. I am proud to belong to a nation which has sheltered the persecuted and the refugees of all religions and all nations of the earth. . . .

The present convention . . . is in itself a vindication, a declaration to the world of the wonderful doctrine preached in the Gita: "Whosoever comes to Me, through whatsoever form, I reach him; all men are struggling through paths which in the end lead to me." Sectarianism, bigotry, and its horrible descendant, fanaticism, have long possessed this beautiful earth. They have filled the earth with violence, drenched it often and often with human blood, destroyed civilization and sent whole nations to despair. Had it not been for these horrible demons, human society would be far more advanced than it is now. But their time is come; and I fervently hope that the bell that tolled this morning in honor of this convention may be the death-knell of all fanaticism, of all persecutions with the sword or with the pen, and of all uncharitable feelings between persons wending their way to the same goal.

—*Swami Vivekananda*

Desikachar developed a system that emphasizes designing poses and breath practices suited to each individual. Perhaps partly because one student at a time is instructed, this style hasn't gained widespread acceptance in the United States. By contrast, Iyengar's brand of yoga is often practiced in the United States today. Sickly as a child and young adult, Iyengar worked diligently with Krishnamacharya to overcome all illness. Later, while working with students who had lost their limbs, he developed a style of yoga that incorporates many props and requires very specific alignment details. Today in his nineties, Iyengar (see figure 1.11) remains a powerful force in yoga.

As for Pattabi Jois, he taught a system of flow yoga in a specific sequence of poses, building inner heat and emphasizing breathing patterns, the gaze of the eyes (*drishti*), and energetic lifts (*bandhas*). Indra Devi, who emphasized the joy of yoga and was revered for her compassion and personal charisma, took yoga all over the world, especially to South America.

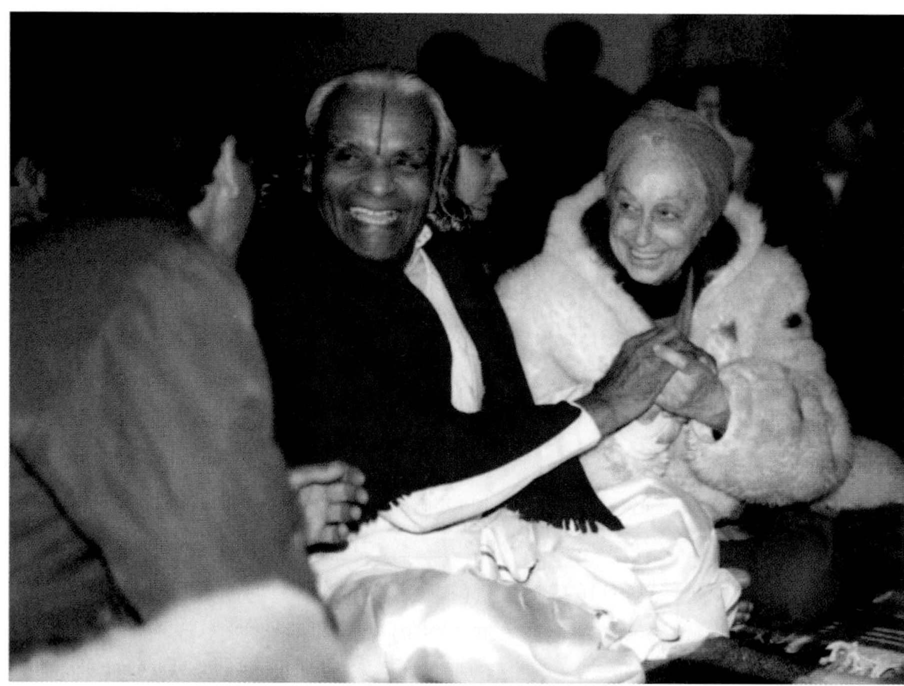

Figure 1.11. B.K.S. Iyengar with his student and friend Vanda Scaravelli

YOGIC TEXTS THAT MARK THE PERIODS

To taste the flavor of each era, let's look at excerpts of texts from each period. From the Vedic period comes the line from the *Rig Veda*, where yoga is first mentioned: "Seers of the vast illumined Seer yogically control their minds and intelligence."[5] As seen in this excerpt, thousands of years ago yoga was more about the mind than the body. When most people think of yoga, they think primarily of physical poses, yet the first detailed writings about poses didn't occur until the fourteenth century.

Also from the Vedic period, the following passage from the Upanishads, a favorite of William Butler Yeats, describes the innate perfection of the world and cosmos working in unity, and hints at the much later perspectives of Tantra.

All is perfect, so perfectly perfect!
Whatever being lives, moves
And breathes on Earth
At every level from atom
To galaxy is absolutely perfect in its place
Precise and choreographed.
Because "That" flows from the Glory of God,
The Lord,
The Self,
Consciousness,
The Source,
Awareness, Peace, and Love,
And is therefore perfect.
When you have surrendered your ego
To "That"
You will find true happiness.
Never ever envy the place of
Any other man or woman.[6]

The epic period (see figure 1.4) is rich with dramatic stories so exciting and intriguing that in India children read them as comic books. Following is an excerpt from the Bhagavad Gita, in which Krishna, as an incarnation of Vishnu, describes to the warrior Arjuna the necessity of being true to his authentic self, a message worth embracing in the modern world:

It is better to do your own duty
badly, than to perfectly do
another's: you are safe from harm
when you do what you should be doing.[7]

The classical period (see figure 1.6) is defined by Patanjali's Yoga Sutras, considered the first book of yoga and the finest distillation of yogic philosophy. We will look closely at this text in the next chapter as it lays out a framework for yoga practice. Here we will focus on his discussion of the dualistic nature of the universe: "Thus, the supreme state of Independence manifest while the gunas reabsorb themselves into Prakriti, having no more purpose to serve the Purusha. O, to look from another angle, the power of pure consciousness settles in its own pure nature."[8] In this passage and elsewhere, Patanjali describes a dualistic world comprised of *Prakriti* and *Purusha,* matter and spirit, with liberation attained by overcoming matter. Consciousness of the *Purusha* is unchangeable, and by absorbing the reflection of it, the mindstuff, *Prakriti,* becomes conscious of the true self.

The oldest existing commentary on the Yoga Sutras is by the revered sage Vyasa. He is credited with writing *Yoga-Bhashya* (*Discussion on Yoga*) around the fifth century CE.

The tantric period (see figure 1.7) is very important since most yoga students practice hatha yoga, which emerged from Tantra. The tantric teachings of the postclassical period are more difficult to excerpt as they are challenging to understand even when explained by a teacher. In fact, some people say the only way to truly learn Tantra is with a guru. The following is an excerpt from the principal tantric text, *Shiva Sutras*: "When the mind is united to the core of consciousness, every observable phenomenon and even the void appear as a form of consciousness."[9]

Some important ideas from the tantric period, according to Rod Stryker, perhaps the preeminent American teacher of Tantra yoga, are: people are capable of infinite bliss and have an infinite capacity to learn. These ideas highlight our ability for continued growth without limitations, providing a positive foundation of fearlessness and joyfulness for yoga practice. Stryker also describes Tantra yoga as offering many strategies for liberation, including herbology, gemology, astrology, alchemy, *kirtan* (devotional chanting), visualization, ritual, contemplation, and Ayurveda.[10]

Interestingly, even though the Lotus Pose is pictured in ancient seals and specific yoga poses, or asanas, were initally named in about 450 CE, written instructions for many yoga postures other than seated poses were first recorded only around 1350, in the *Hatha Yoga Pradipika*. Following is an excerpt describing a specific posture: "Place the right ankle next to the left buttock and the left ankle next to the right buttock. This is called Gomukhasana, and resembles the face of a cow."[11]

The *Hatha Yoga Pradipika* also emphasizes the great benefits of practicing yoga, as in the following passages: "He who constantly practices Uddiyana bandha as taught by his guru, so that it becomes natural, even though he is old, becomes young"[12] and "The yogi that remains even for half an hour with his tongue turned upwards [placed at the hole in the palate] is freed from poisons, disease, old age and death."[13] The *Pradipika* contains four chapters: "Asana," describing sixteen poses; "*Pranayama* and Cleanses"; "Mudra and Bandha"; and "Eternal Bliss."

Both an earlier and a later text describing hatha yoga are still influential today. One, the *Goraksha-Paddhati* (*Tracks of Goraksha*), written in the eleventh century, states that there are 8,400,000 asanas, 84 of which are useful. The *Gheranda Samhita* (*Gheranda's Collection*), recorded in the late seventeeth century as a continuation of the *Pradipika*, describes thirty-two poses.

The fact that yoga poses were described only relatively recently is puzzling. Teachers and scholars believe that either the poses were so much a part of the everyday life of Indian people that recording them would be like writing down what we learn in kindergarten, as one yogi put it,[14] or it was thought that poses should only be taught to students directly by a guru.

The late appearance of detailed descriptions of poses perhaps reinforces the fact that yoga is most concerned not with the body but with quieting the mind so we are able to witness consciousness and eventually attain enlightenment. While practicing yoga, we are reminded of the importance of the spiritual aspects of life and learn to cultivate our role as observer so we don't become upset by daily ups and downs. In fact, one of the most helpful instructions from the Yoga Sutras is the following:

> *When you are disturbed*
> *By unwholesome*
> *Negative thoughts or emotions,*
> *Cultivation of their opposites*
> *Promotes self-control*
> *And firmness*
> *In the precepts.*[5]

This practice of imagining opposites with the intention of maintaining equanimity despite what occurs is very useful. I often use this idea for teaching and in daily circumstances. For example, if a student comes up to me after class and raves about the session, saying it completely shifted her experience of the day, I'm pleased to have helped someone but also know that being egotistical is a trap. So I remember it is yoga that actually helped the student. I also consider how I would feel if a student said it was the worst class they'd ever taken and work to feel equally at ease with myself in that case. Or if I'm running my usual two-mile loop when a car drives by and a young man makes a rude remark, I try to remain calm and imagine how I would feel if his comment were instead a compliment.

The modern period gave rise to numerous texts describing poses. Many are listed in the bibliography.

TYPES AND STYLES OF YOGA

Before looking at the styles of yoga derived from the teachings of Krishnamacharya and his students, it is helpful to understand the difference between types and styles of yoga. Types of yoga are described in ancient texts and include the following:

Jnana yoga, a practice dedicated to liberation through knowledge and wisdom, involves both learning via the mind and learning beyond the mind. It includes studying texts, thinking about ideas, and ultimately developing personal wisdom, which comes through not only the intellect but an inner guide as well.

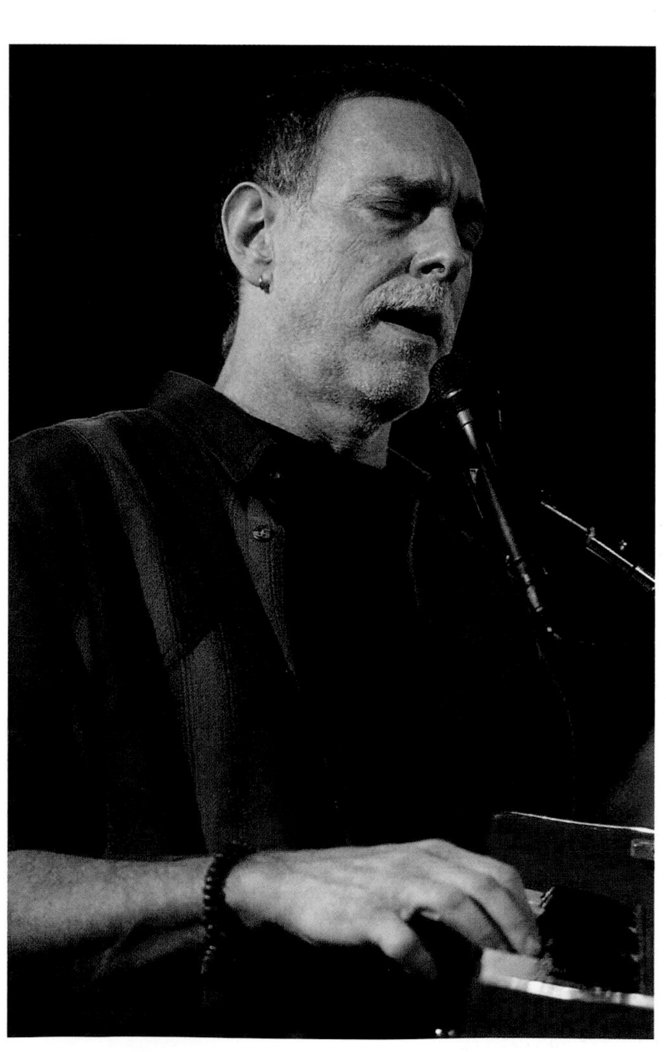

Figure 1.12. Krishna Das

Bhakti yoga is the practice of devotion as a path to enlightenment. It is sometimes called a heart-centered path that entails no longer trying to attain enlightenment through thinking and instead opening to love of the Divine. Some bhakti yogis revere a specific guru in addition to the Divine, while others just focus on general love of the Divine. Krishna Das (see figure 1.12) is a well-known bhakti yogi who espouses *kirtan*. For a firsthand description of devotional chanting, see "Sages Say."

Karma yoga is the path of doing good deeds in the world without regard for outcome or reward. Mother Teresa's work can be seen as an example of practicing karma yoga. Generally it is easier to perform the good deeds than to be unattached to the fruit of such service—for instance, being disappointed when we don't receive acknowledgment for our actions. An excellent way to practice karma yoga is to create community through yoga, such as via a yoga studio, and thus build a platform for performing good deeds. Yoga studios across the country hold events to raise money for local charities. For instance, after 9/11 yoga teacher Lisa Schrempp organized a fund-raising event in Tucson, Arizona, called 108 Sun Salutations for World Peace.

Sages Say

When we see the beauty of our own being, we are seeing the beauty of the Being that is the One of which we are all a part. And when we turn toward that One, love is the natural reaction of the heart.

God or Guru is an endless ocean of love, truth, and presence. First we may hear the distant roar of the crashing waves of the ocean and we're drawn to that sound. As we get closer, we can smell the ocean air and taste the sweet moisture. When we reach the beach and see the ocean for the first time, we're transfixed by the vastness and beauty. We run and we dive in and enjoy the freedom that comes from this ecstasy. Finally we merge with that ocean of love and somehow find ourselves back on the shore, returning to ourselves so that we can share the experience with others.

Those who have returned have given us these names of God. These names are the sound of the surf of that Ocean of Love. They hold the power to help us find our way back to that ocean. We don't have to create anything; we don't have to manufacture any feelings. We can't make it happen. It already is. All we have to do is remember. Everyone has their own path to this beach, to the ocean, but we all wind up in the same place. There is only One.

Satsang is where people gather together to remember, to turn within and find their own inner path to the One. When we gather together to sing like this, we are helping each other find our own paths. We all must travel this path by ourselves because each of us is our own path. All these paths wander on in their own way, but in truth we are all traveling together, and until the last of us arrives we will all keep traveling. So let's sing![16]

—*Krishna Das*

Since then, hundreds of participants in Tucson alone have raised money for outreach programs to assist those in need. On each occasion, yogis practiced the salutations with the intention of creating world peace as well as raising funds. Such events not only bring the tangible benefit of support for worthy causes but unify people physically, mentally, and spiritually. In addition, yogis sometimes teach yoga for free at drug rehabilitation clinics, detention centers, and senior centers as a way of practicing karma yoga.

Mantra yoga is the practice of chanting sounds with specific vibrations for help in life. The chosen mantra could be an affirmation we have either developed ourselves or been given by a teacher—a word or phrase we speak repeatedly, especially when our minds wander to negative self-talk.

Sanskrit mantras evoke a particular power, as each sound creates vibrations in the physical body that can lead to transformation in the energetic body. Following is an example of how one yogi uses mantras to gain wisdom:

> *Two years ago I decided to engage in a forty-day practice, chanting 108 times each night to Saraswati (goddess of wisdom, education, music, and poetry), meditating, and abstaining from alcohol and sex. During that time, a strange sense of clarity began to creep into my daily life. It was mostly a sense of perspective. I began to see how much of my energy had been needlessly consumed by a destructive relationship. At the end of my tapasya, I ended the relationship, feeling self-righteous and indignant, and spent many weeks taking care of myself: nourishing myself with a strong practice, wonderful friends, and new activities. I learned to play the violin and wrote reams of poetry. I felt a happiness bordering on giddiness. I learned, essentially, what it meant to love my self. But alas, that wasn't the end of the lesson. A prayer for wisdom, after all, is a pretty tall order.*
>
> *In time, I missed my partner, and once again sought his company. I inadvertently became involved in a tangled web of overlapping relationships, as he had neglected to tell me that he had begun to see other people while we were apart. My first instinct was to scream out in rage, taking refuge in self-righteous indignation. But this provided no relief, save the luxury of claiming some sort of victim-status or martyrdom, which is a shallow consolation, at best.*
>
> *Turning to my practice, I chanted again to Saraswati and meditated. I began descending through several layers and spirals of feelings—anger, sadness, betrayal, nostalgia, laughter, joy, profound love, and beneath all of these, peace. I began to understand on a deeper level that nothing is ever truly clear-cut. Our love and our hate and our pain and our wounds and our laughter are all inextricably mixed up*

together. And that we create them all, like lesson plans tailor-made for our own enlightened path. That our knowledge outlines our experiences, and gives them a shape we can name and recognize, but that the subtle blending of every color of emotion and confusion and acceptance are what lend to the depth we call wisdom.

I had been warned that chanting brings about change, and that this change may not take a form that I find comfortable. The mantras bring about these changes through resetting our vibrations, subtly changing our energy, like magnets, so that we attract what we need, regardless of what we think we want. We don't, after all, get stronger by looking at big muscles; we get stronger by lifting heavier and heavier weights. And we don't gain wisdom by reading someone else's words; we gain wisdom by letting go of all that we think we know and finding the humility to learn everything anew. The answers to my prayer will keep coming in various forms for as long as I open to receiving them.

Chanting is powerful practice. But beware: it doesn't change the circumstances of your life; it changes you.[17]

Nada yoga invokes the healing power of sound. An example is the vibrational healing done by Richard Rudis, also known as Sonam Dorje or Meritorious Thunderbolt, at a gong bath (see figure 1.13), where a gong is played with multiple mallets while students lie on the floor and experience the vibrations in their bodies.

One student wrote the following poem describing nada yoga:

Gong Bath

Bathed in the song of the gong
I know that I have
many years to live,
a new life
etched in circular sounds,
exploding hexagonal stars,
and a reluctant pain deep in my shoulders.
It is faith that brings us together,
our karma, the gong priest said,
to be members of a one-time sangha
in which the will to heal
may be born

in the sound that is all sounds,
the sound that goes on forever.
One more chance
to live in a state of grace,
brought back to my true self
by the memory of chanting,
the sweet high voice in the dark hall,
the earthy call of chorus and drum
inviting me to follow them home.[18]

Hatha yoga means forceful, or active, yoga. Most of the various styles of hatha yoga practiced today can be traced back to Krishnamacharya and his students. The yoga B.K.S. Iyengar brought to America includes the use of props to aid in doing poses for healing. Following is an excerpt from his book *Light on Yoga*:

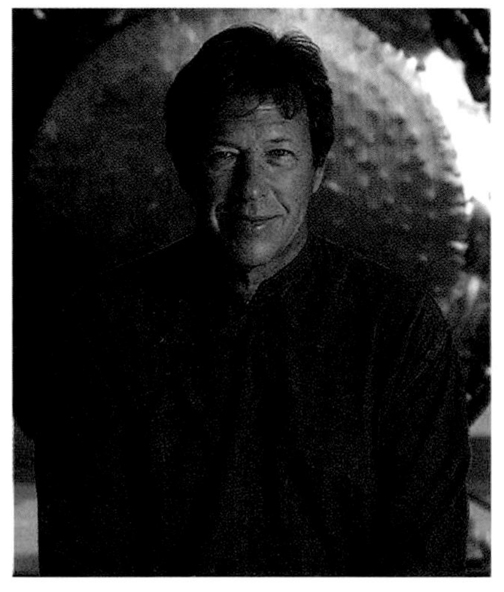

Figure 1.13. Richard Rudis (a.k.a. Sonam Dorje or Meritorious Thunderbolt) at a gong bath

> *By performing asanas, the* sadhaka *[student] first gains health, which is not mere existence. It is not a commodity which can be purchased with money. It is an asset to be gained by sheer hard work. Forgetfulness of physical and mental consciousness is health. The yogi frees himself from physical disabilities and mental distractions by practicing asanas. He surrenders his actions and their fruits to the Lord in the service of the world.*[19]

Iyengar is well-known for his precision in teaching and, especially in his earlier days, for hitting students in poses so that they better understand them. (According to the classical interpretation of yoga, the body and spirit are separate, implying that a teacher's use of force to aid students in perfecting their poses is considered an act of love that helps them reach a spiritual perspective.) Iyengar is revered and loved by many for his teaching and healing. One of his most esteemed and respected students, Patricia Walden, reflects on her teacher in "Sages Say."

Many teachers worldwide practice Iyengar yoga in conjunction with their own rigorous certification programs. Teachers who began with Iyengar yoga and then developed their own approaches include Erich Schiffmann and John Friend. Schiffmann's book, *The Spirit and Practice of Moving into Stillness*, and his teachings of deep listening and trusting articulate the connection between poses and life off the mat. Friend named

Sages Say

Nothing could have prepared me for B.K.S. Iyengar. With his love of yoga, he was the prince of passion and the king of charisma. In my first class with him, he boomed out, "If you keep your armpits open, you won't get depressed"; and from the feeling in my rising, opening chest, I knew exactly what he meant.

There was fire in his presence, a fire that lit the light of yoga in me and changed my life. He was direct and unequivocating, with a fierceness of spirit that implied he could face any challenge.

It is extraordinary and challenging to have Guruji as a teacher, to learn from him year after year and to experience his genius, generosity, and guidance. His passion for excellence and unrelenting interest in yoga are contagious; and those qualities, along with his courage and will power, inspire my life, my practice, and my teaching.

I bring this lesson to my students: if we stay with our chosen path and develop the discipline to go through difficulty, our efforts will transform us.

The greatest gift a teacher/guru can give a student is genuine interest: such genuine interest can transform and shape a student's life beyond measure. Guruji is my link with tradition. He shows me what is possible with practice and represents to me a living example of Sutra I.14—"Yoga is successful when practiced with devotion, uninterrupted, over a long period of time."

I remember one of the first lessons I learned from him: "When confronted with difficulty, take an action, no matter how small." Anything is possible, if you act (and reflect) with love and devotion.

Through his challenging style, Guruji has taught me to face difficulty with wide open eyes, to refine myself through the play of passion and discipline, and to feel secure in his method. As a result I feel joy in my practice—and free in my love for teaching.[20]

—*Patricia Walden*

his style Anusara (Flowing with Grace) and emphasized alignment principles along with the inherent beauty and sacredness of the body.

Kundalini yoga, or yoga of awareness, brought to the West by Yogi Bhajan in 1968, focuses on meditation and on stimulation of the glandular and nervous systems to heighten creative potential. The practice consists of simple postures, *pranayama*, mantras, music, and meditation to teach relaxation, self-healing, and elevation for purposes of gaining inner vitality to compensate for the adverse effects of stress in life.

Ashtanga vinyasa yoga synchronizes a breathing method called *ujjayi* breath with a progressive series of postures so the body produces intense internal heat and a purifying sweat that detoxifies muscles and organs. Ashtanga vinyasa yoga involves a series of set postures so you know exactly which ones will be taught and in what sequence. The first series, called the primary (yoga *chikitsa*), detoxifies and aligns the body; the second series, called the intermediate (*nadi shodhana*), purifies the nervous system; the third series (*sthira bhaga*) integrates the other practices. The name of this form of yoga can create confusion as Ashtanga is the name of the famous eight-limbed path of yoga described by Patanjali in the Yoga Sutras. Pattabhi Jois's Ashtanga vinyasa yoga, on the other hand, is a style of hatha yoga that originated with the sage Vamana Rishi in the *Yoga Korunta*, an ancient manuscript said to contain lists of many different groupings of asanas, as well as teachings on vinyasa, *drishti*, *bandhas*, mudras, and philosophy.

Ashtanga vinyasa yoga has been taught by Pattabhi Jois and his followers, including his grandson, Sharath, and other family members, at the Ashtanga Yoga Research Institute in Mysore, India, where Sharath continues the tradition. Teachers worldwide who have studied in Mysore include Richard Freeman, Tim Miller, and Beryl Bender Birch. There are also teachers who began with Ashtanga vinyasa yoga and then developed their own style apart from the postures, such as Sharon Gannon and David Life with Jivamukti Yoga School. Pattabhi Jois is famous for saying, "Practice. All will come. Yoga is ninety percent practice and ten percent theory."[20] Yet in his book *Yoga Mala* he quotes liberally from the Upanishads as well as the *Hatha Yoga Pradipika*, saying the following about breath:

> *If the asanas and the* Surya Namaskara *(Sun Salutations) are to be practiced, they must be done in accordance with the prescribed vinyasa method only. As the sage Vamana says,* "Vina vinyasa ygena asana din na karayet *(O yogi, do not do asana without vinyasa).*" *When*

yoga is practiced with a knowledge of its proper method, it is quite easy to learn, but practiced without such knowledge it becomes a very difficult undertaking.[21]

T.K.V. Desikachar, son of Krishnamacharaya, teaches an individual style of yoga with emphasis on breath and personal exploration. Another teacher with training in this area is Gary Kraftsow. Desikachar says about his father:

My association with my father was very long. I observed him teaching others at different stages of his life from 1960 to almost the end of his life. He was teaching different people in different ways according to their needs, their age, their health and so on. This taught me a lot of things. Further, for those thirty years I was exposed to many aspects of his teaching. I had the real thing day after day, so I could absorb much of his teaching and at the same time I could always go back to him with questions and case studies. In that way he would help me with my teaching.[22]

Vanda Scaravelli, who studied privately with both Iyengar and Desikachar, eventually established her own syle of yoga practice that integrates alignment principles with breath, focusing on three primary foundations: the breath, the spine, and gravity. She is recorded in a video interview doing full wheel backbends at the age of eighty-five, admonishing her listeners to live fully, enjoy life, and come to yoga with fullness of the breath. She says in her book *Awakening the Spine*:

There is a way of doing yoga poses that we call "asanas," without the slightest effort. Movement is the song of the body. Yes, the body has its own song from which the movement of dancing arises spontaneously. . . . The liberation of the upper part of the body . . . produced **by acceptance of gravity** *in the lower part of the body . . . is the origin of lightness and dancing is its expression. This song, if you care to listen to it, is beauty. We could say that it is part of nature. We sing when we are happy, and the body goes with it like waves in the sea.*[23]

Indra Devi (see figure 1.14), Krishnamacharya's first female student, was born in Riga, Latvia, but lived in India for twelve years. Although Krishnamacharya initially resisted, he eventually accepted her as a student and came to believe that women would be instrumental in the revitalization of yoga, which proved prescient since as many as 80 percent of all yoga practitioners today in the West are women. Indra Devi is often called Mataji and "The First Lady of Yoga."

Indra Devi opened her first yoga school in Shanghai, China, in 1939. After World War II, she continued studying yoga in the Himalayas then, following the death of her husband, moved to the United States. There she founded a yoga studio in Hollywood, where she taught stars of the day such as Gloria Swanson, Jennifer Jones, Ramón Novarro, and Olivia de Havilland. In 1953, she married a renowned doctor and humanitarian, Sigfrid Knauer, and continued spreading yoga throughout the United States and Mexico via conferences, radio, and television.

Over the next several decades, Indra Devi took yoga worldwide. She went to the Soviet Union in 1960, subsequently becoming known as the woman who brought yoga to the Kremlin. She conducted a meditation in Vietnam in 1966 and traveled frequently to India. In 1985, she moved to Argentina, where she taught yoga to thousands and set up the Indra Devi Foundation, spreading yoga throughout South America, as well as holding seminars and classes in the United States and Europe. Over the years, she published a number of books, including *Forever Young, Forever Healthy*, as well as *Yoga for Americans* and *Yoga: The Technique of Health and Happiness*.

Indra Devi practiced what she taught, and as a result she remained active and vital later in life. Even after reaching the advanced age of 100 she continued a yoga practice that included strong twists, forward folds, and sitting in Lotus position. Indra Devi exemplified the yogic principles of love and liveliness until her death at 102.[24]

Many other styles of hatha yoga are practiced in America, including Kripalu, which focuses on poses with breathing yet less emphasis on alignment; Bikram, which follows a preset asana sequence; and Integral Yoga, in the tradition of Sri Swami Satchidananda. All these variations have essentially the same goal: to guide students toward liberation and peace.

Students of yoga should explore the various types and styles to see which appeal to them. Of course, students may be attracted to different types and styles of yoga at various times as their needs or philosophies change. For example, my first experience with yoga was practicing poses to reduce stress while working as a manufacturing supervisor. When the yoga teacher told us to lie down and close our eyes at the end of class, I immediately fell asleep as I was exhausted. Unfortunately, because the teacher ridiculed me for sleeping, I didn't return to yoga for a number of years. When I did, I practiced yoga mostly to counteract the effects of bike riding, running, and parenting without a spiritual component. Later, I discovered Ashtanga vinyasa yoga and, in connecting to my breath, found a deeper meaning to the poses. As I continued practicing, the nondualistic approach to hatha yoga became very appealing to me. I then added other types of yoga to my practice, including mantra yoga and nada yoga. All along, I deepened my practice of karma yoga and jnana yoga, both of which dated back to a passion for learning and social action I had cultivated during my youth.

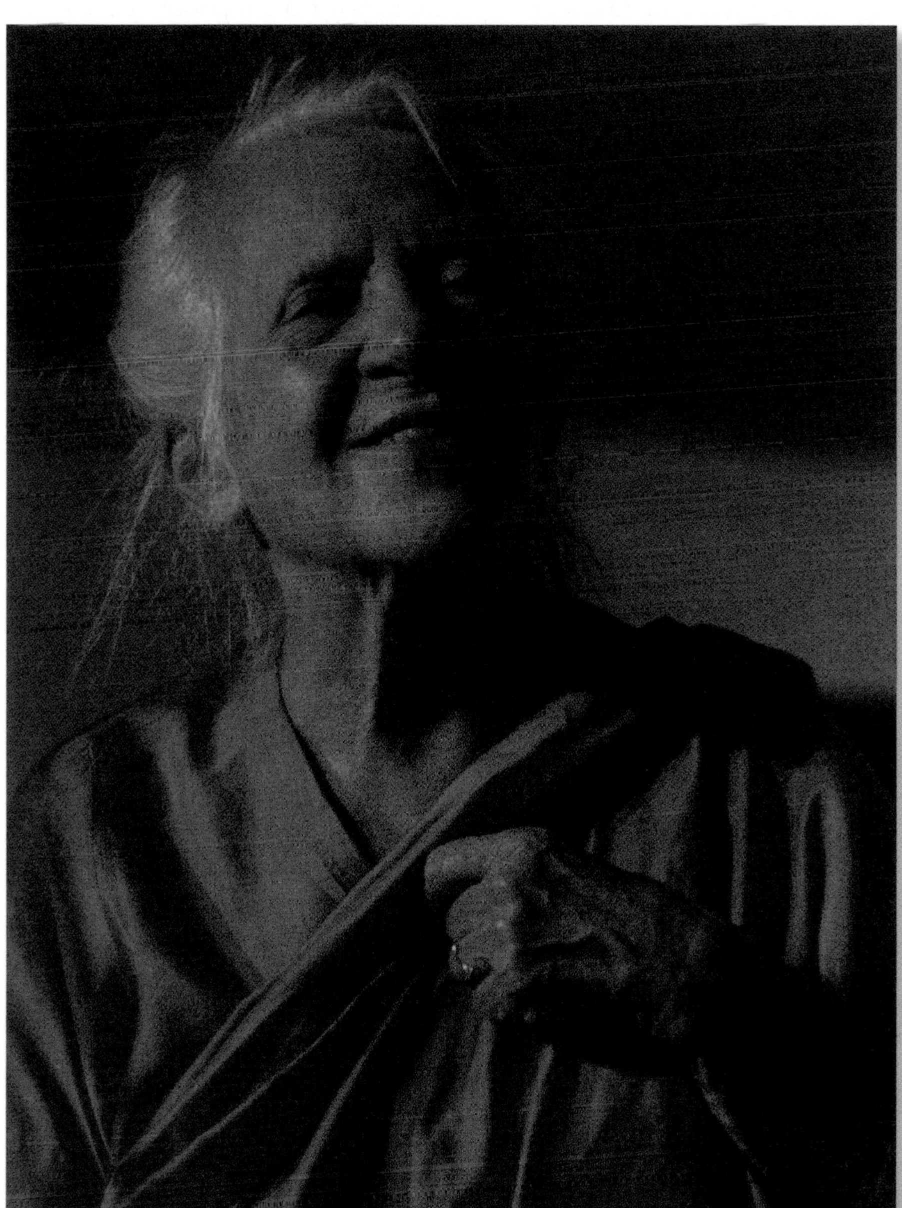

Figure 1.14. Indra Devi (a.k.a. Mataji)

Richard Freeman, the esteemed Ashtanga vinyasa yogi, said in a workshop that all the styles of hatha yoga are just models of reality. And since they are models they have intrinsic flaws, as nothing can completely capture reality. The trick is to find the flaws in the model you are using and decide if it still works or if you want to look for another model.[25]

Consider what sort of yoga teacher or approach might best suit your needs and philosophy. For example, when a teacher says, "Find the pose and breath, looking for how to more completely embody your own perfection," consider how this reflects a different philosophy than when a teacher says, "Put your foot in precisely this position and stay in the pose as long as you can, and then stay longer, allowing your mind to calm as you push your body through the fluctuations."

Watch the video *Yoga Unveiled* to reinforce the historic ideas of yoga and to connect them to the sounds and images of India.

Read the ancient texts online at freeyogabooks.com and other Web sites.

CHAPTER TWO

The Foundational Texts of Yoga

Two foundational texts of yoga, the Yoga Sutras and the Bhagavad Gita, offer a platform on which we stand in yoga. As a result of reading them in multiple translations and considering modern commentaries, we can ultimately find their meaning in our own lives.

THE YOGA SUTRAS: LAYING OUT THE PATH

Studying the foundational texts of yoga assists us in understanding the philosophy behind the practice and gives us invaluable knowledge for enhancing any physical yoga practice, such as work with poses or breathing. The first book of yoga, the Yoga Sutras, written by Patanjali (see figure 2.1) between 200 BCE and 200 CE, is the entry point to the wisdom of yoga. Patanjali describes yoga's practices and benefits in 196 short instructional verses that inspire readers to explore their meaning via teachers and life experience.

As with most early texts, the Yoga Sutras were originally an oral tradition. At the time of their composition, students of yoga, consisting of men and nonhouseholders only, would memorize the entire work in Sanskrit and then explore its meanings.

We will first examine passages from classical translations of the Yoga Sutras and their possible meanings. Then we will consider some contemporary nonliteral poetic renditions that aim to inspire readers. Today's technology also makes many other versions available. For instance, the entire Yoga Sutras are online on many Web sites, some of which offer sound files so you can hear the verses.[1] When selecting from among the

Sanskrit Gem

***Sutra* means thread, as in the medical term "suture," a stitch to close a wound. A sutra is also a style of writing used in many ancient Indian texts.**

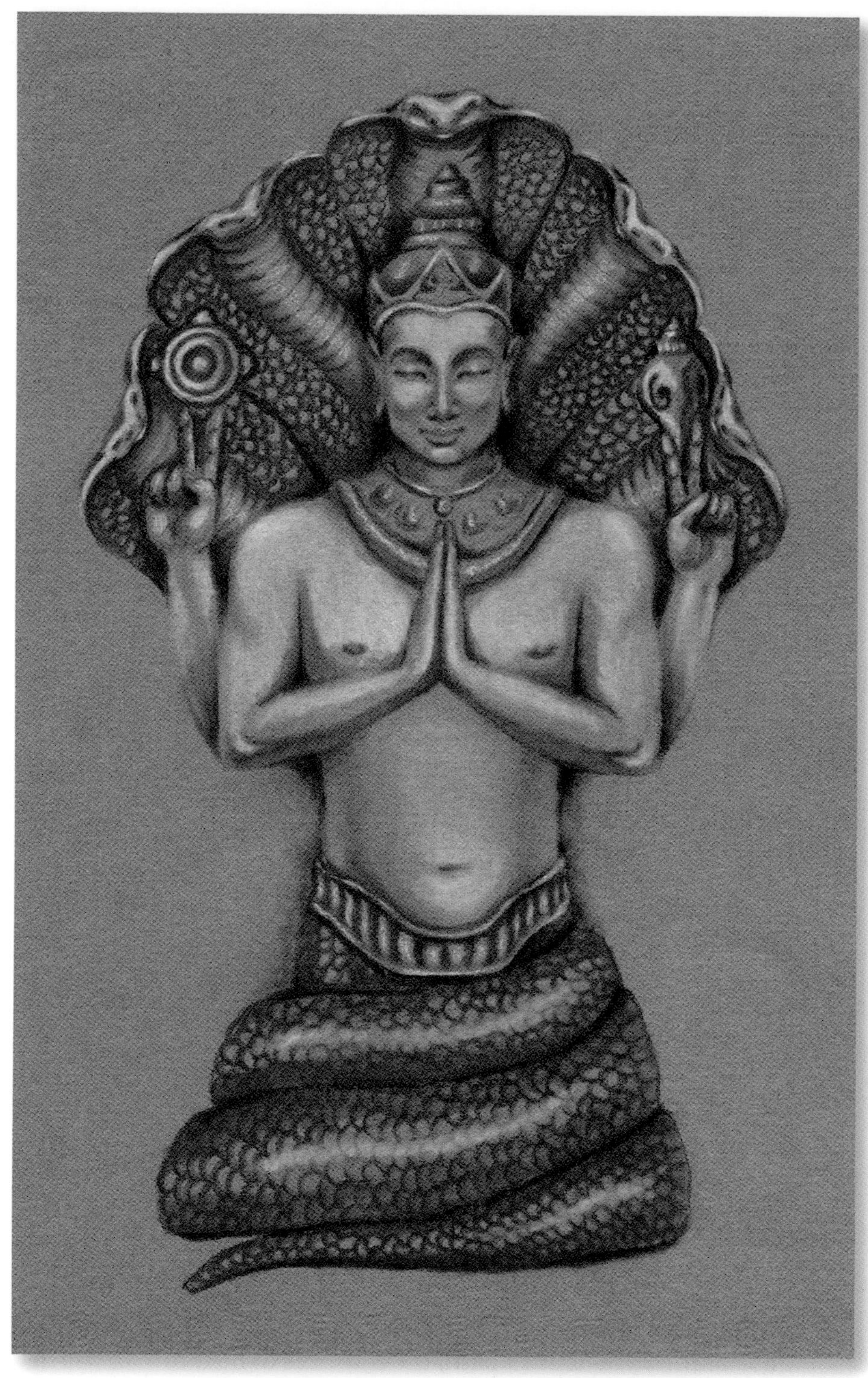

Figure 2.1. An artist's interpretation of Patanjali, regarded as author of the Yoga Sutras

many translations of this work available today, it is important to find one that inspires and motivates you.

The Yoga Sutras are composed of four chapters, or *padas*, meaning feet. Feet figure centrally in yogic thinking. Since we stand on our feet, they are our main connection to earth and reflect the way we use our body. When we practice poses, asanas, we focus on the way we use our feet, especially but not only for standing poses. Further, to sit at the feet of a teacher means we are humbling ourselves to learn. The four *padas* of the Yoga Sutras are the following:

1. "Samadhi Pada—Merging with Divine Self," 51 verses. This chapter describes a path to self-knowledge through creating a quiet mind that leads ultimately to *samadhi*, or ecstasy. It details obstacles to overcome and takes into account individual diversity and the use of multiple paths to the same goal. For example, to paraphrase verses 34–39: You can lessen the obstacles (to self-knowledge) by forcibly exhaling, then retaining the *prana* during the pause following the exhalation; or another way to steady the mind is by binding it to higher, subtler sense perceptions or by contemplating the luminous light arising from the heart, which is the source of true serenity, or by making the mind's object a self-realized being who has transcended passion and attachment, or by the knowledge arisen from dreams or from the dreamless state of deep sleep, or by persistent meditation in harmony with your religious heritage.[2]
2. "Sadhana Pada—Creating Spiritual Practice," 55 verses. This *pada* specifies ways to reach enlightenment through yoga. It examines five fundamental causes of suffering: ignorance of the true self; egotism; attachment to pleasure; aversion to pain; and clinging to life out of fear of death. It reminds us that it is possible to avoid suffering and embrace happiness in the future. Then, beginning with verse 28 it introduces the eight-limbed path of yoga and describes the first five in detail.
3. "Vibhuti Pada—Manifesting Divine Power," or "On Supernatural Abilities and Gifts," 56 verses. This *pada* discusses the last three limbs of the eight-limbed path, the practices of meditation, which are collectively called *samyama*. It describes how to practice *samyama* and the uplifting benefits, such as absolute freedom, the ability to move consciousness anywhere through space, and the power to move the body as fast as the mind.

Sanskrit Gem

Sam **means full, complete, and** ***yama*** **means control.**

we want to focus and on what, as well as become completely absorbed in the present. The first *pada* is rich with passages about the benefits of objectivity, or nonattachment:

The ultimate state of nonattachment
Arises from self-realization,
In which there is indifference
To the primordial forces of desire,
As everything
And everyone
Is experienced as one's
Own True Self.[12]

Yoga's ability to foster greater awareness by teaching us how to observe the mind and body is reflected in a memorable experience I had while teaching. A student mentioned that she hadn't been feeling well and didn't know if she would be able to participate in class but would try. After class I asked how she felt, and she replied, "I don't know if I feel any better really, but I feel better about the way I feel."

In general, the eight limbs are strategies for opening to our inner reservoir of peace. The first two limbs guide our behavior toward ourselves and the world. The third limb opens the body through physical poses, the fourth cultivates breathing, and the fifth teaches withdrawal of the senses. The remaining limbs teach us how to gradually master meditation.

To help keep the eight limbs of the Ashtanga path clear in your mind, refer to the Ashtanga map shown in figure 2.2, which is further delineated in table 2.1. The first two limbs, *yama* and *niyama*, form the foundation of the eight-limbed path. They provide the guidelines for inner work fundamental to all external transformations in our lives. The *yamas* give specific guidelines for dealing with our minds and interacting with the world in an ethical and peaceful way. The *niyamas* help us

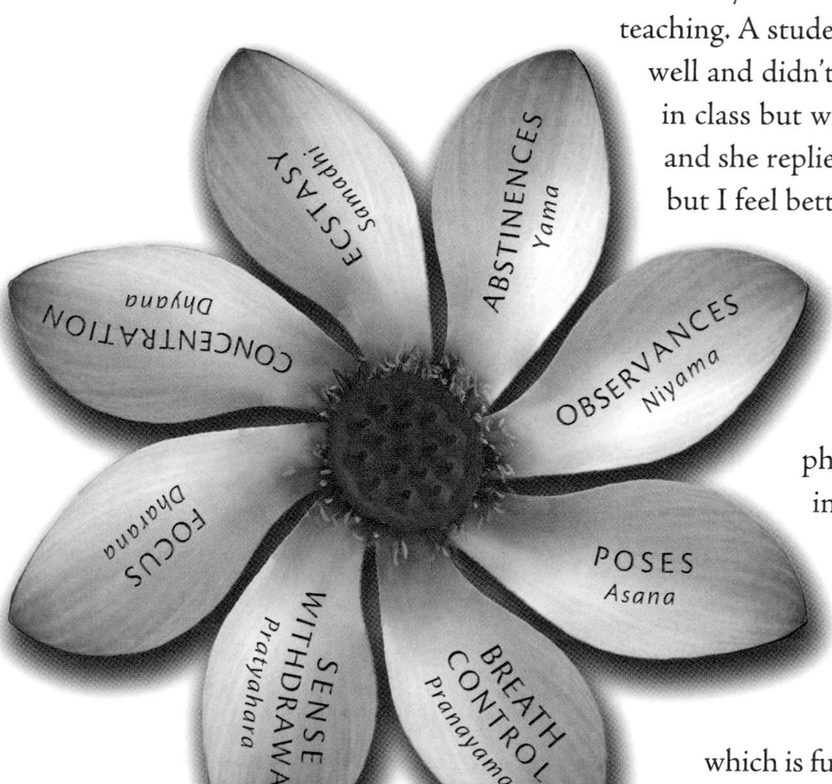

Figure 2.2. Ashtanga map: The Eight Petals of Yoga

cultivate orderliness and cleanliness, contentment, commitment, self-study, and finally letting go of the idea that we have control and surrendering to the universe. For example, a yoga student reported that when she had a difficult interaction on the phone with a customer service representative, initially she was angry. Then she began working with the first two limbs and contemplated whether she may have been attached to some particular outcome. Eventually able to practice these concepts while negotiating on the phone, she found she could remain unattached to the results of her interaction.

The third limb, asana, describes how to be happy and peaceful in our bodies. Interestingly, in the Yoga Sutras no specific poses are described but instead instructions are given about the general attitude and overall goal of yoga practice—to attain steadiness and happiness. Not until hundreds of years later do detailed descriptions of poses appear in texts. While this third limb focuses on poses that help us become stronger, more flexible, and more balanced, it also benefits us emotionally and spiritually. A key to increasing the awareness necessary to reap these benefits is using the breath to become a witness to sensations resulting from the poses. Total transformation isn't usually immediate, although change can be surprisingly fast. One thing is certain, according to my experience: each time you step on the mat you will know that when you step off it you may not have solved your problems but you will have gained a more positive, universal perspective.

The fourth limb, *pranayama*, details how to control our life force, *prana*. In becoming more conscious of breath, we are able to move energy in new places in the body and achieve lightness of mind, not taking everything so seriously. Specific *pranayama* practices are given in the text, such as forcibly exhaling and then holding the breath to diminish obstacles to self-knowledge. A yoga student and professional golfer reports that she uses the breathing practice she learned in yoga classes to relax and thus enhance her performance during tournaments. She says that at this point in her career she doesn't need to improve her golf technique but rather to quiet her mind.

The fifth limb, *pratyahara*, demonstrates ways to withdraw the senses in order to achieve balance and peace. Sense withdrawal is actually something we practice unconsciously—for example, when being unaware of sounds while reading. The text suggests, however, that by *consciously* tuning out sensory input we can quiet the mind, such as when we want to limit exposure to marketing messages or diminish the din of a restaurant or the noise of children to focus on our partner. One student reported that practicing *pratyahara* during winter holiday season by reducing her exposure to advertising eliminated stress and increased awareness of her inner self, helping her remain calm and contented.

The six, seventh, and eighth limbs, called collectively *samyama,* focus on various levels of meditation and subtle experiences of the mind. The ultimate paths to enlightenment, they are discussed in detail in the third *pada,* although it is sometimes hard to distinguish among them. As a whole, while practicing *samyama* by remaining completely absorbed in the object of meditation, we can increase our ability to relax when life is challenging and chaotic.

The eight limbs of Ashtanga yoga can be practiced sequentially, simultaneously, or iteratively. As such, rather than thinking of them as hierarchical, it is best to regard them as concentric rings that build on one another. We can enter the practice wherever we are able, perhaps first by focusing on poses at a yoga studio or gym, and later concentrating on the first two limbs to build a foundation for the rest of the path—leading to increased awareness of how to live in the world and gain peace and enlightenment through meditation. Then, too, when we are having trouble with one limb we can explore another to keep advancing in our practice. For example, if we can't find balance in a pose we can focus on breathing. If we are feeling agitated even after practicing poses, we might work with *santosha,* contentment, or just sit quietly in meditation.

The last three limbs can be practiced in combination with some poses, such as a balance pose. For example, first focus your eyes on a spot (*dharana*), then meditate (*dhyana*) with great energy on it so that you steady your pose and your mind. Finally, you may be so connected to that spot it seems as if you have merged with it, an experience that could be described as a flash of *samadhi,* or enlightenment. *Samadhi* doesn't have to occur in a remote location; if you've been so immersed in a task that you didn't realize time had passed, you've had an inkling of *samadhi.* With attentiveness, we can find moments of *samadhi* during each day, and over time experience more and more such moments of ecstasy and bliss.

The fourth, last *pada* lays out a path to liberation available once we have mastered the cessation of thoughts that prevent clarity of perception. Here is verse IV.31 followed by T.K.V. Desikachar's interpretation:

> *"When the mind is free from the clouds that prevent perception, all is known.*
> *There is nothing left to be known."*
> *The sun shines. All is evident. There is no need for artificial light.*[13]

1. Yama	Universal observances, self-control for social harmony, attitudes toward the environment:		
		Ahimsa	Nonviolence, love
		Satya	Truth, compassion
		Asteya	Nonstealing, generosity
		Brahmacharya	Moderation, boundaries for the creative life forces
		Aparigraha	Nongreed, nongrasping, awareness of abundance
2. Niyama	Personal observances, attitudes toward ourselves:		
		Sauca	Orderliness, cleanliness, simplicity, purity
		Santosha	Contentment, being at peace with oneself
		Tapas	Fire of commitment, self-discipline
		Svadhyaya	Self-study, sacred study
		Isvara-pranidhana	"I give up"; honoring the Divine
3. Asana	Poses, body exercise		
4. Pranayama	Breath control		
5. Pratyahara	Sense withdrawal, detachment		
6. Dharana	Focus		
7. Dhyana	Concentration		
8. Samadhi	Ecstasy; also bliss, pure consciousness, enlightenment		

TABLE 2.1

Having attained such clarity of perception, we may experience ecstasy and liberation.

Now let's consider some concepts of the *yamas* and *niyamas* and what they mean in daily life. To begin, due to the great variety of interpretations and translations of key concepts in these first two limbs, table 2.2 can be used as an aid to selecting a translation of the Yoga Sutras that inspires you and guides you in assessing your experiences.

Of the *yamas* (see figure 2.3), abstinences, perhaps the most important is the first one, *ahimsa*, nonviolence, or abstaining from violence, beginning with the self, which is the foundation of yoga. To understand how this concept relates to the self, watch your thoughts and notice how frequently you are violent toward yourself by criticizing yourself or sending yourself discouraging messages, often unconsciously. Then consider how you can transform your negative criticism to positive thoughts, giving yourself the kind of loving support you would extend to a beloved friend or family member.

Ahimsa is often cited as the basis for yogis being vegetarians, a claim disputed by scholars. In the context of food, nonviolence may mean not killing an animal for food or instead finding foods that have been cultivated in a nonviolent way.

The second *yama* instructs us to seek *satya*, or truth, right communication, and integrity. Practicing *satya* involves recognizing what is in keeping with our sense of integrity and maintaining an objective approach to life so that upsets do not prevent us from seeing and acting on the truth. Searching for a balance between nonviolence and truthfulness can be an aspect of many life experiences. For example, we could be completely nonviolent toward ourselves by staying in bed all day, but that probably would not be truthful to our goals in life.

SENSE WITHDRAWAL
Pratyahara
FOCUS
Dharana
BREATH CONTROL
Pranayama
CONCENTRATION
Dhyana
POSES
Asana
ECSTASY
Samadhi
OBSERVANCES
Niyama
ABSTINENCES
Yama

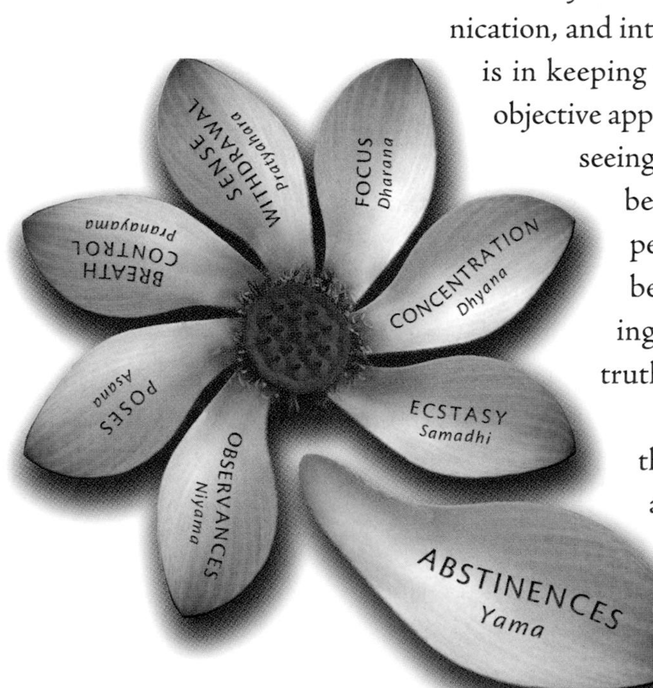

Figure 2.3. The first limb of Ashtanga yoga, yama

To assess your tendency to compromise in this way, observe if you suppress your truth to get along with other people by, for example, watching TV with friends when you would rather take a bath, or going to lunch with coworkers when you would prefer sitting quietly outdoors. Another aspect of *satya* is acting in accordance with your values as you face challenges in life such as keeping a nonviolent demeanor while talking on the phone to a distant service representative who continually puts you on hold and doesn't address your requests.

The next *yama* is *asteya,* or not stealing, noncovetousness, and generosity. When we think of not stealing, we usually think of not stealing physical items from others. But stealing also applies to taking people's time and energy—for example, staying on the phone with someone long after they have said they need to get off. Another approach to *asteya* is the practice of generosity, giving of ourselves in small ways that could make a difference in another person's life, like thanking someone for some action on our behalf.

The *yama* after that is *brahmacharya,* which means moderation, balance, and protection of our creative life forces. Some older translations defined *brahmacharya* as abstention or celibacy. While the latter may have been appropriate for Patanjali's audience, today's yoga students are more inclined to interpret this *yama* in terms of establishing boundaries. Many people have been taught to concern themselves so completely with how others are doing that they need to cultivate boundaries on their own time and energy. Learning to balance giving with not giving beyond what we can to protect our life force often means saying, "No, I'd like to do that, but I don't have the space right now in my life." When we start to see how such boundaries nurture us, we feel empowered in a new and satisfying way.

The last *yama* is *aparigraha,* which means both nongrasping and awareness of abundance and fulfillment. It involves not holding on to our thoughts, expectations, and things. For example, if we are focused intently on the acquisition of new objects as a shortcut to happiness, *aparigraha* suggests understanding the underlying emotional causes for attachment to physical objects and seeing if we can create the same feelings without purchasing the items.

While on the mat practicing poses, you might notice yourself grasping at the perfection of some pose as seen in a photograph or holding on to some trait of your body that corresponds to an external definition of beauty. It's important to notice grasping while on the mat because injury can result when you seek an ideal instead of being with yourself just as you are in the moment.

Aparigraha also means gaining awareness of abundance and focusing on our inherent sufficiency instead of deprivation. Lynne Twist, a Project Hunger worker who has raised money from the wealthiest people to help the poorest, comments on the tendency of people in modern societies to perceive what they have as insufficient. She writes in her book, *The Soul*

	Christopher Isherwood, Swami Prabhavananda[14]	*T.K.V. Desikachar*[15]	*Mukunda Stiles*[16]	*Nischala Joy Devi*[17]
Yama	Abstention from evil-doing	Our attitudes toward our environment	Self-control for social harmony	Reflection of our true nature
Ahimsa	Abstention from harming others	Consideration for all living things, especially those who are innocent, in difficulty, or worse off than we are	Nonviolence	Reverence, love, compassion for all
Satya	Abstention from falsehood	Right communication through speech, writings, gesture, and actions	Truthfulness	Truthfulness, integrity
Asteya	Abstention from theft	Noncovetousness or the ability to resist a desire for that which does not belong	Freedom from stealing	Generosity
Brahmacharya	Sexual abstinence	Moderation in all our actions	Behavior that respects the Divine as omnipresent	Balance and moderation of the vital life force
Aparigraha	Abstention from greed	Nongreediness or the ability to accept only what is appropriate	Freedom from greed	Awareness of abundance, fulfillment

TABLE 2.2

	Christopher Isherwood, Swami Prabhavananda[14]	*T.K.V. Desikachar*[15]	*Mukunda Stiles*[16]	*Nischala Joy Devi*[17]
Niyama	Various observances	Our attitudes toward ourselves	Precepts for personal discipline	Evolution toward harmony
Sauca	Purity	Cleanliness, or keeping our bodies and our surroundings clean and neat	Purity	Simplicity, purity, refinement
Santosha	Contentment	Contentment, or the ability to be comfortable with what we have and what we do not have	Contentment	Contentment, being at peace with oneself and others
Tapas	Mortification	The removal of impurities in our physical and mental systems through the maintenance of such correct habits as sleep, exercise, nutrition, work, and relaxation	Self-discipline and purification	Igniting the purifying flame
Svadhyaya	Study	Study and the necessity to review and evaluate our progress	Self-study	Sacred study of the Divine through scripture, nature, and introspection
Isvara-pranidhana	Devotion to God	Reverence to a higher intelligence or the acceptance of our limitations in relation to God, the all-knowing	Devotion to the Lord of Yoga	Wholehearted dedication to the Divine

TABLE 2.2 CONTINUED

of Money, that we swim in a sea of feeling that we don't have enough. We wake up thinking we don't have enough time, we didn't get enough sleep, we don't have enough money. She urges us to shift our thinking so we consider whatever resources we have as sufficient. And she teaches that we all have many resources, both inner strengths and gifts and, on the outside, friends, family, and community.[18] To test this idea for yourself, assess whether you wake up in the morning thinking of what you lack rather than the inner and outer resources you already have.

The *niyamas* (see figure 2.4), observances, consist of five key principles. The first *niyama* is *sauca*—maintaining cleanliness, keeping things in order, and getting rid of whatever no longer serves us, including certain ideas. Practicing *sauca* can help you gain inner tranquility by keeping your living space neat and clean, for example, clearing cutter off your desk before work, removing items that are not used from your home, or eliminating from your mind negative thoughts that make you feel anxious or undermine your self-esteem.

The second *niyama* is *santosha*—contentment, cultivating happiness and peace with yourself and others, and being comfortable with what you now have. One way to do this is by observing your experiences of contentment and noting their causes. You may notice that even though you've been brought up to believe that some tasks are grueling you nevertheless find contentment doing them. For example, even though you resented raking leaves for your parents as a child, now you may observe that it actually makes you feel contented to rake leaves on a sunny, crisp fall day.

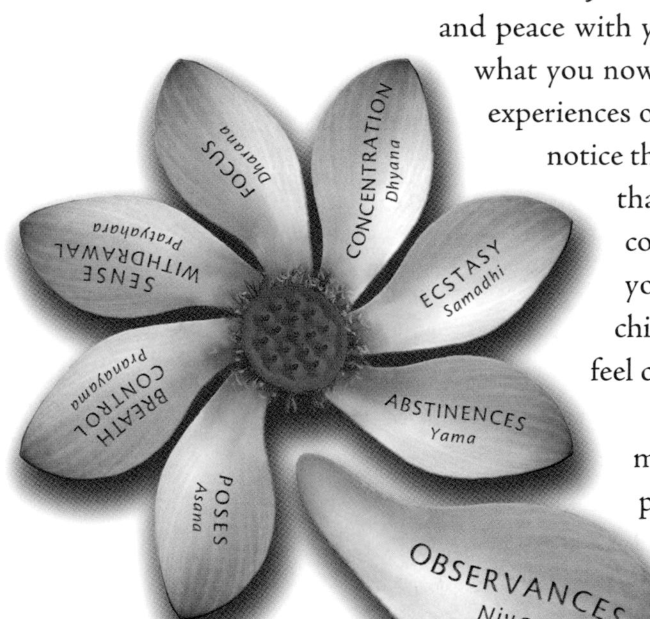

Figure 2.4. The second limb of Ashtanga yoga, niyama

Practicing *santosha* while doing yoga poses can make them come alive by giving you an attitude of playfulness and detachment. A more subtle way to practice *santosha* is by observing how often your lips are pursed and your forehead is furrowed, then smiling more and noticing how this simple act makes you feel. Some say that a sign of enlightenment is a slight smile.

The third *niyama* is *tapas*—inner fire for self-discipline, passion for the work of yoga, and purification. We need both energy and focused intention to live consciously in the world, and must learn how to ignite our inner fire and modulate the flame so we don't burn too fast or too hot. The yogic goal of awakening to our inner bliss is supported by both the energy of the flame and the self-discipline to use it consciously. Yoga offers poses and breathing practices to help with *tapas*, but we also need to employ sleep, relaxation, fun, and self-discipline as "correct habits," says T.K.V. Desikachar.[19]

The fourth *niyama* is *svadhyaya*—self-study, introspection, and study of informative texts. To practice *svadhyaya*, we can study the great scriptures of yoga or any other works that focus on a path to enlightenment. Most important, we can study ourselves, becoming the ultimate guru of our own experience by identifying our patterns of behavior on and off the mat. For example, by observing ourselves in poses we may notice a tendency to mentally wander off during class or feel agitation. Or we may see a pattern in the way we awaken each morning or interact with our children. Being able to discern our patterns of behavior is critical to self-knowledge, and choosing to keep them or change them is necessary for growth.

The last *niyama* is *isvara-pranidhana*—wholehearted dedication or surrender to the Divine. An alternative translation is "I give up." This is applicable, for example, in considering solutions to problems. When I can't determine the best one, I practice *isvara-pranidhana*, saying to myself, "I give up. I've done all I can do, and now I'm trusting that the universe will take care of the next step." Of course, this doesn't mean just sitting on your mat and waiting for the universe to resolve problems but instead realizing that you are not in control of situations and need to let go.

Another way to practice *isvara-pranidhana* is to dedicate your poses, meditation, or activities in your life to others in the world who need help. For example, you could say to yourself, "I dedicate my yoga practice today to children everywhere who are hungry for food or love"; or "I dedicate my meditation today to the people of Burma who are oppressed"; or "I dedicate these poses to the young girls of Egypt who are being forced to undergo genital mutilation." The idea is to set intention at the beginning as an offering to the universe, which can help create a positive attitude for inspirational yoga practice.

These first two limbs of the eight-limbed path embody the foundational concepts used when approaching the rest of the six limbs, both on and off the mat. Each of the remaining six limbs is discussed in later chapters, the third limb in chapter 6, the fourth limb in chapter 4, and the last four limbs in chapter 5.

Here is how one student worked with the first two principles:

As I've been paying closer attention to my actions, reactions, thoughts, patterns in life, I've been seeing more places in which ahimsa and satya can be practiced. These two yamas can very clearly be applied to my yoga practice on the mat: being honest about the general condition of my body; knowing that I have limits, exploring them, accepting them, and not feeling as though I've failed because of them.

Off the mat, too, there are many opportunities to apply these yamas. Sometimes I can't think straight or even sleep because I have so much anger toward other people. A few nights ago, I started looking at the situation from an honest (satya) perspective and realized that much of my anger was really directed toward myself, though it was much easier to place it outside of me. I was annoyed at myself for behaving in certain ways. Then I knew that if things were to change I'd have to break the pattern and let go of my anger. In other words, satya would have to be put into action to avoid any type of conflict, including conflict with myself.

The other thing I realized was that after being honest about where my anger was placed I'd have to practice ahimsa toward myself by not being so hard on myself and laughing more about things I take seriously.

In short, I see that if I practice ahimsa and satya in my daily life—to prevent reactions, break patterns, speak the truth in a loving manner—many conflicts and tensions can be avoided. And practicing these yamas myself will inevitably have an impact on those outside of me because my outlook will be softer, more open and honest.

Focus on one of the ten concepts of the *yamas* and *niyamas* for a specific period of time—a day, week, or month—making it the underlying principle of your life. Remind yourself of it as you awaken in the morning, as you go to sleep at night, and at various times during the day. Be mindful of how you integrate the concept into the events of daily life, how you perceive yourself in relation to it, and what you are learning as a result.

Study more of the Yoga Sutras by reading a translation that appeals to you. Following is a list of possibilities: *Yoga Sutras of Patanjali* by Mukunda Stiles, *The Secret Power of Yoga* by Nischala Joy Devi, *How to Know God* by Christopher Isherwood and Swami Prabhavananda, *Yoga Discipline of Freedom* by Barbara Stoler Miller, *The Essence of Yoga* by Bernard Bouanchaud, *Light on the Yoga Sutras of Patanjali* by B.K.S. Iyengar (see bibliography). Also consider reading *How Yoga Works* by Geshe Michael Roach and Christie McNally, a fictionalized account of a young woman in India long ago teaching her captors the principles of the Yoga Sutras.

THE BHAGAVAD GITA: A CALL TO ACTION

The Bhagavad Gita is translated variously as *Song of the Beloved, Song of the Blessed One, Song of the Glorious One, Song of God,* and *Song of the Divine*. A long, eighteen-chapter poem written in about the fifth century BCE as part of the *Mahabharata,* the Bhagavad Gita is a dialogue between a noble warrior, Arjuna, and his charioteer, Krishna, a divine teacher and incarnation of the god Vishnu.

The story is set on a battlefield where combat is about to take place between two factions of a family with a long history of convoluted deceptions, violence, and retribution. Arjuna has come ready to do battle against an enemy who is also a family member. In the moment before the battle, Arjuna has a crisis of conscience, aghast at the prospect of killing his kin, and asks Krishna for advice. To bring him to his senses, Krishna reveals to him the true nature of the world. What follows is a discussion of the meaning of yoga, the purpose of life, and how to live it. Ultimately Krishna states that yoga is a path imbued with action, wisdom, and clarity.

The fact that the Bhagavad Gita is, on the surface, a story about warfare may at first make it difficult for some modern-day yogis to embrace. If the first precept from the Yoga Sutras is nonviolence, they may question how this story could be concerned with yoga. But after studying the Bhagavad Gita it becomes clear that the story is a metaphor for being a warrior facing battle on the inner battlefield, struggling with integrity and truth.

The pivotal moment of decision is portrayed like most such moments people have experienced, not on a literal battlefield with chariots and armor but instead perhaps in families, relationships, or workplaces. For example, perhaps after years of grappling with some difficult conflict you have come face-to-face with a decision that will affect the outcome of the situation.

One yoga student recounts such a pivotal moment in her marriage of fifteen years. She and her husband had gone to therapists and religious counselors since the beginning of their marriage, and yet her spouse still habitually became enraged at her, berating her and calling her demeaning names in front of their young children. Meanwhile, she was working hard through yoga to face her own role in the drama. Her "warrior" moment of decision came one night when she and her children were huddled in a locked room, holding out against her husband's threatened violence, where she was able to witness the scene as if she were seeing it from the perspective of another person watching from above. As a result, she asked God for help—just as Arjuna, in his moment of despair, asks Krishna for advice—vowing to herself that when she awoke in the morning she would know what to do. When the sun rose, the decision was obvious to her, and without engaging in conflict or accusations she ended her marriage. She reports years later that yoga developed her perspective and her warrior self, and since then she has had a special affection for the Warrior Pose.

Sanskrit Gem

Dharma has many meanings, including a person's purpose or duty, the rules of proper conduct, and the principle or law that orders the universe.

A principal theme to which the Bhagavad Gita repeatedly returns is: Figure out your purpose or duty (*dharma*); act on it with all your energy; and then release any attachment to the outcome:

> *You have a right to your actions,*
> *But never to your action's fruits.*
> *Act for action's sake.*
> *And do not be attached to inaction.*[20]

And again:

> *Though the unwise cling to their actions,*
> *watching for results, the wise*
> *are free of attachments and act*
> *for the well-being of the whole world.*[21]

Parenting offers a good example of this lesson from the Bhagavad Gita. Parents have been entrusted to raise children and do it with all their energy. They search for the right response to problems, listen carefully to their children and their own hearts, and do what they can in a heartfelt way. Then once the children leave home, parents have to release any attachment to how the children interact and succeed in the world. If they remain attached, only suffering will follow, according to the Bhagavad Gita.

In numerous life circumstances, we can practice this pattern of considering the path of action, doing it with all our energy, and then releasing attachment to the outcome. For example, we might carefully choose a gift for a friend, give it with all our heart, and then release attachment to any prescribed outcome, not becoming upset if the friend isn't thrilled with the gift.

Another theme of the Bhagavad Gita is the two approaches to life described by Krishna: the path of action (karma yoga) and the path of learning (jnana yoga). Let's look at this section using two translations:

In this world there are two main paths:
The yoga of understanding
For contemplative men; and for men
Who are active, the yoga of action.[22]

In this world there are two roads of perfection,
as I told thee before, O prince without sin:
Jnana Yoga, the path of wisdom of the
Sankhyas, and Karma Yoga, the path of
action of the Yogis.[23]

The Bhagavad Gita stresses that different approaches are appropriate for various types of individuals. For example, one yogi may be perfectly happy to study great texts, meditate on their meaning in life, and worship his chosen deity, whereas another yogi may be content to study much less and spend more time practicing acts of service in the world, such as feeding the hungry, teaching yoga gratis to homeless people, or volunteering in a voter registration drive. Practically, we can't always choose just one of these two approaches, although we may have a preference for it. But despite these different approaches the Bhagavad Gita makes clear that the underlying idea remains the same: find your purpose or duty; do it with all your energy; and release attachment to the outcome.

Krishna also discusses karma and jnana yoga. Concerning karma (action) yoga he states:

> *It's better to do your own duty*
> *Badly, than to perfectly do*
> *Another's: you are safe from harm*
> *When you do what you should be doing.*[24]

Regarding jnana yoga he says:

> *Nothing in the world can purify*
> *As powerfully as wisdom;*
> *Practiced in yoga, you will find*
> *This wisdom within yourself.*[25]

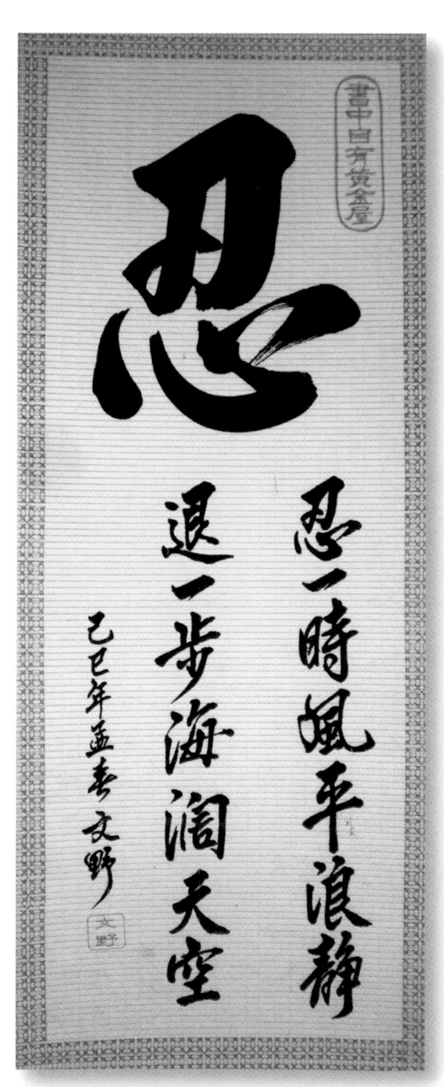

書中自有黃金屋
忍
忍一時風平浪靜
退一步海闊天空
Figure 2.5. Chinese wall hanging depicting equanimity

Further, the Bhagavad Gita defines yoga as equanimity or composure. It instructs us not to be blown around by positive and negative thoughts and emotions brought by life experiences. Instead, it advises us to maintain distance as an observer and not be attached to the need to control outcomes. This is clearly expressed in the following important verse:

> *Self-possessed, resolute, act*
> *Without any thought of results,*
> *Open to success or failure.*
> *This equanimity is yoga.*[26]

Having equanimity means maintaining balance when the external world presents challenges. A famous Chinese saying (see figure 2.5) urges individuals to remain as calm as a large boat on the sea no matter how high or turbulent the waves may be. In yoga practice, we work to maintain such equanimity physically, mentally, emotionally, and spiritually. For instance, if you feel discouraged that you cannot master a particular pose, you might say to yourself: "How would I feel if I could do the pose perfectly? How would I feel if I couldn't even do what I'm now doing? Can I imagine both states and then attain one in which I'm completely at ease in any event?"

Since the Bhagavad Gita was originally part of an oral tradition, the way it sounds is also important. Consequently, you may want to read it aloud or listen to it read. Deepak Chopra has recorded a CD of the Bhagavad Gita, and you can find other readings of it online. There are also new translations that may appeal to you more than the older ones.

The Bhagavad Gita has inspired readers for generations, including Ralph Waldo Emerson, Henry Thoreau, and Mahatma Gandhi. For example, in 1868 Emerson wrote the following to Emma Lazarus, author of the inscription on the Statue of Liberty: "And of books, there is another which, when you have read, you shall sit for a while and then write a poem—[it is] the 'Bhagvat-Geeta,' but read it in Charles Wilkins' translation."[27]

Years later, in a letter to Max Müller on August 4, 1873, he confessed:

> *I owed . . . a magnificent day to the Bhagavat Geeta. It was the first of books; it was as if an empire spake to us, nothing small or unworthy, but large, serene, consistent, the voice of an old intelligence which in another age and climate had pondered and thus disposed of the same questions which exercise us. Let us not now go back and apply a minute criticism to it, but cherish the venerable oracle.*[28]

Mahatma Gandhi said the following about the Bhagavad Gita:

> *The Bhagavad-Gita calls on humanity to dedicate body, mind and soul to pure duty and not to become mental voluptuaries at the mercy of random desires and undisciplined impulses.*
>
> *When doubts haunt me, when disappointments stare me in the face, and I see not one ray of hope on the horizon, I turn to the Bhagavad-Gita and find a verse to comfort me; and I immediately begin to smile in the midst of overwhelming sorrow. Those who meditate on the Gita will derive fresh joy and new meanings from it every day.*[29]

Read one of these recommended translations of the Bhagavad Gita: *Bhagavad Gita: A New Translation* by Stephen Mitchell and *The Bhagavad Gita* by Juan Mascaró. You can also find the text online.

To understand how Arjuna came to this moment, create his family tree with notes describing the conflicts. (Most translators and commentators on the Bhagavad Gita include this history in the introduction, as do Ram Dass and Juan Mascaró in the books cited above.)

Read Ram Dass's *Paths to God: Living the Bhagavad Gita*, a book based largely on a workshop he gave in summer 1974 at the Naropa Institute in Boulder, Colorado. This excellent volume illuminates the concepts of karma yoga, bhakti yoga, and jnana yoga in an inspiring way that helps in applying them to daily life. For example:

> *Whatever karma it is that brought you to this point, it's now your dharma to work with it. It's now your task to work with being in the situation of reading this book, and confronting these questions. You ask, "What exactly does that mean? What do I have to do about all this?" Well, that's something you're going to have to work out for yourself. We each have our own path. I don't know what yours is—I can hardly figure out my own. What I can predict, though, is that for you, as for Arjuna, it will probably include giving up some cherished notions about yourself, some ideas about who you are and where you're going.*[30]

CHAPTER THREE

Vibration As Tool

SANSKRIT: THE LANGUAGE OF VIBRATION

Vibration is an important yogic tool for creating energetic transformations in and ultimately beyond the body. And Sanskrit, the original language of yoga, is mantric, meaning it is specifically designed to vibrate in the body.

In yoga, the sounds of Sanskrit vibrate the body through the wheels of energy known as the chakras and along the center channel, the *sushumna nadi*. Vibration may occur through use of the Sanskrit names for poses while doing them, through chanting before or afterward, and by practicing the poses. This chapter focuses first on how vibration occurs in the body, the way Sanskrit vibrates the body, how the language is written, and a few key yogic words in Sanskrit. Then the energy centers and specific Sanskrit mantras for transformation are discussed.

Today's quantum physicists and ancient yogis agree that we are more space than substance. For thousands of years yogis have used Sanskrit sounds to consciously vibrate that space, thereby connecting to the pulse of the cosmos. And recent scientific discoveries substantiate the understanding of living tissue as vibrating. In fact, videos of a live cell under a microscope reveal that it is vibrating to some rhythm.

In 2001, the nanotechnologist Jim Gimzewski, Distinguished Professor with the UCLA Chemistry and Biochemistry Department, learned that when living heart cells are put in a petri dish with appropriate nutrients they continue to beat. Since sound is vibrations traveling through the air, he wondered if all cells might pulsate and make noise. To find out, he built a tiny amplifier and held an atomic force microscope against the membrane of a yeast cell so that, like a record needle, it would record

Sanskrit Gem

***Mantra*—composed of *man*, meaning to think or *manas* meaning mind, and *tra*, meaning without or protection—signifies a chant with meaning beyond the reach or protection of the mind.**

any movement and translate it into sound. He discovered that a cell wall rises and falls a distance of three nanometers—the equivalence of about 15 carbon atoms stacked up—1,000 times a second so the cell seems to "sing." According to *Smithsonian Magazine*, the frequency of the yeast cells tested has always been in the same high range, "about a C-sharp to D above middle C." Sprinkling alcohol on a yeast cell to kill it raises the pitch, while dead cells give off a low, rumbling sound that Gimzewski says is probably the result of random atomic motions. He also found that yeast cells with genetic mutations make a slightly different sound than normal yeast cells, giving rise to hope that the technique might be applied to diagnosing diseases such as cancer, which is believed to originate with changes in the genetic makeup of cells. Gimzewski calls his new science "sonocytology," though he's not sure whether the cells are really making the noise or absorbing vibrations from elsewhere, including the microscope itself.[1]

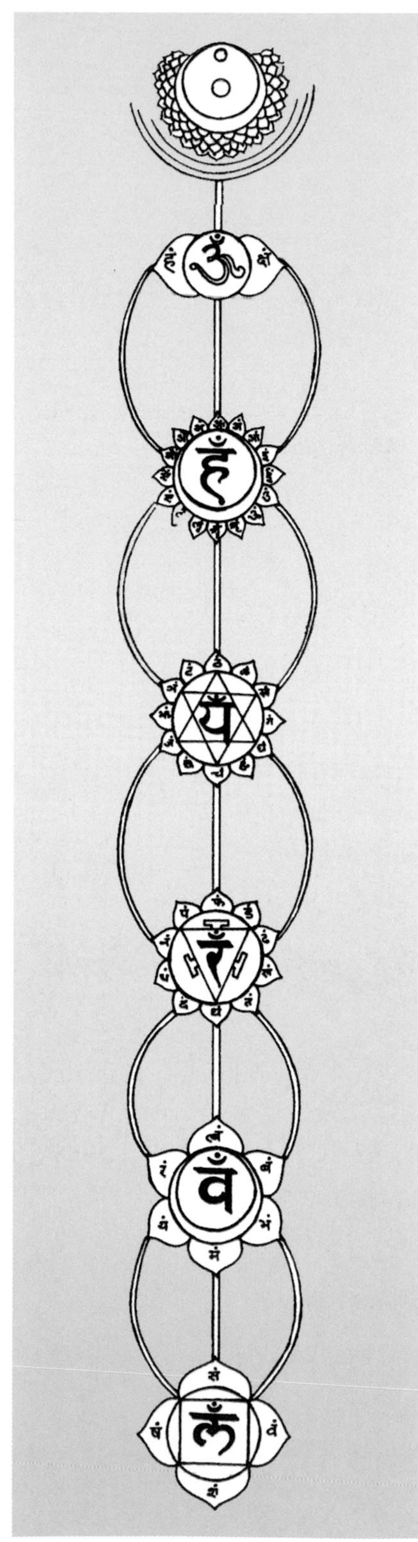

Figure 3.1. Chakra petals with Sanskrit letters

In practicing yoga we increase both our awareness of vibration and our understanding of Sanskrit as a vibrational tool. We practice "focused listening" so we feel our body vibrating. Then we open our body, mind, and spirit to eliminate blockage or confusion in order to become a more effective conduit for vibrating energy.

The sounds of Sanskrit vibrate the *sushumna nadi* by activating the wheels of energy, or chakras. Ancient seers became aware of chakras when, during meditation, they saw swirling wheels of energy moving in the body along the center of the torso, from the base of the spine to the top of the head. The seers visualized these vortices as flowers with petals on which the fifty letters of the Sanskrit alphabet vibrated when the language was spoken (see figure 3.1). Each of the fifty letters of Sanskrit vibrates a specific part of the body.

Each chakra is associated with a particular "seed syllable" that contains the essence of powerful information for growth and transformation, just as tiny redwood seeds hold the potential to become towering redwoods. The chakras and the vibrating seed syllables associated with them are shown in figure 3.2.

The most famous seed syllable is *Aum* (see figure 3.3). It is composed of three sounds—ahhh, oooo, mmmm—that vibrate in the body, ahhh at the back of the throat, oooo in the center of the mouth, and mmmm at the lips. Chanting this seed syllable, which is often done at the beginning and end of yoga practice, connects us to our own vibration and to the energy of the cosmos.

The power of this syllable is described early in the Upanishads.

Yama replied:

That word to which all Vedas point,
To which all austerities lead,
Which all men and women desire
Who thirst after righteousness,
Which they try to live
As spiritual seekers.
That word is AUM.
That eternal sacred syllable
Signifies the Absolute
Supreme Brahman.
He who comprehends
The sound and meaning of
AUM
Truly understands Self-Realization.
AUM is the best support,
AUM is the highest support.
He who chants this support
Is magnified.[2]

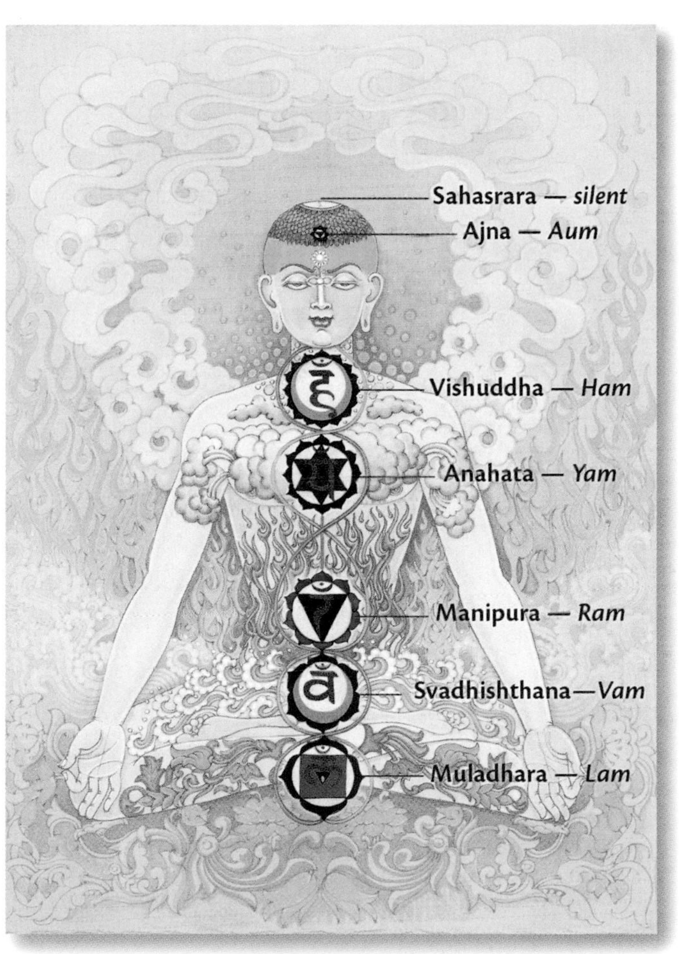

Figure 3.2. The chakras and their seed syllables

Aum is also praised in the Yoga Sutras:

The sound denoting
That Self is
the eternal vibration Aum,
which manifests the
grace of the
divine presence.
By constantly repeating
the sacred sound
with great respect and love
and reflecting
upon its meaning,
one attains spiritual wealth.[3]

Sanskrit Gem

Chakra means wheel.

Chanting the seed syllable *Aum* heightens the awareness of vibration not only in the chakras and the *sushumna nadi* but elsewhere in the body and in the external world. *Aum* can also be thought of as mimicking the ongoing cycle of life—beginning, continuing, and ending, or birth, preservation, and death—associated with the three Hindu deities known as Brahma, Vishnu, and Shiva.

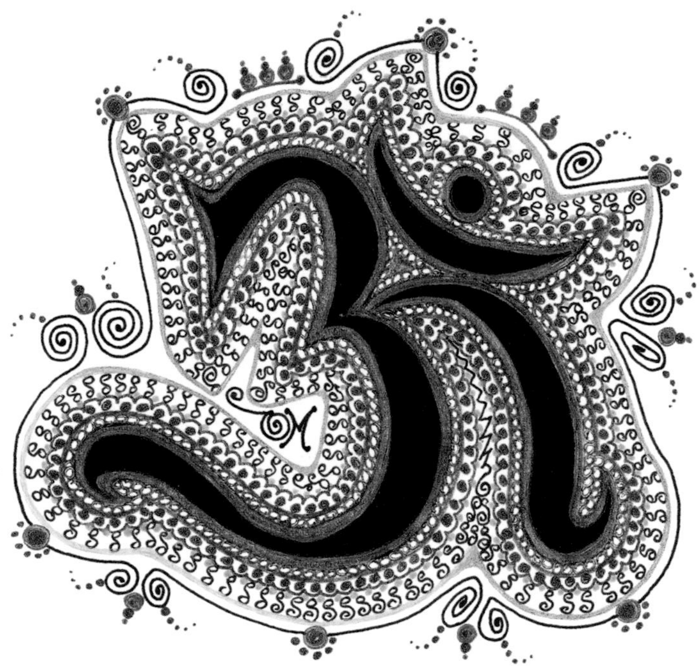

Figure 3.3. An artist's drawing of the seed syllable Aum

Sanskrit Gem

Devanagari, the Indian alphabet used to write Sanskrit, combines the words *Deva*, which means god, brahman, or celestial, and *nāgarî*, which means city or sacred script of the city, and expresses visual beauty.

The letters of Sanskrit are written in Sanskrit Devanagari. For purposes of being a yoga student or teacher, it is useful to learn to recognize and write a few keys words in Sanskrit Devanagari, such as *Aum*, *yoga* (literally "yoke" or "union"), and *namaste* (literally, "I bow to you," or more poetically, "From the still quiet place in me I bow to the quiet still space in you, and when we are both in that place we are one"), a salutation acknowledging the yogic principles of respect for others and the unity of humanity, usually accompanied by putting the hands together at the chest and bowing slightly as shown in figure 3.4.

YOGA AND ENERGETICS

An essential aim of yoga entails cultivating and managing energy in the body. And among the body's multiple layers, as understood by ancient practitioners, is an energetic layer known as *pranamaya kosha*, which contains pathways, called *nadis*, that circulate like rivers. This occurs in what is called the subtle body, or astral body, which exists in a dimension not often seen or acknowledged in our culture. Every day, we sense others' vibrations even if we are not consciously aware of it. For example, when we walk into a room crowded with people and get a feeling that the space is positive or negative, we are reading their energy. To become more aware of your ability to read such energy, notice, when you are in a yoga class, at a mall, or some other location, the energy others project and the energy you have as a result.

While the sounds of Sanskrit vibrate the *sushumna nadi* and the chakras, yoga poses and breath development open up the *nadis* of the body. The *sushumna nadi* begins at the base of the spine and forms the trajectory of the ascending Kundalini *shakti*, latent energy that, once unleashed, can rise to the crown of the head. On either side of the *sushumna nadi* is an energetic pathway—on the left is the *ida*, characterized by the feminine cooling qualities of the moon, and on the right the *pingala*, associated with the masculine warming qualities of the sun. These two pathways spiral up the spine, intersecting along the *sushumna nadi* and forming the vortices of energy called chakras, located along the center spine.

One of the great gifts of the Tantra yoga movement (see discussion in chapter 1) was the expanded use of vibration in yoga by refining this

Sanskrit Gem

Pranamaya kosha **combines the words *prana*, meaning life force, *maya*, meaning full of, and *kosha*, meaning layer or sheath, and represents the layer comprising the expansion of our vital energies.**

Sanskrit Gem

Sushumna **means, literally, "She who is most gracious," and *nadi* means conduit.**

Sanskrit Gem

Ida **means pale, and *pingala* means reddish.**

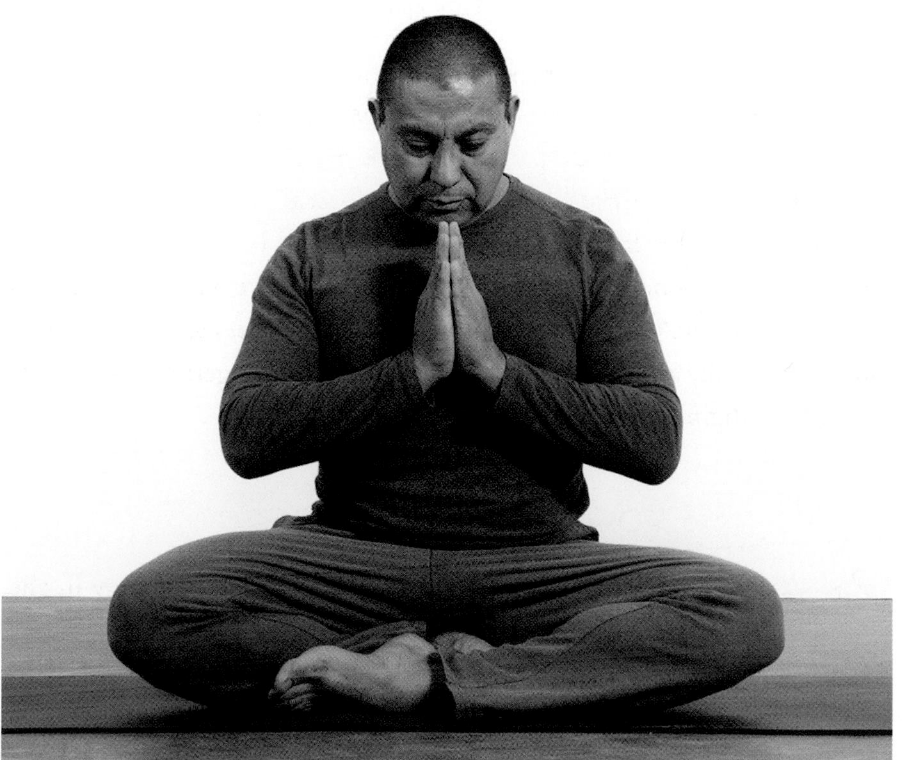

Figure 3.4. Namaste gesture

model of the Kundalini energy moving along the chakras while spiraling up through the *sushumna nadi.* All the poses of hatha yoga are designed to free up this energy so it can rise in the body. When it flows freely up the two pathways alongside the *sushumna nadi,* the body, heart, and mind are completely open and in sync, making it possible to attain bliss and liberation—the goal of yoga.

Altogether, seven key chakras can be vibrated: *Muladhara, Svadhishthana, Manipura, Anahata, Vishuddha, Ajna,* and *Sahasrara* (figure 3.2). The qualities attributed to each chakra vary according to different traditions. Also, correlations are made between the chakras and physical aspects, especially involving the endocrine system. To discover what each chakra means to you, chant the seed syllable associated with it as you meditate on it.

Sanskrit Gem

Mula means root, and *adhara* means supporting.

Some basic traits are the following. The first chakra, *Muladhara,* the root chakra located at the base of the spine, is associated with the seed syllable *Lam,* the earth, the color red, the sense of smell, and the feeling of being grounded. As you chant *Lam, Lam, Lam* nine times, visualizing this chakra in red, ask yourself: Do I feel supported by life? Do I have a sense of being grounded? Over time, as you practice chanting and asking these questions you may notice that your answers change. If you discern from your own body knowledge that this area is in need of attention, you might work with the chakra through specific poses.

Sanskrit Gem

Sva means self, and *adhishthana* means base.

The second chakra, *Svadhishthana,* a few finger widths below the navel and above the root chakra, is associated with the seed syllable *Vam,* safety, water, the sense of taste (literally or aesthetically), the color orange, and sexual desire. As you chant the seed syllable *Vam, Vam, Vam* nine times, visualizing this chakra in orange, ask yourself: Am I living the life I desire? Are my passions being fulfilled? Do I know my tastes?

Sanskrit Gem

Manipura means jeweled city.

The third chakra, *Manipura,* is the solar plexus, located between the navel and the rib cage. It is associated with the seed syllable *Ram,* power to affect the world (physically and psychically), fire, the sense of sight, and the color yellow. The organs of digestion, sometimes called the second brain,[4] have complexity and intelligence, as they contain 100 million nerves along with sensory and motor neurons and information-processing circuits that use the major neurotransmitters dopamine, serotonin, acetylcholine, nitric oxide, and norepinephrine. On the subtle plane, we can connect to the power of this chakra to attain enlightenment. As you chant *Ram* nine times, visualizing this chakra in yellow, ask yourself: In what ways do I feel powerful in the world? In what ways do I lack power, physically or otherwise? In what ways would I like to cultivate more power?

The fourth chakra, *Anahata*, or the heart chakra, is located in the center of the body near the heart and associated with the seed syllable *Yam*, air, the sense of touch, and the color green. The heart chakra is about love and compassion for ourselves, then for others. To be "unstruck" doesn't mean we don't acknowledge the pain in our lives—perhaps anger and sadness from childhood or a divorce—but that in spite of it we can lovingly accept ourselves and feel compassion for others. As you chant *Yam* nine times, visualizing this chakra in green, ask yourself: Can I experience freedom unfettered by past pain? What prevents me from feeling love and compassion? Would forgiving myself and others be helpful in attaining love and peace?

Sanskrit Gem

***Anahata* means unstruck.**

The fifth chakra, *Vishuddha*, is located at the throat and associated with the seed syllable *Hum*, finding your voice (literally as well as creatively), space, the sense of hearing, and the color blue. As you chant *Hum* nine times, visualizing this chakra in blue, ask yourself: Is my life right now the most creative expression of my inner self? If anything were possible and I weren't concerned about the opinions of others, how would I live? What is the most expansive vision I could have for myself?

Sanskrit Gem

***Vishuddha* means pure.**

The sixth chakra, *Ajna*, located at the third eye—between and slightly above the eyebrows—is associated with the seed syllable *Aum*, intuition, inner wisdom, and the color indigo. As you chant *Aum* nine times, visualizing this chakra in indigo, ask yourself: Do I listen to the guidance of my intuition, my "inner guru"? You can also ask your inner guru for clarity regarding a specific question, such as whether to stay in a job, a relationship, or a home. Ask the question, chant, and wait for a response, remaining alert for answers from any source, internal or external, as you go about your daily life.

Sanskrit Gem

***Ajna* means command.**

The seventh chakra, *Sahasrara*, is the crown of the head, visualized as a thousand-petal lotus and the connection between self and the universe. This chakra is associated with no seed syllable, only silence. After working with the other chakras and feeling open along the *sushumna nadi*, meditate on the crown chakra and ask yourself: How do I connect to the world? How do I experience the souls of other beings? Where do I end and others begin, in an energetic sense, and what is our common purpose?

Sanskrit Gem

***Sahasrara* means thousand-spoke wheel.**

You can practice chanting the seed syllables for each chakra (*Lam, Vam, Ram, Yum, Hum, Aum*) as a way of working with the Kundalini energy rising up through the body. Usually this is best done after an asana and *pranayama* (breath control) practice as the body is more open then, making it easier to sense these subtle vibrations.

Another effective use of chanting Sanskrit seed syllables associated with chakras is to focus on the area that corresponds to a problem. For example, a student who was feeling physically and psychologically weak chanted *Ram* 108 times after doing yoga poses to activate the *Manipura* chakra. Over time, she began chanting *Ram* during the poses and even mentally on other occasions when she felt low, resulting in the immediate return of her strength.

MANTRAS FOR TRANSFORMATION

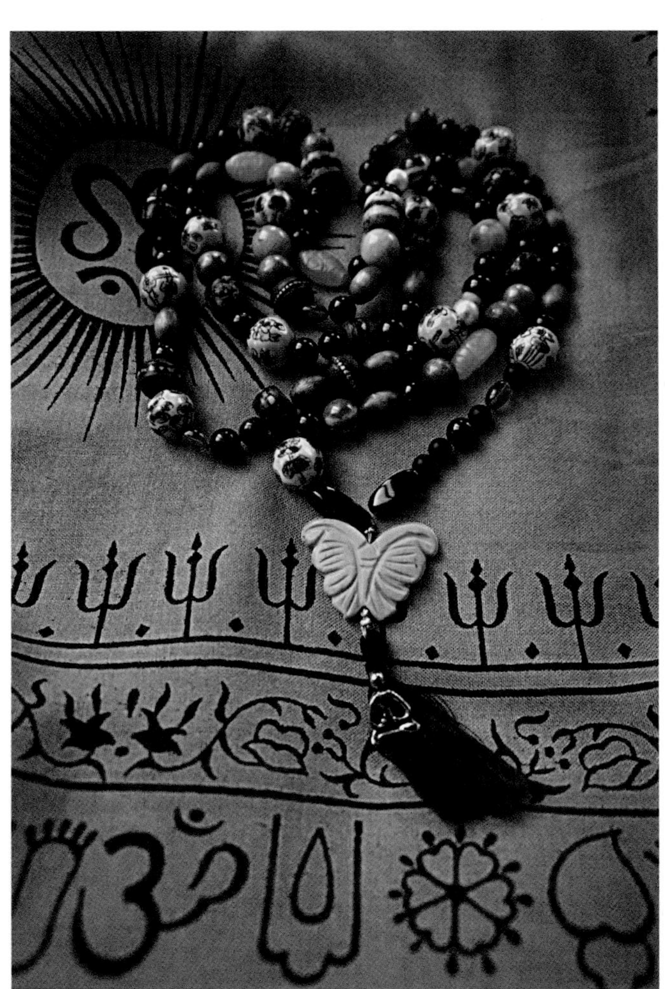

Figure 3.5. Mala, used to count chant iterations

In addition to chanting Sanskrit seed syllables, there is an ancient yogic practice of chanting mantras for help with any situation, such as healing, transformation, finding a job or lover, or pursuing an educational endeavor. Vedic masters who have studied this tradition in India teach powerful chanting methods in America. One such teacher, Thomas Ashley-Farrand, has written many books and produced CDs to help students embrace this ancient tradition of Sanskrit mantra practice.[5]

When I began studying yoga, I was skeptical about the power of chanting. But as the energetic channels of my body opened, first through asana practice, then *pranayama*, and finally meditation, I was drawn to chanting since by then I had experienced vibration through yoga in a number of ways.

Chanting is usually done with a *mala*, a garland of 108 beads (see figure 3.5), though the Sikh tradition uses a *mala* of 108 knots tied in a string of wool. Chanting sometimes takes place with a fraction of that, such as a half *mala*, 54, or a quarter *mala*, 27. For the significance of the number 108, see "Sages Say."

When I began chanting I purchased a full *mala* and chanted a simple mantra 108 times twice a day—*"Aum, Shrim Maha Lakshmyai Swaha"*—following the pronunciation guide from a CD by Thomas Ashley-Farrand. *Aum* and *Shrim* are both

Sages Say

- Both 9 and 12 have spiritual significance in many traditions, and 9 × 12 = 108. Also, 1 + 8 = 9.
- The number 108 reflects a multiple of the powers of 1, 2, and 3: 1 to the first power (1 × 1) = 1; 2 to the second power (2 × 2) = 4; 3 to the third power (3 × 3 × 3) = 27. 1 × 4 × 27 = 108.
- The number 108 is a Harshad number, an integer divisible by the sum of its digits. (*Harshad*, from Sanskrit, means great joy.)
- It is believed that if one is able to be so calm in meditation as to have only 108 breaths in a day, enlightenment will come.
- There are said to be 108 *marmas* in the subtle body. *Marmas*, or *marmasthanas*, are energy intersections like chakras but formed by the convergence of fewer energy lines.
- Some yogis believe that a complete counting of the repetitions of the *mala* amounts to 100. The remaining are said to cover errors or omissions, or be an offering to God and guru.
- The sacred Ganges River spans a longitude of 12 degrees (79 to 91) and a latitude of 9 degrees (22 to 31). 12 × 9 = 108.
- In astrology, there are 12 houses and 9 planets. 12 × 9 = 108.
- The diameter of the Sun is 108 times the diameter of Earth. The distance from the Sun to Earth is 108 times the diameter of the Sun. The average distance from the Moon to Earth is 108 times the diameter of the Moon.
- Tantra estimates the average number of breaths per day at 21,600, of which 10,800 are associated with solar energy and 10,800 with lunar energy. 108 × 100 = 10,800. 2 × 10,800 = 21,600.
- The number 108 is used in Islam to refer to God.
- In Chinese astrology, there are 108 sacred stars.

seed syllables; *Maha* means great or big; *Lakshmi* is the female manifestation of prosperity and abundance; and *Swaha* means honoring. I committed to a forty-day practice, with the intention of chanting for more prosperity to help me fund an educational course for my eldest daughter. On the second day, while cleaning out a drawer I found a decades-old gift of a Krugerrand, a gold coin at the time worth about $750, and immediately identified the discovery as an outcome of the mantra practice. A few weeks later I learned of a $7,000 scholarship for state residents that would pay for my daughter's tuition. As a result of these initial experiences, I came to respect the power of chanting.

By sitting quietly, perhaps after a physical yoga practice or at the beginning or end of the day, bringing full attention to our breath, setting a clear intention of purpose, and bringing all of ourselves to the chanting, we can experience the transformative power of this practice. Through the miracle of vibration, understood so long ago by ancient yogis and now being evaluated by modern science, while chanting we can connect to ourselves at our most basic energetic level and appreciate who we truly are.

LAYERS OF EXPERIENCE

Yoga also offers a model from the Upanishads that expands our view of ourselves and helps us navigate our experiences. According to this model, the human organism has five *koshas*, layers or bodies of consciousnss, ranging from dense to subtle (see figure 3.6). The outermost layer is the physical body, or *annamaya kosha*, which has miraculous abilities for healing and transformation.

Sanskrit Gem

Anna means food, *maya* means full of, and *kosha* means sheath or layer.

For example, a student came to yoga with sometimes incapacitating back pain from spinal stenosis, causing pinched nerves. He attended therapeutic yoga classes and private yoga instruction weekly, and after several months was able to sit almost pain free. Then, due to a change in schedule, he was unable to practice yoga for a couple months, and his condition worsened. When he resumed his practice of yoga, however, he returned to a nearly pain-free life. Another student who experienced persistent low back pain found some relief by doing poses and complete relief only after chanting for releasing obstacles over several weeks.

The second layer of experience is the *pranamaya kosha* (see also chapter 4), or energy body. Breath practices affecting this layer can improve the physical body, as I experienced in taming asthma.

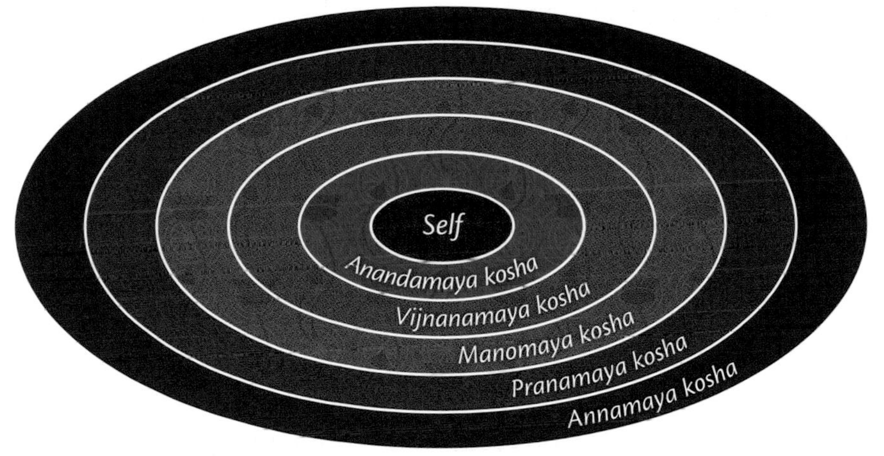

Figure 3.6. The five layers of consciousness, called koshas

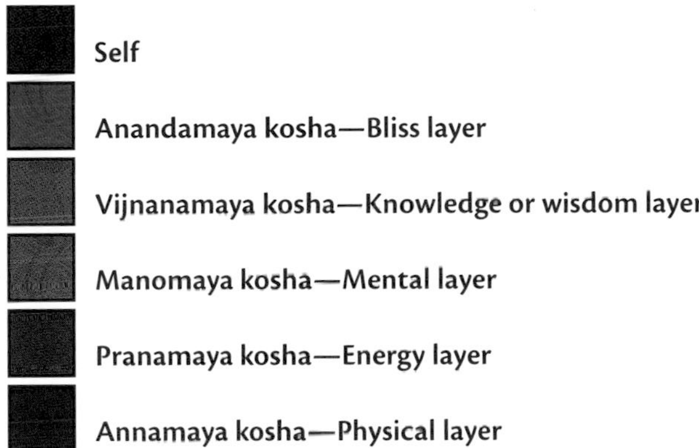

The third layer is the *manomaya kosha*, or mental body, and is composed of two qualities, *manas* and *buddhi*. *Manas* is the rational mind we use in daily life, while *buddhi* is intellect.

The fourth layer is *vijnanamaya kosha*, or the intellectual body. *Vijnanamaya kosha* is the place from which, having absorbed knowledge and understanding from the third layer, we can make judgments with wisdom.

The fifth, and subtlest, layer is *anandamaya kosha*, or bliss body, the place of ecstasy and peace, where all things become one.

Although the practices described in this chapter—chanting seed syllables and mantras, and viewing experience through the lens of *koshas*—may appeal to you either immediately or after considerable yoga training, cultivating vibration as a tool can be a powerful way to relate to the body, mind, and soul. Even in the early stages of practice it can bring about a deep transformation.

Sanskrit Gem

Mano means mind.

Sanskrit Gem

Vi is intensity for all experiences, and *jnana* is knowledge, intellect, wisdom.

Sanskrit Gem

Ananda means bliss.

Practice writing *Aum*, *yoga*, and *namaste* in Sanskrit Devanagari as shown in figures 3.7 and 3.8.

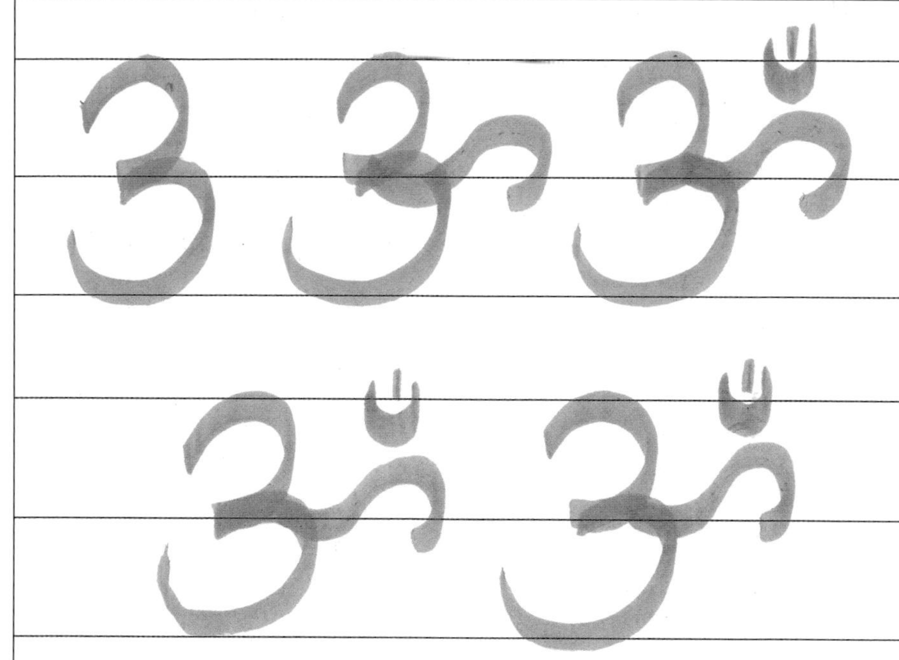

Figure 3.7. A tracing of *Aum* in Sanskrit Devanagari

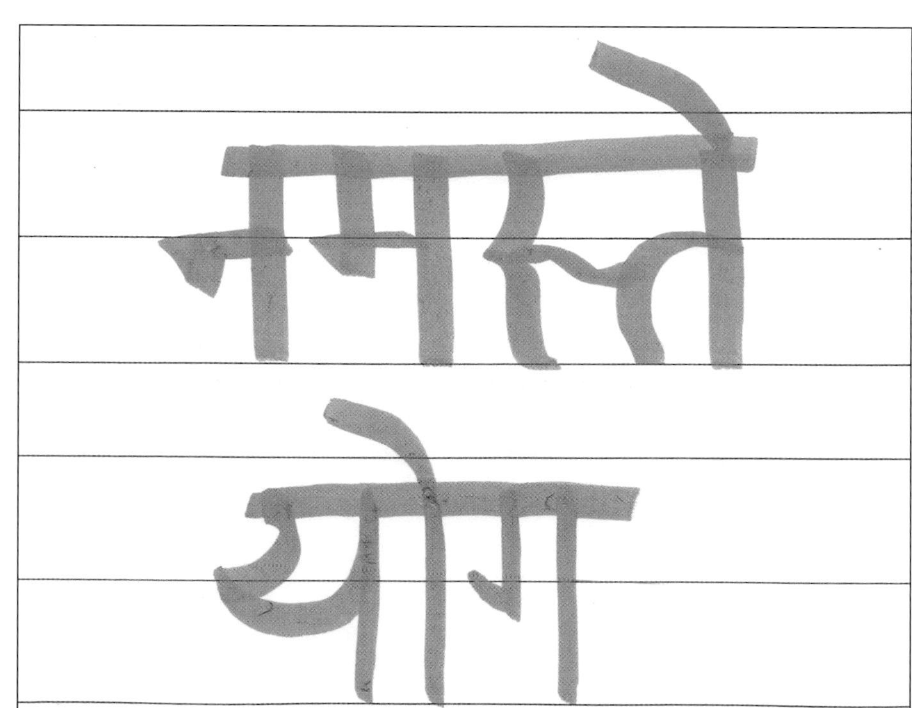

Figure 3.8. Tracings of *namaste* (top) and *yoga* (bottom) in Sanskrit Devanagari

After chanting the seed syllables for the chakras, create your own chakra chart with your personal vision. You could make a collage, drawing, or mobile using the Sanskrit Devanagari seed syllables, pictures from your past, images you envision, or abstract shapes. Figure 3.9 shows one yogi's chakra creation.

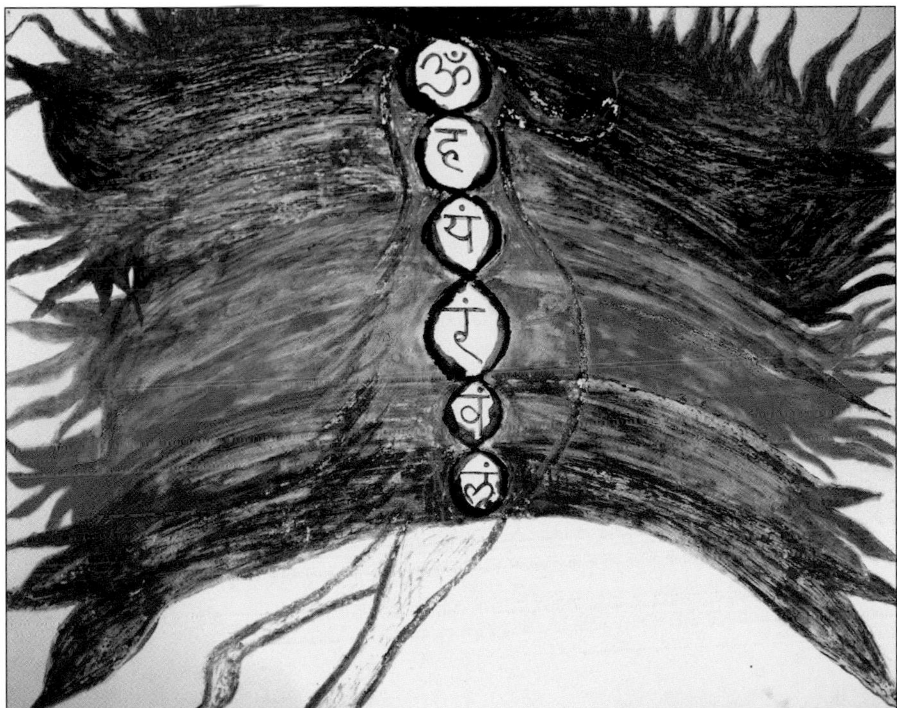

Figure 3.9. A student's chakra chart

Explore and cultivate experiences that make you feel vibration, such as Sanskrit mantra chanting, beat music, the sounds of nature, or the buzz of a large sporting event. Become aware of how the vibration affects your sense of power and well-being.

Choose a seed syllable or a phrase for a personal mantra to say whenever your mind wanders off to some undesirable concept. Then, instead of trying to avoid thinking of something that is upsetting or that you've decided to minimize in your life, chant the mantra until your thoughts change.

PART II

ON THE MAT

The focus of this *pada* is yoga practice on the mat, beginning with the fourth of Ashtanga yoga's eight-limbed path. Some individuals say that you have to learn the limbs sequentially and not work on the fourth limb (*pranayama*) until the third (asana) is mastered: "Pranayama is the conscious, deliberate regulation of the breath replacing unconscious patterns of breathing. It is possible only after a reasonable mastery of asana practice."[1] Certainly, practicing poses opens the body and mind, making meditation easier, but I've found it is also useful to bring all the concepts of the other limbs to the mat while practicing poses, including *pranayama* and the last four limbs, concerned with meditation.

Consequently, this *pada* begins with chapter 4, "Breath, Bandhas, and Mudras: The Subtle Realm," which includes a description of the fourth limb, *pranayama*, along with five specific practices. The importance of the time of year for practicing is discussed, as well as the soft palate. The three *bandhas*, or energetic holds, are described, and finally the use of mudras, or gestures, usually of the hands, is shown.

Chapter 5, "Meditation for Beauty and Bliss," focuses on the last four of the eight limbs of yoga, which are concerned with going ever deeper into the inner realm. The fifth limb, *pratyahara*, or sense withdrawal, is described, and then *dharana*, *dhyana*, and *samadhi*, the sixth, seventh, and eighth limbs, are discussed, which constitute progressively more refined forms of meditation. Specific meditation techniques follow.

Chapter 6, "Poses for Freedom," brings the teachings of all the limbs to the practice of poses on the mat. The purposes and benefits of poses are discussed, as well as advice from ancient texts on how to do poses. General principles are given for poses, followed by commentary on seven categories of poses. The chapter also includes information on the importance of setting intentions before practice, as well as the use and development of core strength with both classical poses and neo-asanas. Finally, basic anatomy useful for understanding the poses is described.

CHAPTER FOUR

Breath, Bandhas, and Mudras: The Subtle Realm

THE FOURTH LIMB: PRANAYAMA, BREATH CONTROL

For thousands of years, yogis have taught that our life force, or *prana*, can be guided through breath practices to become a very powerful tool for liberation. Most of our breaths are unconscious, yet breathing techniques can be cultivated to offer us many physical and spiritual benefits, including *samadhi*, or ecstasy. *Pranayama* (see figure 4.1) isn't only about inhaling oxygen and exhaling carbon dioxide; it concerns breathing specifically to influence the flow of *prana* in the *nadis*, or energy channels, ultimately to awaken our being to its potential.

The benefits of breath regulation are beginning to be understood by Western science—for example, the role of slowing the breath to regulate high blood pressure[1] and help with heart disease[2] and other chronic illnesses. When we slow our breath and breathe consciously, our central nervous system quiets down, our heart rate drops, and our entire body relaxes in a measurable way. This also enhances our mental state, resulting in less nervousness and anxiety. The spiritual benefits of *pranayama* are stated in many ancient yogic texts, including the Yoga Sutras:

As a result
of this pranayama,
the veil obscuring the radiant
supreme light of the Inner Self
dissolves.
And as a result,
the mind attains fitness
for the process of contemplation
of the True Self.[3]

Figure 4.1. The fourth limb of Ashtanga yoga, *pranayama*

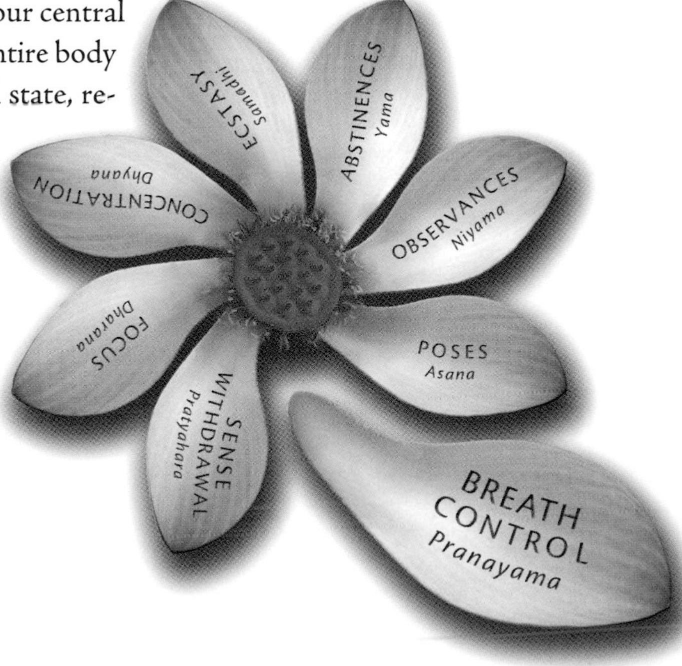

For many yoga students, regulating the breath is more challenging than doing poses. Yet breath control is the most potent tool we have to connect to our authentic inner self. On the mat, in life, and whenever we are nervous or scared, or the mind is wandering aimlessly, the most expedient way to return to calmness is through breathing deeply and consciously.

Consciously focusing on breathing is also the most important practice for working with poses. While the Yoga Sutras describe a stepwise path—that is, asana before *pranayama*—*pranayama* informs all yoga poses, as they begin, continue, and end with the breath.

Three-Part Yogic Breath

For all the practices detailed here, breathe through your nose with your mouth closed, unless you are ill and need to open your mouth slightly. To begin breath practice, lie down in what Vanda Scaravelli has called "Lying Release" and breathe with consciousness of the breath, spine, and gravity—the triumvirate of breathing. As you inhale, the belly lifts, the rib cage expands, then the upper chest fills; and as you exhale, the upper chest descends, then the rib cage, and finally the lower belly (see figure 4.2). We can call this a wave of breath. Just as ocean waves rise to a crest and fall, so breath waves rise and fall in the body.

Vanda Scaravelli's work is based on this wave of the breath:

> *There is a way of doing yoga poses that we call asanas without the slightest effort. Movement is the song of the body. Yes, the body has its own song from which the movement of dancing arises spontaneously. In other words, the liberation of the upper part of the body produced by the acceptance of gravity in the lower part of the body is the origin of lightness, and dancing is its expression. This song, if you care to listen to it, is beauty. We could say that it is part of nature. We sing when we are happy and the body goes with it like waves in the sea.*[4]

Once you have a feel for moving the breath through the body, you can work with the specifics of three-part yogic breath:

Begin by putting your hands on your belly. Then inhale into your belly and exhale from your belly, noticing how your pelvic bowl tilts up and down.

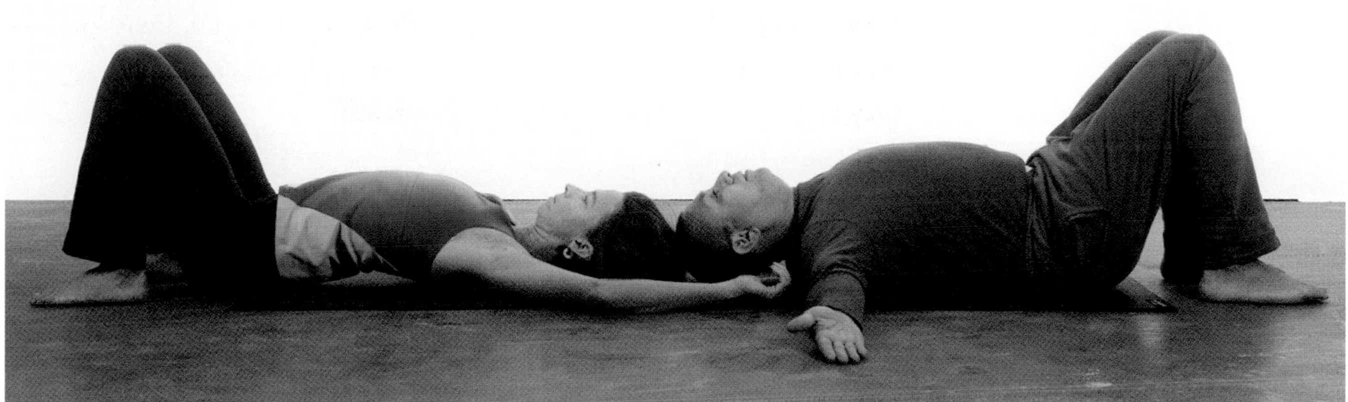

Figure 4.2. Lying Release inhale (left) and exhale (right)

Next, move your hands to your rib cage and feel your ribs expand as you inhale and contract as you exhale. Notice that your ribs actually move in all directions—up to the sky, out to the side, and down to the floor.

Now move your hands so they rest on your clavicles, or collarbones, and feel the clavicles rise slightly and spread as you inhale and fall slightly as you exhale.

Once you have felt breath move separately into each of the three areas, begin breathing into each one sequentially, inhaling into your belly, making your rib cage flare out, then your upper chest lift, then exhaling as your upper chest sinks down, your mid-torso descends, and finally your belly moves down. Continue practicing this three-part yogic breath at the beginning of your *pranayama* work to reinforce the complete movement of the spine with the breath.

When we first begin to observe our breath, usually the mind resists, saying things like, "This is incredibly boring" or "Don't you have something more important to do?" So the first challenge is to not act on such thoughts but instead simply observe them and refocus on the experience of connecting to your breath. Then, as you become conscious of breathing, focus on the sensations in your body without being judgmental. For example, perhaps you notice stiffness in your lower back, tightness in your left shoulder, or a gripping feeling in your throat. Such an assessment will increase your awareness of possible blockages to the free flow of life force in your body. Becoming aware of sensations in the body, both subtle and gross, with an open mind is the key to conscious yoga practice.

Ujjayi: Victory Breath

Sanskrit Gem

Ujjayi means victory.

Ujjayi, or victory breath, is a type of yogic breathing that creates a resistance against which the breath flows, building stamina in the heart and lungs. Apart from these physical benefits, *ujjayi* can calm the mind and emotions, giving rise to a sense of lightness and peace since it helps us feel part of a greater whole, as if being in an infinite ocean of breath.

This type of breath, which sounds like a hissing or low rumbling, is controlled by slightly contracting the back of the throat, the epiglottis. When you swallow, you'll feel a small movement in this area, closing off the lungs so that the saliva from your mouth goes down to your stomach and not to your larynx or voice box.[5] You control the epiglottis when you gargle and when you whisper.

To practice *ujjayi*, begin in a comfortable seated posture (see figure 4.3 for options) and say, "Ha," out loud. Feel the contraction and the air move in the back of your throat. Now close your mouth and try to say, "Ha," which will sound more like humming. Inhale normally through your nose and then constrict the back of your throat as you exhale. You'll begin to hear a hissing sound. Keep practicing the exhale, and then when you are comfortable with that, begin contracting your epiglottis on the inhale as well. If the inhale is difficult, do it only a few times, then relax. Don't ever strain when practicing *pranayama* or any kind of yoga.

Sanskrit Gem

Sama vritti means full complete breathing.

Now that you have a tool for regulating the speed at which the breath moves, with *ujjayi* practice you can find your inner beat and count beats for the inhale and exhale. Initially you can work toward making the inhale and exhale the same length, called *sama vritti*. As you inhale, count slowly one, two, three, pause; then as you exhale, count one, two, three. Practice at the number that corresponds to the fullest inhale and the most complete exhale, moving in the direction of making the two numbers equal. When you have mastered this, you may want to practice extending the exhale longer than the inhale and see how that feels. Variations with different ratios of inhale to exhale may also be explored.

Kumbhaka: Breath Retention

Retaining the breath is a practice mentioned in the first book, verse 34, of the Yoga Sutras: "That calm is retained by the controlled exhalation or retention of the breath."[6] Practicing *kumbhaka*, breath retention, has many physical benefits, including strengthening the heart, building lung capacity, and providing relaxation. There is even a form of *kumbhaka* designed to help individuals with asthma, which includes retention after the exhale, strengthening the lungs. This can provide asthma sufferers with an immediate bronchodilator and a more long-term, holistic approach to their problems.

Sanskrit Gem

***Kumbhah* means pot, either full or empty.**

Kumbhaka confers mental, emotional, and spiritual benefits by helping us cultivate detachment and by connecting us to cosmic energy. For example, when we practice breath retention our mind will eventually go on red alert with thoughts that we are about to die. At that point, taking a breath as a conscious action rather than a reaction to fear calms our thoughts and emotions and links us to the greater pool of energy called *mahaprana* (the great *prana*), or cosmic energy.[7]

To practice *kumbhaka*, begin in a comfortable seated posture. Relax your eyes, gazing down or closing them. If *ujjayi* breath is comfortable for you, use it, and if not just breathe slowly and rhythmically. Inhale to a slow count of three. You could say to yourself, Om-One, Om-Two, Om-Three. Then pause. Neither inhaling nor exhaling, count again, Om-One, Om-Two, Om-Three.

Watch your mind as you retain your breath. Of course, you can breathe anytime you want, but the idea is not to react to your mind. Notice your mind talking; think to yourself, "Thanks for sharing," then focus again on your sensations. Relax your throat, soft palate, and lungs, and retain your breath from the lowest part of your belly and low spine.

When you are ready, slowly exhale, counting, Om-One, Om-Two, Om-Three. Pause and then inhale counting, Om-One, Om-Two, Om-Three, and continue the cycle, retaining breath only at the top of the inhale. As you become comfortable with the practice, you can increase the duration of breath retention. If you gasp for breath after *kumbhaka*, you have held your breath too long. Find a balance between being nonviolent toward yourself yet honest about your ability, not doing so little that there is no work involved. This is the balance we are always looking for in yoga and in life.

When you are comfortable with retention after the inhale, practice retaining your breath at the end of the exhale: Inhale Om-One, Om-Two, Om-Three, Om-Four, Om-Five or longer, depending on your capacity, pause, then

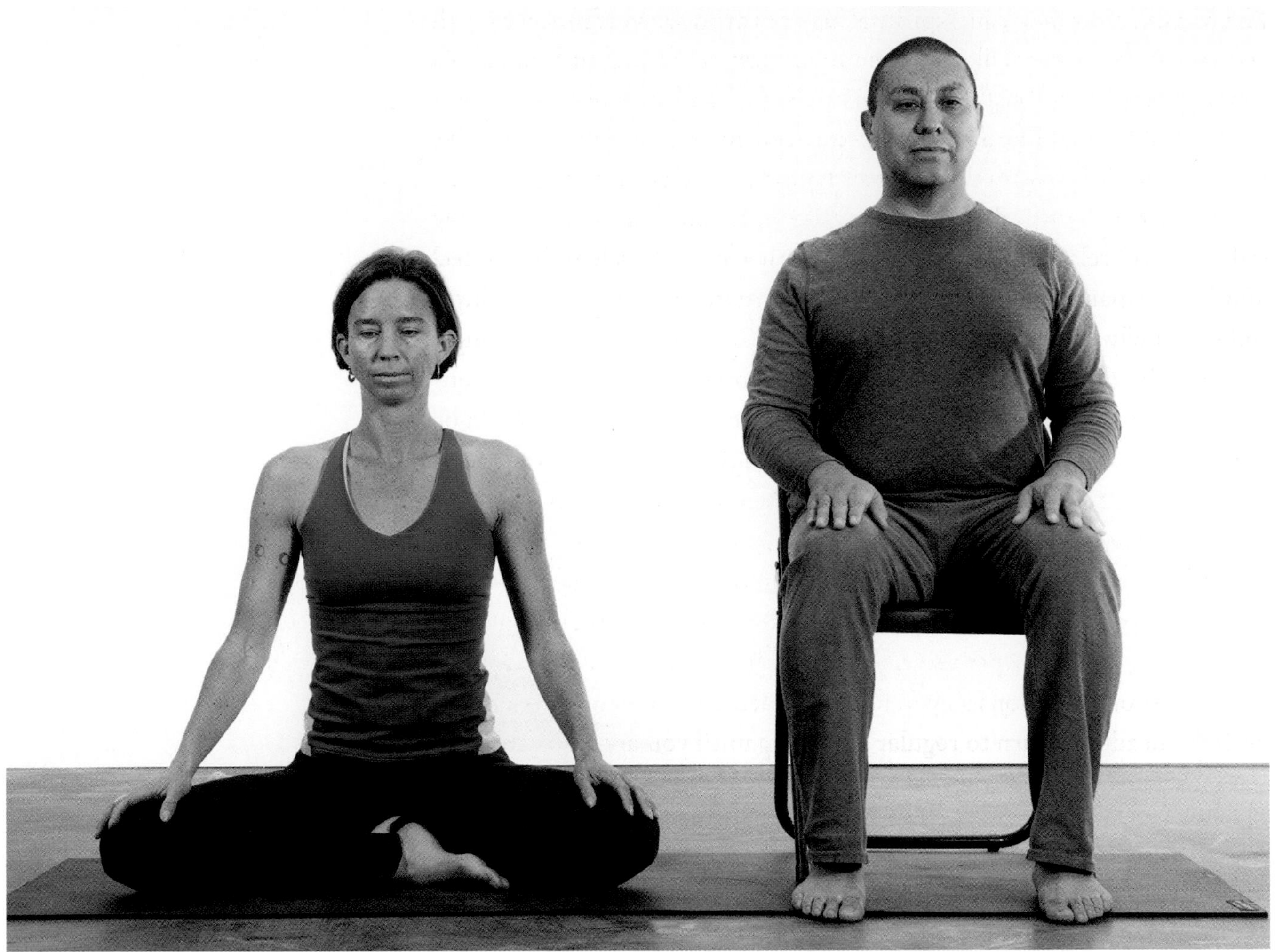

Figure 4.3. Comfortable seated postures for pranayama practice

exhale Om-One, Om-Two, Om-Three, Om-Four, Om-Five, then pause and retain breath Om-One, Om-Two, Om-Three, Om-Four, Om-Five, watching your body and mind. Then release the retention and inhale Om-One, Om-Two, Om-Three, Om-Four, Om-Five, continuing for about ten cycles or until you are no longer able to focus or find calmness while breathing.

Kapalabhati: Shining Skull Breath

Sanskrit Gem

Kapala means skull, and *bhati* means shining.

The meaning of *kapalabhati,* shining skull, suggests how you might feel after practicing it—like your head is radiant. The physical benefits of *kapalabhati* include developing internal warmth; cleansing and opening the sinus cavities; increasing lung and heart strength; and opening the ears.

The mental, emotional, and spiritual benefits are a sense of inner warmth that can be comforting, like a self-embrace; less emotional turmoil; and a calmer mind. This robust *pranayama* can be an excellent way to begin your day on a cold winter morning or as preparation for meditation, as it can feel like cleaning sludge from the heart and mind so you can find inner peace.

Begin in a comfortable seated posture with your hands on your belly and your eyes relaxed, gazing down or gently closed. Inhale fully and feel your belly expand. Then exhale forcibly through your nose and strongly pull your belly back toward your spine. Inhale again easily, and strongly exhale, pulling your belly back. Do this a number of times slowly, continuing to focus on your exhale and belly movement. Inhaling should be easy as you've created a sort of vacuum by completely emptying the lungs.

Once you have the feeling of the exhale and abdominal movement, begin to exhale more quickly and strongly. Count about ten exhales, then inhale fully, returning to normal breathing, and see how you feel. Practice again, perhaps to twenty exhales. After you've practiced this over time, you could try exhaling once per second. Start with three cycles, and modulate the number of repetitions so you feel enlivened but not exhausted. If you feel light-headed, return to regular breathing until you are ready to begin again, perhaps more slowly.

Nadi Shodhana: Alternate Nostril Breathing

Nadi shodhana purifies the *nadis*. This practice, which moves *prana* between the right and left sides of the brain through alternate nostrils, is ultimately excellent for balancing the left and right sides of the brain. Although we need both sides of the brain to function, if they are out of balance they can cause us difficulties. *Nadi shodhana* not only balances the two sides of the brain for better health and functioning but also benefits us physically by opening up the nostrils and the head, often diminishing headaches and confusion. Mentally, emotionally, and spiritually it can bring peace and a sense of connection to cosmic energy.

Since ancient times yogis have known the brain is composed of left and right sides and that balancing the two helps alleviate distortions that disturb our lives, causing stress. Yogis describe the flow of energy up the spine as two waves that feed the different sides of the brain—the right brain, which is the feminine, transformative, holistic, creative moon side, and the left brain, which is the masculine, logical, discerning, sun side.

Sanskrit Gem

***Nadi* means channel, or flow, and *shodhana* means purification.**

Today, using brain imaging techniques, scientists are able to verify such differences between the sides of the brain. One neuroanatomist, Dr. Jill Taylor, even had the remarkable experience of having a stroke in only her left brain and, as a result, being able to feel pain in that side followed by an experience of peace and a cosmic perspective as her right brain took over. She described this as a sense of inner calm while feeling a part of all that is.[8]

To practice *nadi shodhana*, begin in a comfortable seated posture and breathe normally. You can use *ujjayi* breath for this rhythmic three-part yogic breath. Keep your eyes relaxed, gazing gently down or closed. Place your left hand comfortably on your left thigh, with your index finger touching the tip of your thumb, and your palm either up or down. Place your middle and index fingers of your right hand gently on your forehead between and just above your eyebrows. With relaxed hands and fingers, gently close your right nostril with your thumb (see figure 4.4) and inhale fully through your left nostril; at the top of the inhale, pause and close your left nostril with your ring finger.

For a moment, both nostrils are closed and breath is retained. Witness your body, mind, and sensations, then lifting your thumb, open your right nostril and exhale slowly through it. Pause briefly and inhale through your right nostril. At the top of the inhale, pause, close both nostrils, and watch. Then open your left nostril and exhale. Repeat in this fashion—inhaling on the same side and switching sides for the exhale. Always pause briefly with both nostrils closed. As you practice, make sure your shoulders don't get tense and that your arm is relaxed. Repeat five times, then release your hand to your leg and return to normal breathing, watching sensations in your body. Repeat three times.

A variation on alternate nostril breathing is directing your breath with your mind rather than your hand. This can be more relaxing, and you may be surprised at how easy it is to do. Begin in a comfortable seated posture, eyes relaxed and gazing down or closed. Focus your attention on your left nostril as you inhale only through that nostril, pause, then exhale through your right nostril. Inhale through the same side, pause, then exhale through your left nostril. Continue in the same manner, keeping your hands relaxed on your thighs as you move the *prana* between nostrils.

Sanskrit Gem

Ayur **means life, and** ***veda*** **means knowledge.**

Seasons and Pranayama

According to yogic wisdom, we are at one with the world of nature. And so Ayurveda, the science of life, advocates considering our environment and

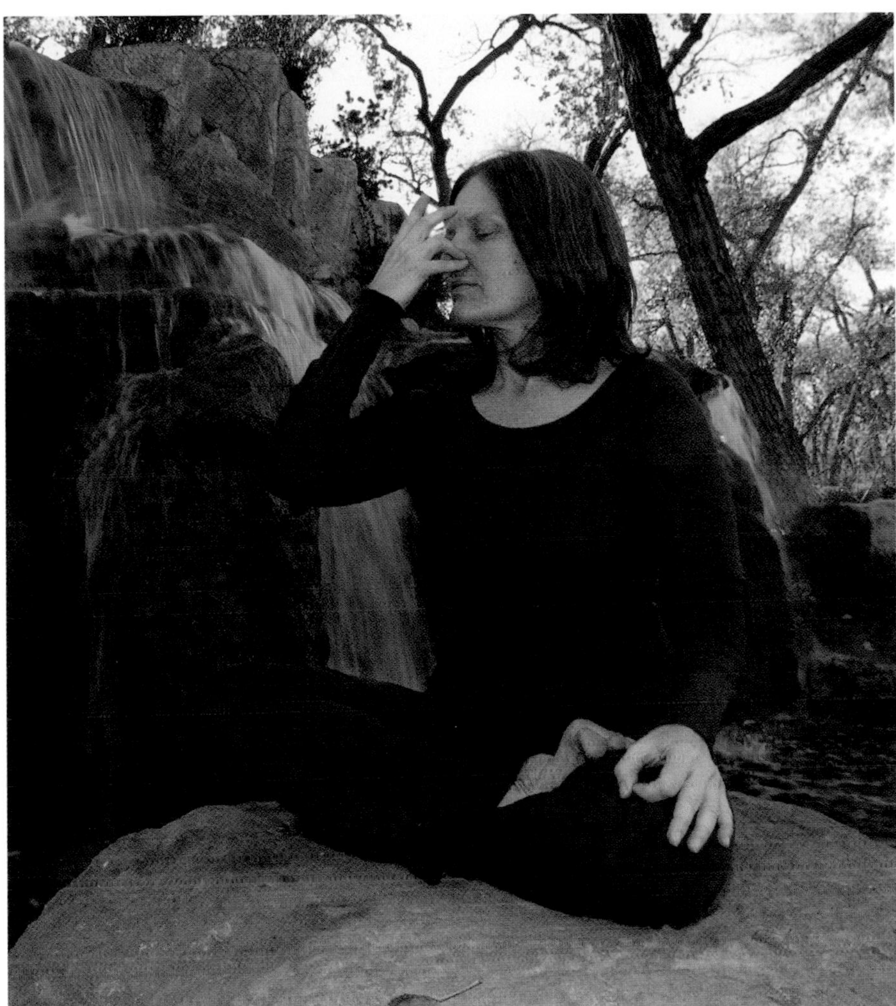

Figure 4.4. Hand position for nadi shodhana

the seasons when designing yoga practice. For example, the hottest days of summer might not be a good time to practice *kapalabhati*, since it is a warming practice more appropriately done during winter. In summer it is better to practice *nadi shodhana*, a more calming and balancing *pranayama*.

The Soft Palate

Relaxation and expansion of the soft palate can trigger relaxation responses in the jaw, eyes, ear canals, head, and eventually, with practice, the entire body. Consequently, practices focusing on the soft palate are good for maintaining tranquility.

Yogis describe three diaphragms of the body: the literal diaphragm, the soft palate, and the pelvic floor. These three diaphragms can be experienced as having a synergistic relationship, so developing our awareness of one enhances our ability to work with the others. The literal diaphragm, a lateral flat muscle attached to the lower ribs, sternum, and lumbar vertebrae (see figure 4.5), moves down as the lungs expand and up as air is exhaled, a movement you can feel in the wave of the three-part yogic breath, described at the beginning of this chapter.

You can experience the soft palate by placing your tongue behind your upper teeth then sliding it back until you feel the hard palate (roof of the mouth) become the soft palate back by the throat. At first you may think that you have no control of such an obscure part of your body as the soft palate, but practice and imagination can teach you how to relax and expand it for calming. Once you have practiced the wave of the breath and your breath moves freely with your spine, you can begin to imagine the soft palate opening softly and expanding. This practice can help you relax in any situation because from the outside it doesn't appear you are doing anything. Physically you benefit from release of tension in the body; mentally and emotionally it feels as if everything is easier, as if a tight wire has slackened; and spiritually you let go of your sense of control and yield to a greater force.

As you practice becoming aware of your soft palate during *pranayama*, you will increase your ability to relax your entire body. For example, practice the following: Sit in a comfortable posture and let your eyes gaze softly down, or close them gently. Begin three-part yogic breathing and feel your soft palate with your tongue. Then let your tongue slide down and relax in your mouth. Now, on both the inhale and the exhale visualize the soft palate relaxing and opening even more, like a parachute gently catching the *prana* and floating ever more open. As you continue, notice how your face and jaw relax, your eyes seem to sink further into your skull, and your ear canals seem to open. Continue breathing and focusing on relaxing your soft palate for about a minute, then return to normal breathing.

You can practice opening the soft palate in asana, *pranayama*, meditation, or any time you feel the need to relax. For example, one student remembered waiting in a doctor's office before a difficult visit following painful surgery. As she waited, becoming increasingly annoyed, she could feel her teeth clenching. Being a yogi she decided to visualize her soft palate expanding. She immediately felt the tension leave her body and her mind calm. Even while talking with the doctor, she intermittently focused on her soft palate, remaining relaxed.

THE BANDHAS AND POWER

Bandhas are subtle energetic holds in the body that can be used to lock *prana* in specified areas and redirect its flow toward the central energetic channel. There are three important *bandhas*, all powerful yet subtle: *mula bandha*, *uddiyana bandha*, and *jalandhara bandha*.

Sanskrit Gem

Bandha means hold, lock, or tighten.

The first lock, *mula bandha*, gives physical support to the organs of the pelvis, especially those involved in elimination and reproduction. One yoga teacher and physical therapist reports using ultrasound machines to monitor the bladder and assess pelvic floor function when *mula bandha* was engaged, finding that the bladder wall changed shape.[9] Considering the common occurrence of prolapsed organs,[10] this lock can benefit many people. Mentally, emotionally, and spiritually, *mula bandha* creates a sense of being grounded and having inner power.

Sanskrit Gem

Mula means root; *uddiyana* means upward flying; and *jalandhara* is derived from the word *jala*, meaning net, and *dhara*, meaning carrying or upward pull.

Mula bandha is engaged by lifting the pelvic floor, between the anus and the genitals, up and into the body. Imagine a straw sucking up energy between the legs to support the entire spine and body. You can practice finding *mula bandha* when urinating by stopping the flow of urine, holding it, and then allowing it to flow again. Skeletal descriptions of *mula bandha* place it where the pubis bone moves toward the coccyx, or tailbone.

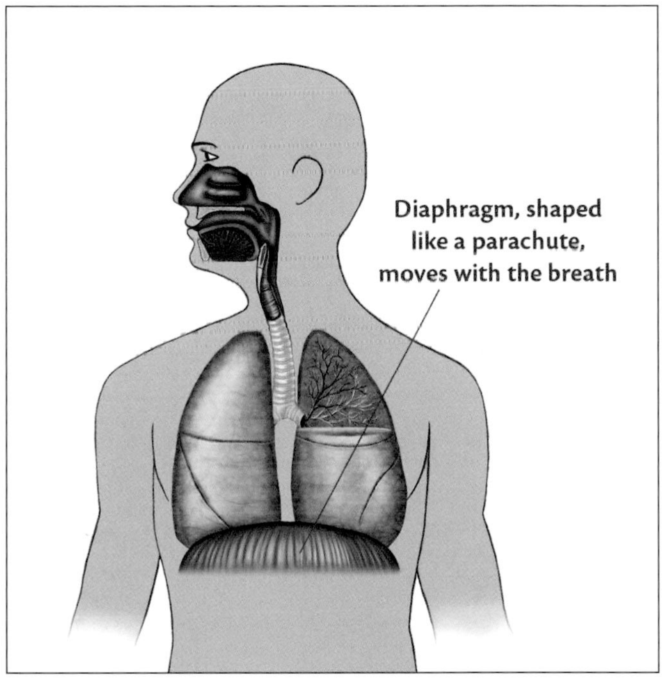

Figure 4.5. Diaphragm

The second lock, *uddiyana bandha*, builds core strength in the body. An ancient text states: "He who constantly practices *uddiyana bandha* as taught by his guru, so that it becomes natural, even though he is old, becomes young."[11]

Physically, the practice can make you feel younger, stronger, and more in control. Mentally and emotionally, it helps you feel less anxious, less timid, and clearer. And spiritually it supports your sense of connection with universal energy. *Uddiyana bandha* is engaged when, as you do *mula bandha*, you lift the lower abdominal muscles up and back almost under the rib cage (see figure 4.6).

The third lock, *jalandhara bandha*, eliminates pain arising in the throat.[12] According to ancient texts, due to a pooling of energy at the throat it may enhance function of the thyroid and parathyroid glands and improve metabolic functions. Mentally and emotionally it is calming, and

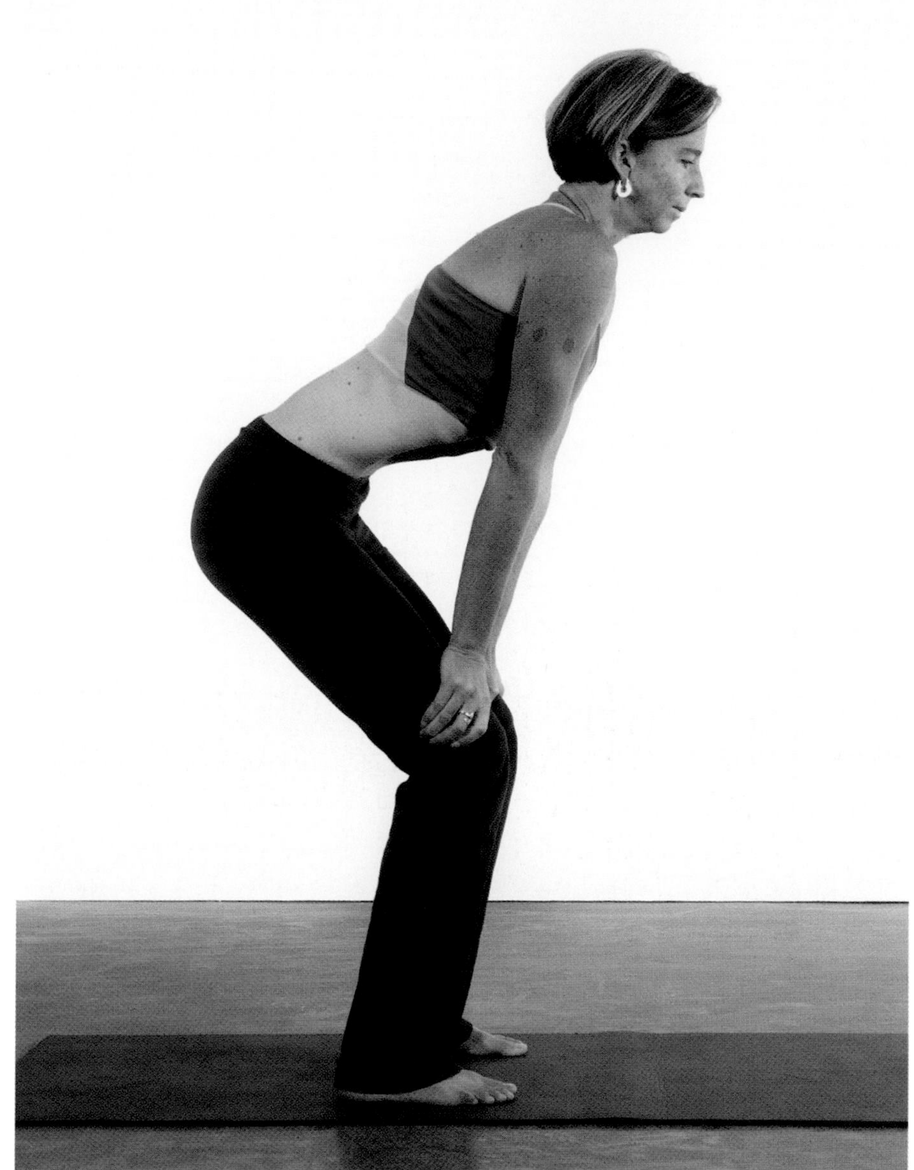

Figure 4.6. Uddiyana bandha

spiritually it aids in self-expression. This is so because while in the lock it's as if you are looking from the Ajna chakra (the third eye, discussed in chapter 3) into your heart, and your mind and heart are speaking to each other. *Jalandhara bandha* is formed by inhaling and lifting the sternum up toward the chin; elongating the head and neck upward; and then exhaling and gently tilting the chin toward the sternum. In this position the chin and sternum are like lovers who want to connect and are moving toward each other as shown in figure 4.7.

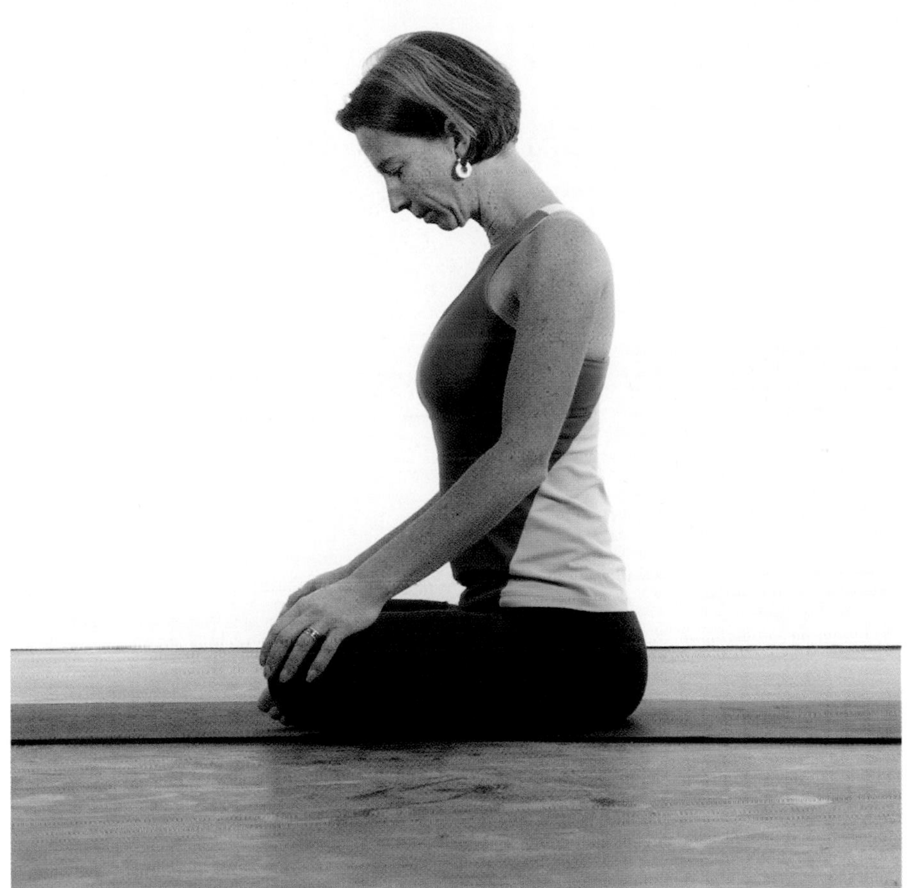

Figure 4.7. Jalandhara bandha

MUDRAS

Mudras are gestures, usually of the hands, that channel energies to the energetic pathways, *nadis,* and chakras, creating specific experiences in the body, mind, and spirit. As such, mudras establish a subtle, nonintellectual connection to the nervous system and the brain. The consistent use of mudras can help break undesirable habitual patterns. The *Hatha Yoga Pradipika* extols the virtues of mudras: "So, the yogi should carefully practice the various mudras to rouse the great goddess (Kundalini) that sleeps, closing the mouth of Sushumna (the doorway to the Absolute)."[13] The ancient text goes on to proclaim that mudras prevent old age and death. Other texts note that mudras help us develop an awareness of the flow of *prana* in the body and redirect it to the upper chakras, resulting in higher states of consciousness.

Sanskrit Gem

***Mudra* means gesture or attitude.**

You can immediately sense the power of mudras by doing the following exercise. While sitting, clench one fist. Next, close your eyes and feel the energy move in your hand, arm, shoulder, neck, back, and head, as well as any other sensation. Then relax your hand and, letting your palm roll faceup, scan your body in the same way, beginning with your hand and moving up your arm, shoulder, neck, back, and head. Notice the physical feeling of vibration and then the feeling of your arm in space. Keep practicing this at various times during your daily routine—such as while talking on the phone or eating a meal—noticing ever more subtle sensations in the flow of energy and becoming aware of how mudras add intention to yoga.

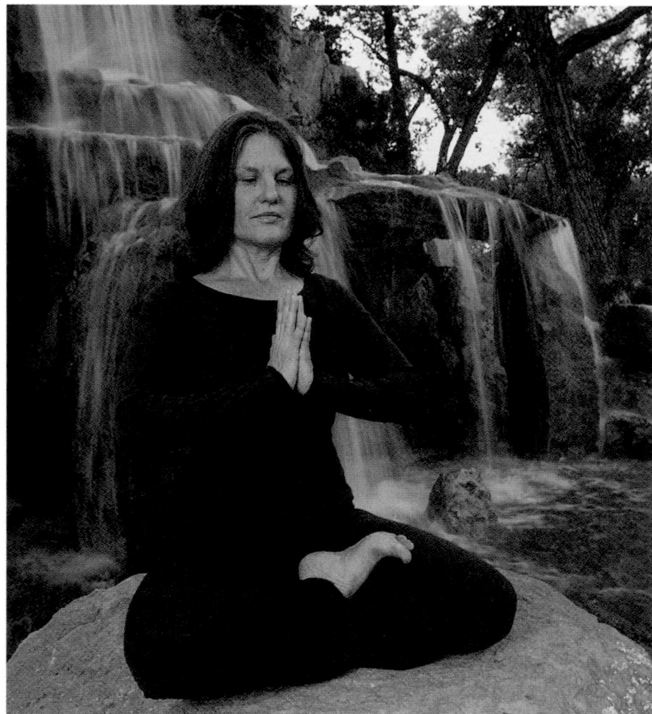

Figure 4.8. Anjali mudra

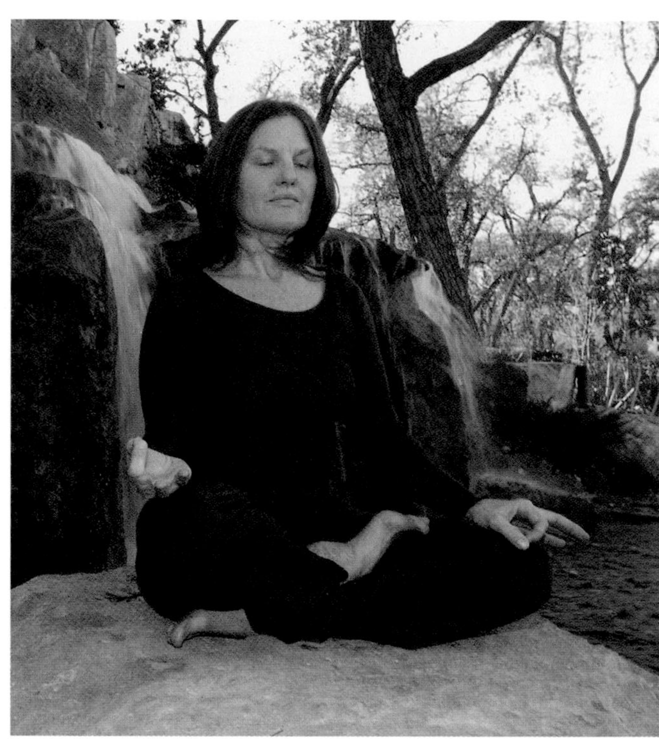

Figure 4.9. Jnana (on right) and chin (on left) mudras

Different mudras are used for a variety of purposes.[14] The prayerful gesture of *namaste*, discussed in chapter 3, is a mudra called *anjali*, which encourages humility and connection to one's divine inner self and to that of others (see figure 4.8). The hands held together signifies the unity of apparent duality, the bringing together of matter and spirit, the right and left sides of the brain, self and cosmos. Some have said that the right hand represents our higher nature, the divine in us, while the left hand

Sanskrit Gem

Anj means to adorn, honor, or celebrate, and _anjali_ is often translated as offering.

represents our lower nature, the worldly in us. If you are uncomfortable making this gesture toward others, you can look in the mirror and make it to yourself, saying, "*Namaste*." Pause, breathe, and repeat. Then release the mudra with your eyes closed and notice any subtle physical sensations in parts of your body, as well as your state of mind. Often this gesture creates a feeling of gratitude, which is the emotion that most readily quiets the mind and produces a state of contentment.[15]

In the earlier discussion of *nadi shodhana* (see figure 4.4), the left hand was in a mudra with the index finger touching the thumb. When the palm faces up, this hand gesture is called *jnana* mudra, and when the palm faces down it is called *chin* mudra (see figure 4.9 for both).

Sanskrit Gem

Jnana mudra means gesture of knowledge.

Sanskrit Gem

Chin mudra means psychic gesture of consciousness.

Other hand mudras are designed to enhance the energy of specific chakras. Using them can be helpful when you feel out of balance. For example, at stressful times, perhaps during a hectic holiday season or an especially busy period in your work life, you might sit quietly in a comfortable position and create the mudra for the root chakra, known as *bhu* mudra, as shown in figure 4.10. If you are feeling frightened or insecure, you might create the mudra for the second chakra, *bhudi* mudra, as shown in figure 4.11.

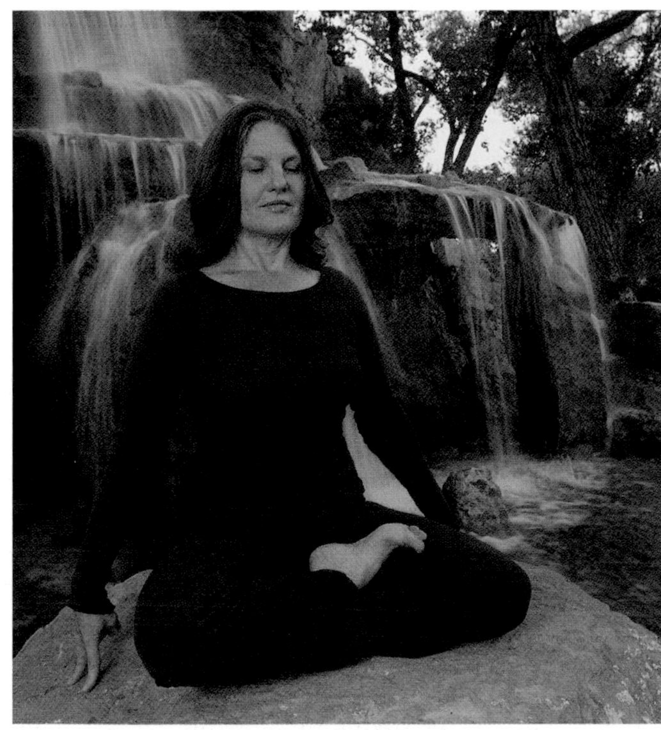

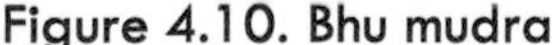

Figure 4.10. Bhu mudra

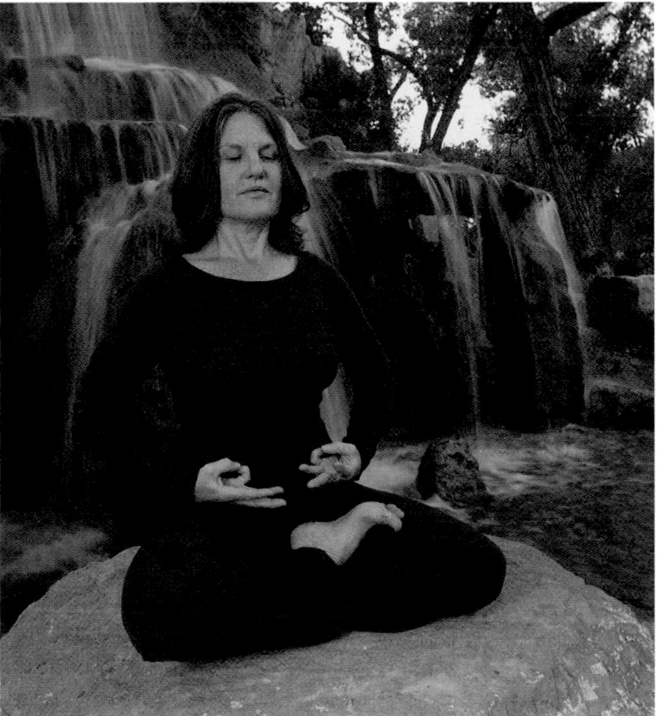

Figure 4.11. Bhudi mudra

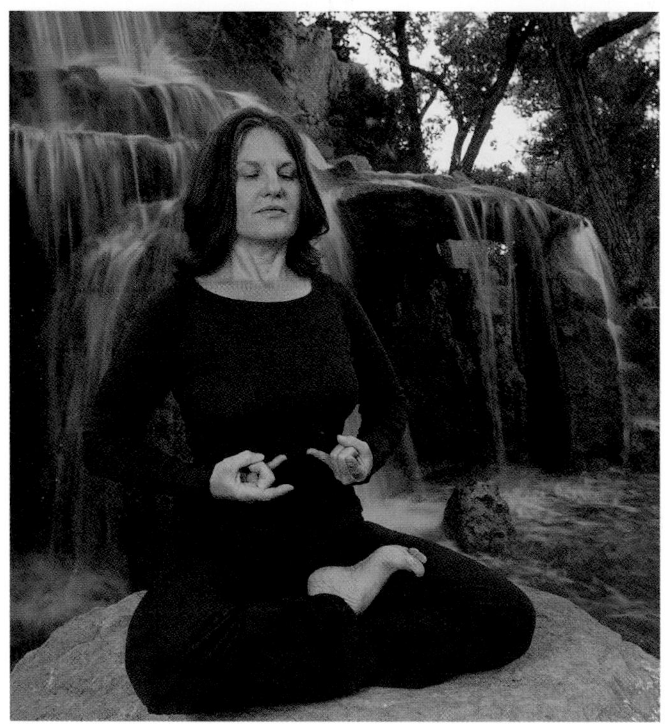

Figure 4.12. Rudra mudra

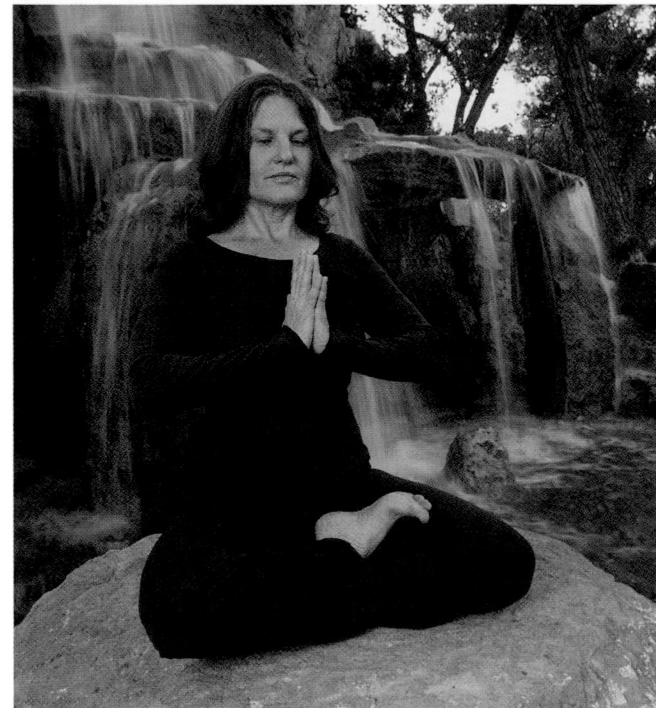

Figure 4.13. Anahata mudra

A Mudra for Each Chakra

Although a number of hand mudras are associated with each chakra, one for each is suggested here, along with directions. Generally, you will want to hold the mudra with relaxed shoulders and your arms at the level of the chakra, unless this is uncomfortable, in which case rest your arms on your legs. Practice long slow yogic breaths as you breathe consciously into the chakra space along the spine. Do ten to twelve breaths at each chakra before moving on, or work with only one chakra at a sitting.

First (root) chakra, *Muladhara—bhu* (earth) mudra: Use your thumb to hold your ring and pinkie fingers in the palm of your hand; extend your index and middle fingers toward the ground to psychically or actually touch it (see figure 4.10).

Second chakra (below the navel), *Svadistana—bhudi* (fluid) mudra: With palms up touch the tip of your pinkie finger to the tip of your thumb (see figure 4.11).

Third chakra (solar plexus), *Manipura—rudra* (fierce form of Shiva) mudra: Touch the tips of your middle and ring fingers to the tip of your thumb. Extend your index and pinkie fingers (see figure 4.12).

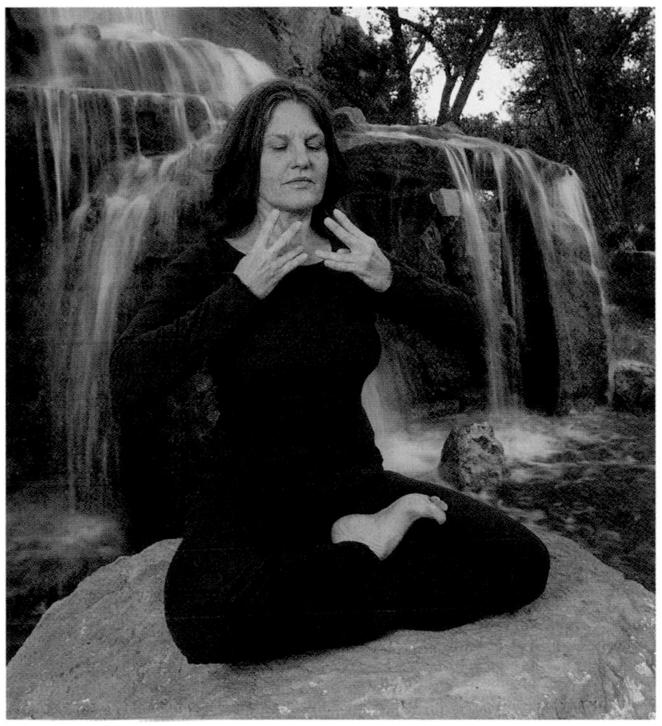

Figure 4.14. Vishuddha mudra

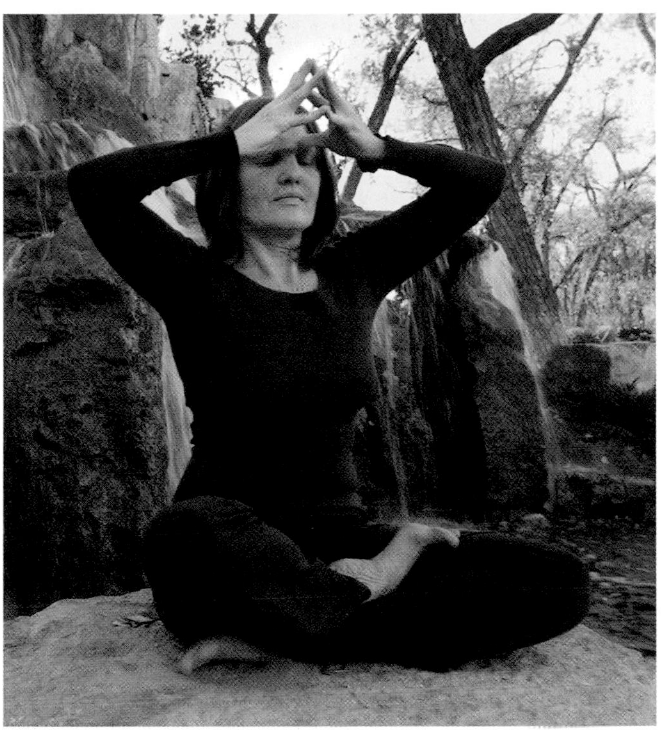

Figure 4.15. Hakini mudra

Fourth (heart) chakra, *Anahata—anjali* mudra: Hold your palms together in front of your heart (see figure 4.13).

Fifth (throat) chakra, *Vishuddha—vishuddha* (purification) mudra: Hold the tip of your thumb to the second rung of your ring finger, applying gentle pressure to its inner edge (see figure 4.14).

Sixth (third eye) chakra, *Ajna—hakini* mudra: Hold your hands in *anjali* mudra, then separate the heels of your hands and palms, keeping your fingertips touching; hold at the level of your heart or third eye (see figure 4.15).

Seventh (crown) chakra, *Sahasrara—padma* or lotus mudra: Hold your hands in *anjali* mudra; then separate your ring, middle, and index fingers from each other. Hold at the level of your heart or at the crown chakra (see figure 4.16). *Padma* mudra resembles the shape of the flower, and we can visualize ourselves opening like the flower to our highest nature. To yogis,

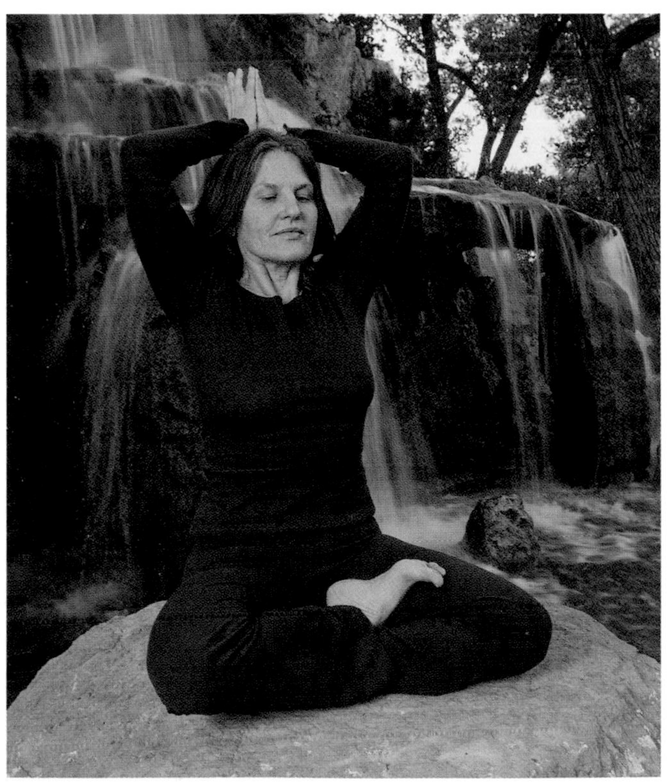

Figure 4.16. Padma mudra

the lotus flower represents expansion of consciousness and enlightenment. The chakras are often visualized as having a particular number of flower petals, and the seventh chakra is called the thousand-petal lotus. Then, too, just as the lotus rises out of the mud and blooms with remarkable beauty so is the Kundalini energy said to rise through the body so that we "bloom" and attain enlightenment.

Garuda Mudra

Sanskrit Gem

Garuda means king of birds.

Garuda mudra symbolizes freedom, unlimited possibilities, a sense of taking flight with exhilaration. Try this mudra when you are looking for inspiration. Begin by crossing your arms with your right arm closer to your chest. Spread your fingers, palms facing you, then hook your thumbs and hold them near your heart (see figure 4.17).

Sanskrit Gem

Maha means great or noble; this mudra is sometimes translated as the great psychic attitude.

Maha Mudra

Perhaps the most powerful mudra is *maha* mudra, which is said to be very healing, according to the *Hatha Yoga Pradipika*:

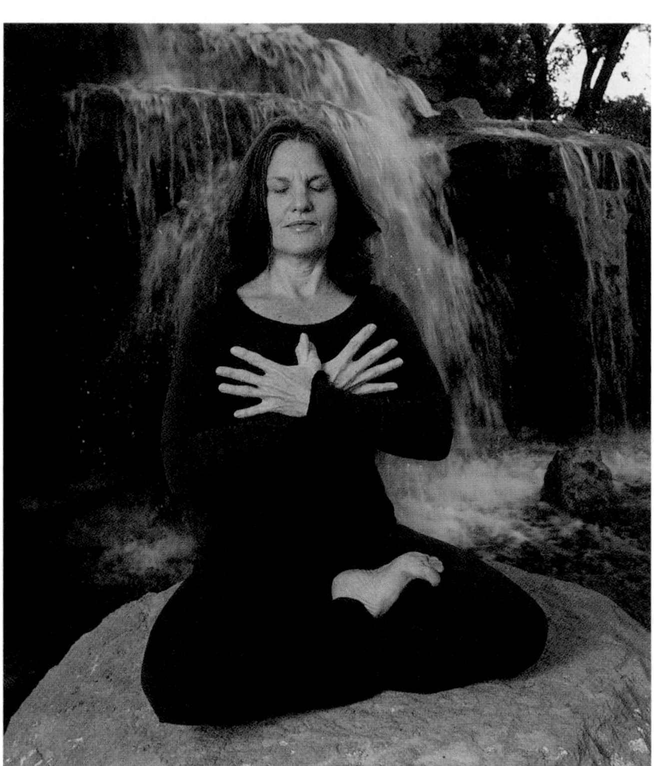

Figure 4.17. Garuda mudra

> *Maha mudra removes the worst afflictions and the cause of death. Therefore it is called "the great attitude" by the ones of highest knowledge. . . . For one who practices maha mudra, there is nothing wholesome or unwholesome. Anything can be consumed; even the deadliest of poisons is digested like nectar. Abdominal disorders, constipation, indigestion and leprosy, etc. are alleviated by the practice of maha mudra. Thus maha mudra has been described as the giver of great siddhis. It must be kept secret and not disclosed to anyone.*[16]

Begin by sitting on the floor with both legs outstretched. Bend the knee of one leg, and put the heel of your hand at the root, or *mula*, the area between the genitals and the anus, so that you are sitting on this heel. Bend forward over the extended leg, holding the foot if you are sufficiently flexible (see figure 4.18).

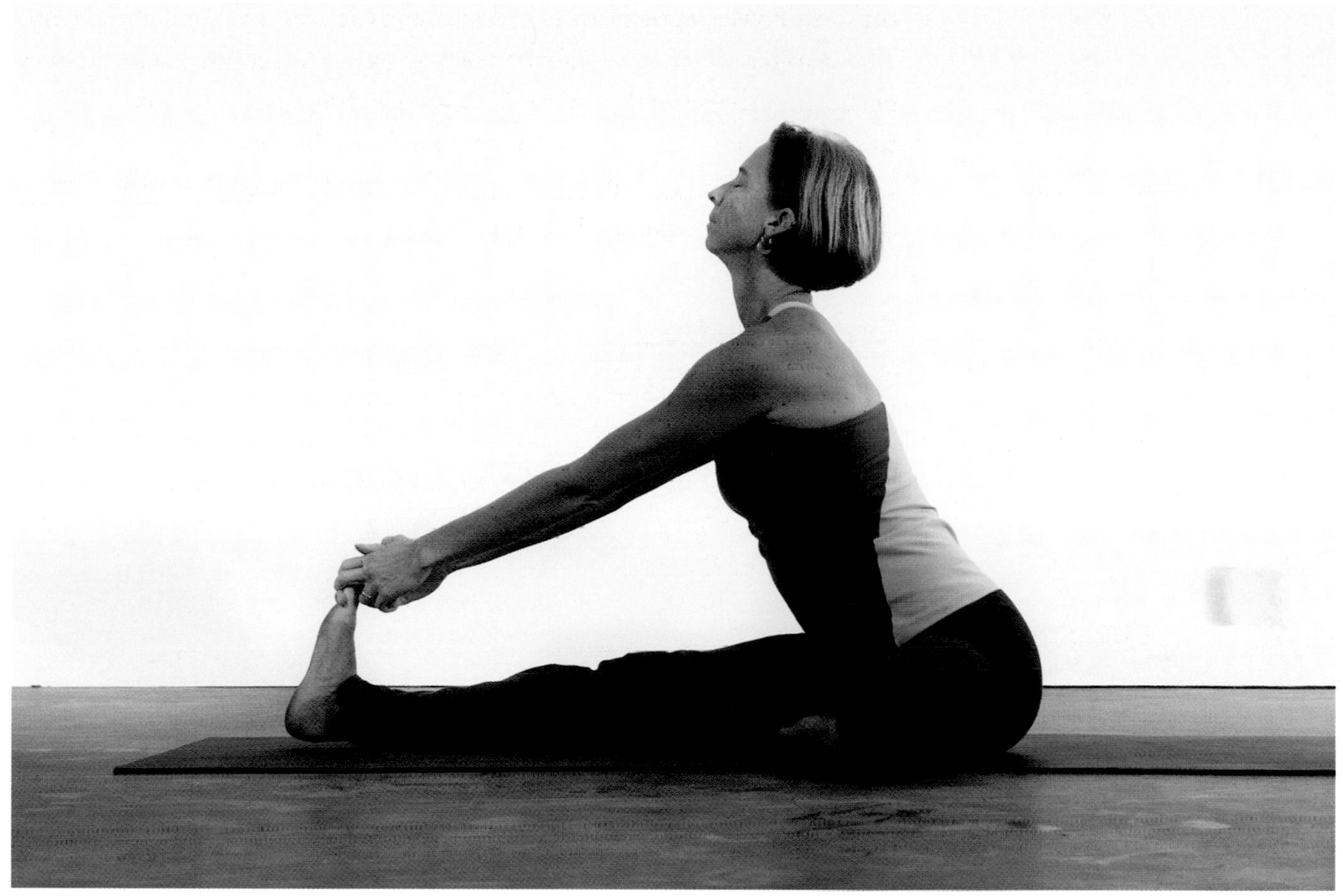

Figure 4.18. Maha mudra

Inhale and, without strain, look toward the third eye (*shambhavi* mudra), engage *mula bandha,* feeding the lift of the *uddiyana bandha.* Then lift the sternum up as you lower your chin to meet it for *jalandhara bandha.* Hold your breath, and either silently repeat the sacred sound of *Aum* or mentally send breath up the *sushumna nadi,* following the breath from the first through the sixth chakra. When you need to breathe, first release the *bandhas,* then inhale. Repeat on the other leg. As your ability improves, you may want to practice a number of repetitions before moving to the second leg.

Practice *nadi shodhana* with the left hand first in *jnana* mudra, then in *chin* mudra. Notice any differences in feeling, perhaps more internal with *jnana* mudra and more external with *chin* mudra.

Practice each *pranayama* for a week after your asana practice while sitting comfortably. Notice how they affect you. Gradually introduce small increases in duration and repetition. Then develop a *pranayama* practice for the season you are in, building inner heat in the winter and cooling the body in the summer. When the next seasons come, develop a practice for each.

Practice each of the three *bandhas*. Begin with *mula bandha*, then do *uddiyana bandha*, and finally *jalandhara bandha*. Practice these at the end of the day for five minutes, sitting comfortably on the floor, a chair, or anywhere you are relaxed. Journal your feelings and sensations after each session.

Choose a mudra that corresponds to a chakra you would like to enhance. For one week practice that mudra at the beginning and end of each day for a few minutes. Keep a journal of how you feel after mudra practice at the beginning of the day, how your day unfolded, and how you feel after practice at the end of the day. When you are comfortable with one mudra, move to another.

CHAPTER FIVE

Meditation for Beauty and Bliss

THE FIFTH LIMB: PRATYAHARA, SENSE WITHDRAWAL

The purpose of withdrawing the senses (see figure 5.1) is to remove ourselves from any attachment to the duality of pleasure and pain, which causes distress. Rather than constantly turning away from what we don't want and craving what we do want, we practice detachment from sensory input to facilitate focusing on our inner world and understanding that we are more than our responses to the exterior world. Then when we are again exposed to the sensory input, we are able to be less reactive because we can remember the neutral space of no input.

The Yoga Sutras say the following about this limb:

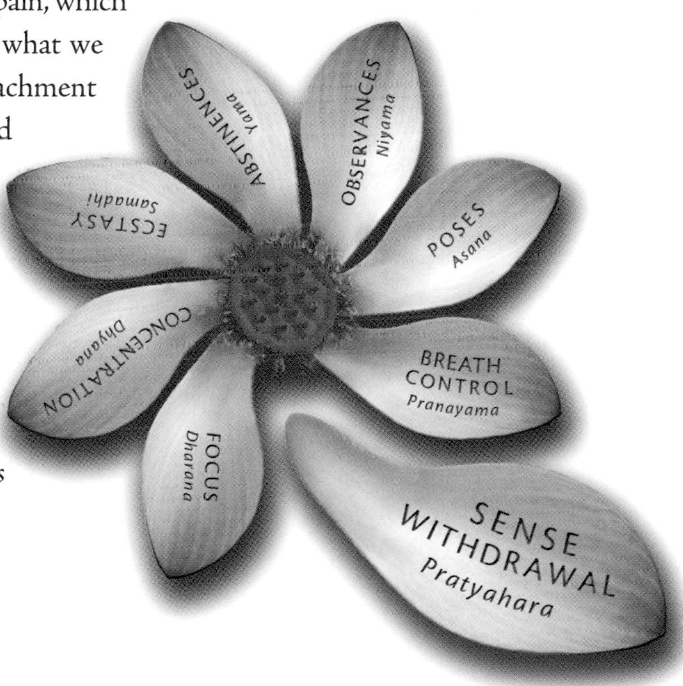

Figure 5.1.
The fifth limb of Ashtanga yoga, *pratyahara*

II.54
When the energy of the senses withdraws
and the impetus
to come into contact
with their objects ceases,
the senses imitate,
as it were,
the essential nature
of pure consciousness.

II.55
From that arises
the highest mastery
over the senses.[1]

When we are able to "boycott" thoughts, feelings, and desires, we become capable of creating a world that most meets our highest aspirations. Then we have mastery over the senses.

At first it may seem like practicing sense withdrawal is a means of suffering instead of enjoying life, but it actually heightens the power of the senses and makes us appreciate them more. Also, practicing *pratyahara* is a means for handling sensory overload that often occurs in modern life. We practice excluding sensory input frequently—for example, shutting out the sounds of a siren while attending an outdoor concert or ignoring another conversation while talking on a phone in the same room. *Pratyahara* turns such daily experiences into a practice that we can use consciously to withdraw from sensory input and gain mastery over the senses.

On the mat you can practice withdrawal of the visual sense by staying focused on your own poses, perhaps even keeping your eyes closed to avoid comparing yourself, either favorably or unfavorably, to others in the room. You may also practice withdrawing some of your aural sense if, for example, the teacher is playing music you don't like or there is a disturbance outside the studio. And you can practice withdrawing your sense of smell if a student nearby has produced gas or body odor, both of which are normal, even desirable, outcomes of asana practice.

Specific mudras can assist in withdrawing the senses—for example, *shanmukti* mudra as shown in figure 5.2. To practice this mudra, sit in a comfortable posture with your spine lifted equally in all directions, grounded on your sitting bones, with your elbows lifted to the height of your shoulders. Then place your thumbs on your ear orifices with just enough pressure to adequately muffle incoming sound but not cause pain. Close your eyes and turn them up toward the top of your head. Put your index and middle fingers lightly on your eyes. With the tips of your fourth fingers, close off your nostrils slightly so that your breath will be slow, long, and deep. Let your pinkie fingers rest gently on your lightly closed mouth in a gesture of no speaking.

Sanskrit Gem

Shan mean six, and *mukti* means mouth.

Stay in this position carefully watching your breath move in your body from the base of your spine to the crown of your head, giving special attention to the sixth chakra, the third eye, the inner eye of knowing. Listen to your inner sounds—the sound of your breath, as well as more subtle sounds. Hold the pose as long as is comfortable. Then release slowly, keeping your eyes closed as you spend time experiencing this mudra. If this practice appeals to you as a calming influence, perhaps in preparation for meditation, after a long day, or when in a crisis, make a commitment to practice it for six months and then evaluate the effects.

You can practice *pratyahara* in the world the next time you go to a mall, a big store, or when your work is stressful. Withdraw one sense, perhaps sound, noticing how just that amount of decrease in sensory input gives you a feeling of ease in an otherwise chaotic environment.

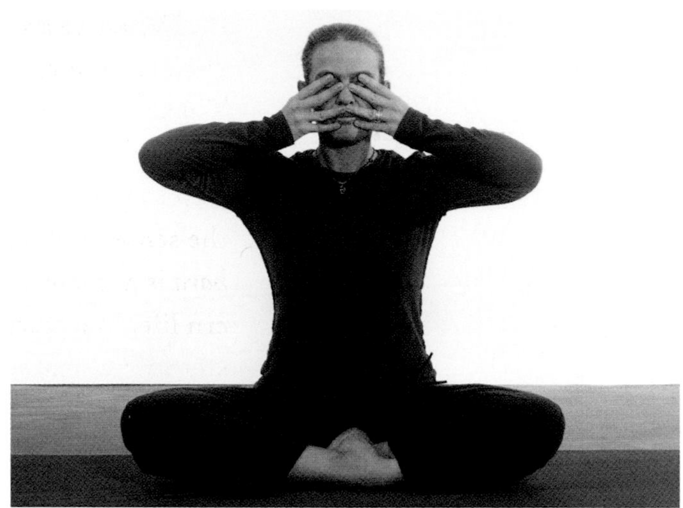

Figure 5.2. Shanmukti mudra

THE FINAL THREE LIMBS: SAMYAMA CONSCIOUSNESS

The last three limbs of the eight-limbed path identify deepening levels of meditation. By combining these last three limbs in a separate *pada*, perhaps Patanjali was indicating that together they take us into substantially different terrain, leading to liberation and happiness in any life situation. Patanjali says that when all three of these limbs are flowing harmoniously with one another we have integrated the full spectrum of the mind's potential and arrive at a place of transcendence, or *samyama*.

The sixth limb—focus, *dharana*—involves directing the mind to attend to one topic or object (see figure 5.3). Often this is done by focusing on the breath, but there are other strategies as well. The purpose of *dharana* is to attain inner ease and bliss, and its benefits are the ability to embrace life completely, no matter what comes our way. Everything learned in the previous limbs helps in achieving this goal.

The first thing most people notice in such focusing is how often the mind is distracted by thoughts. It requires practice to learn to focus a long time with fewer distractions.

After accomplishing this, we move to the seventh limb—concentration, *dhyana* (see figure 5.4). The purpose of this limb is to refine our ability to stay focused for longer and longer periods of time. As we practice this, we begin to feel a continuous sense of staying in the moment. The benefits of the seventh limb are an increased state of well-being, a feeling of deeper relaxation, and calmness.

Sanskrit Gem

Sam **means equally or completely and** ***yama*** **means control, so** ***samyama*** **means the self has attained perfect discipline, or integrated, regulated consciousness.**

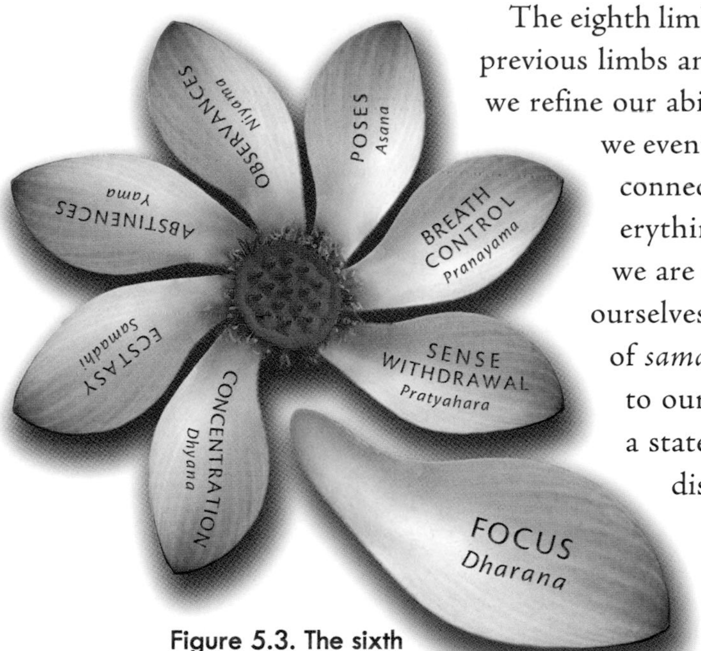

Figure 5.3. The sixth limb of Ashtanga yoga, *dharana*

The eighth limb—ecstasy, *samadhi*—is attained as a result of the previous limbs and so is not practiced directly (see figure 5.5). As we refine our ability to stay focused for very long periods of time, we eventually arrive at a place that seems at once both less connected to the outer world and more connected to everything. We may feel like we have merged with what we are observing as if there were no distinction between ourselves and the object of our focus. Attaining this state of *samadhi* is the goal of yoga, the complete connection to ourselves and the world around us that leaves us in a state of absorption and yet completely unattached to distractions.

Patanjali, in the Yoga Sutras, describes this state in the following way:

III.1
Contemplation
is
the confining
of thought
to one point.

III.2
Meditation
depends upon this
foundation for directing thoughts
into a continuous flow
of awareness.

III.3
Being absorbed in Spirit
is that consciousness
whose object is
void of form or goal
and only the
essence of the object
remains
shining forth.

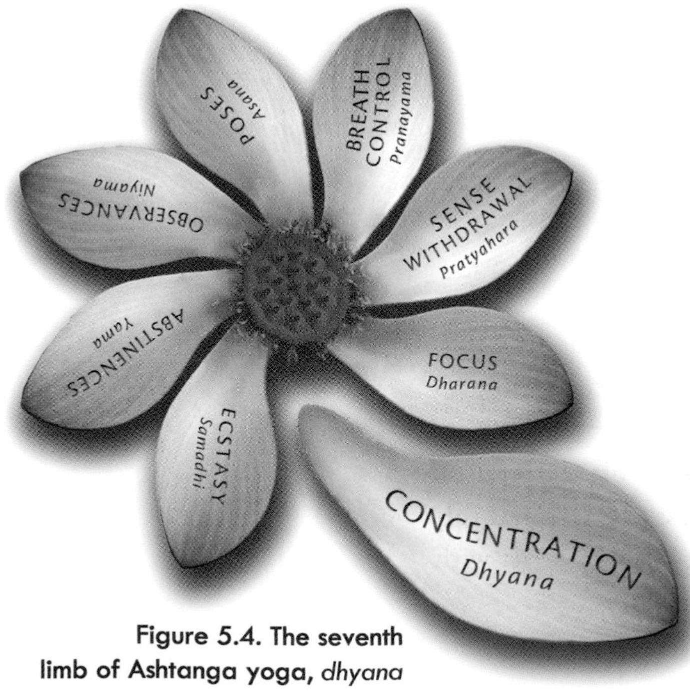

Figure 5.4. The seventh limb of Ashtanga yoga, *dhyana*

III.4
Samyama
occurs when these three processes
flow together harmoniously,
integrating the full spectrum
of the mind's potential.

III.5
By mastering this,
the light of
transcendental insight
dawns.[2]

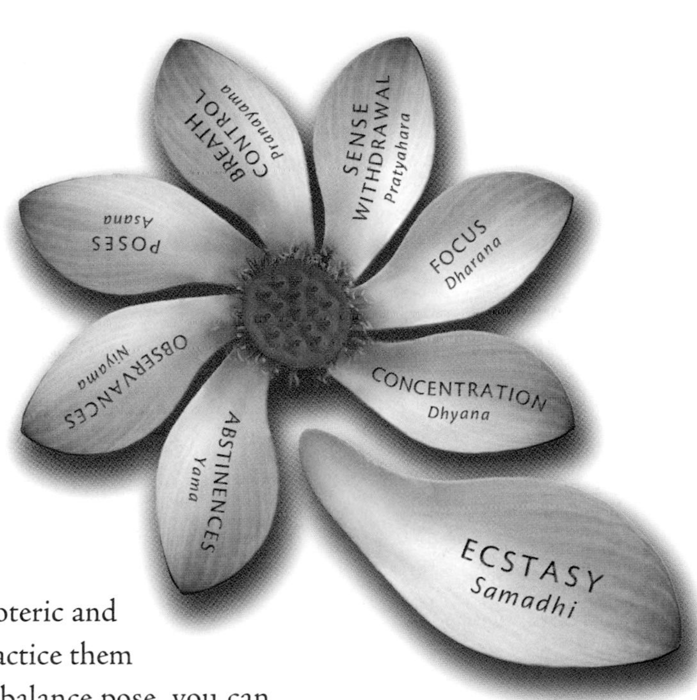

Figure 5.5. The eighth limb of Ashtanga yoga, *samadhi*

Although these last three limbs may sound esoteric and unrelated to the physical realm, it is possible to practice them on the mat while doing asanas. For example, in a balance pose, you can focus so intently on a spot on the floor (*dharana*) that the rest of the room fades away (both *pratyahara* and *dhyana*). Perhaps for just a moment while holding the pose you may be so connected to the spot that time seems to stand still, you cease being able to distinguish between yourself and the spot, and experience a momentary sense of complete joy (*samadhi*). If you have ever been so absorbed in a task that time seemed suspended, you are already familiar with such a feeling.

MEDITATION STRATEGIES

There are many specific strategies for developing these three limbs. You may want to explore those described in this chapter to find the best approach for you as meditation is about practice, not theorizing.

To realize the benefits of meditation, once you find a method that works stay with it for a while, perhaps six months, before moving on to another method. Prior to each session, you might read a short inspiring text to begin focusing within. Consider setting a timer to fifteen minutes, gradually advancing toward twenty minutes, to assess your general tolerance for meditation. If this is too long, you might prefer to start with five minutes. Once you've been practicing for a month or more, you'll probably look forward to meditation and want to increase the time you spend doing it.

It's never too late to begin meditating. My father, Harry Hirschl, agreed to try meditation at age eighty-two, and for him, reading a short inspirational text before sitting has made a world of difference. He reads from Thich Nhat Hahn's *Peace at Every Step*, then sits for ten to fifteen minutes five mornings a week; after meditating he does five asana poses. The practice has helped calm him, and the readings often stay with him throughout his day. He says of the meditation-asana practice:

> *Meditation and yoga have made a clear and positive difference in my life. Meditation helps me think about myself and the world around me in a very positive and almost mystical way. I'm heavily oriented toward Jewish values, and the readings fit into that and cause a new light to shine on what I think is important. For instance, while trying to help a group at my temple and finding that my presentation wasn't being received, I suddenly became frustrated and then angry, thinking,* This isn't working so I'll just get off the committee. *Fortunately, my meditation practice convinced me to exit graciously, without anger or upset and without burning bridges or alienating anyone. As for yoga, it has made me more flexible than I've been in a long time. And while before I had low back pain, now I'm basically free of it.*

Meditation: Follow the Breath

Focusing on, or following, the breath is the most direct method of connecting with the inner self since then we literally exchange air between inside and outside ourselves. The purpose of this meditation is to turn the attention inward, and the benefit is quieting the mind and relaxing the body. As you work with this method, you may discover moments when you can follow your breath at work, in a meeting, or while interacting with your children.

To practice: Sit in a comfortable position and close your eyes gently (see figure 5.6). Then inhale slowly, following your breath from the bottom of your spine up toward your third eye. Pause, neither inhaling nor exhaling. Then exhale, following your breath as it moves from your third eye down your spine. At the end of the exhale, pause again, noticing the space between breaths. As soon as you observe that your mind is distracted by thoughts, smile, without getting perturbed, and bring your focus back to your breath and body sensations. Avoid getting caught up

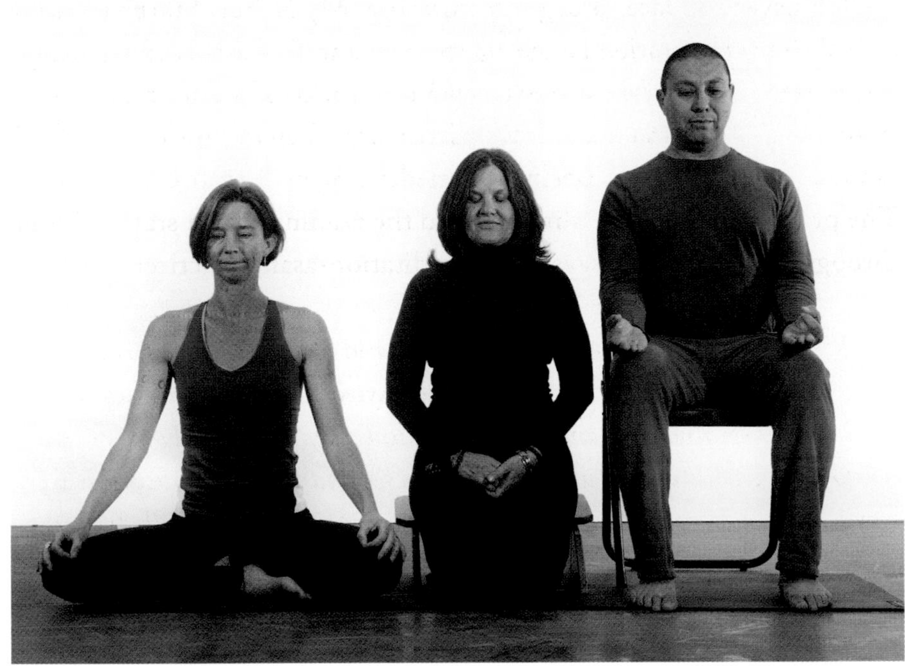

Figure 5.6. Comfortable seated postures for meditation practice

in self-criticism, such as saying to yourself, "I'm such a loser I can't even meditate," as this is just another thought. Instead, regard passing thoughts as if they are fluffy clouds passing by as you look out an airplane window. Whenever you are distracted by thoughts during meditation or daily events, it may help to remember this image, smile, and say to yourself, "There goes another cloud!"

Meditation: Counting

Some students find meditation easier using counting down as a way to focus on the breath and the body. To practice: Sit comfortably, either on the floor, on a cushion or prop, or on a chair. Close your eyes or gaze softly at a single point on the ground. Inhale slowly and say to yourself some number, then count down to zero. You can experiment with counting down on the exhale as well as the inhale. If you get lost in a thought, start at the beginning again, without slipping into self-criticism, or just start again at the last number you remember. When you get to zero, if the timer hasn't gone off you can either start over at fifty or just sit quietly and watch your breath as described in the first meditation practice.

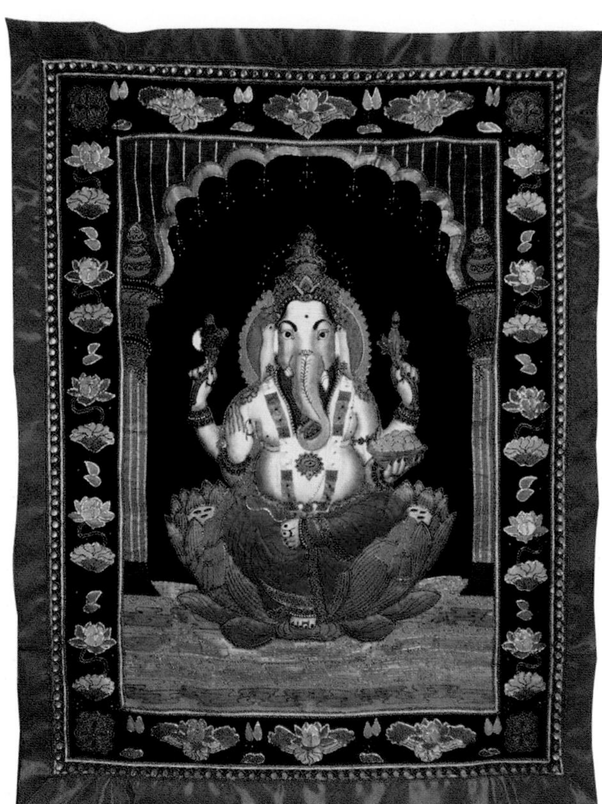

Figure 5.7. Sample image of Ganesha, remover of obstacles, for meditation

Meditation: So Hum, Repeating a Mantra

Another method for meditating is to silently repeat a mantra or seed syllable (see chapter 3: "Vibration As Tool"). The purpose of using a mantra, especially one composed of a meaningful word or phrase, is to have a focus for your mind when it wanders off, helping you return to the present. As a result, you may be able to stay focused longer.

There is an ancient Sanskrit mantra meditation practice called *So hum*, which means "I am that," or "I am that I am." To practice: Sit in a comfortable position and silently say *"So"* on the inhale and *"hum"* on the exhale. Either count the number of times you say the mantra or just breathe slowly and continue until the timer goes off, or longer, then quietly watch your experience. Feel free to instead repeat a phrase that has personal meaning.

Meditation: Trataka, Gazing at an Object

Another approach, called *trataka*, is to focus the eyes intently on an object. The purpose of this practice is to employ more of your senses and thus focus more easily or have a substantially different experience. A benefit is that by emphasizing a visual dimension you may see colors or shapes, feel an expanded freedom, or be transported in a new way. You can create your own image or object for gazing meditation, or find one that inspires you (see figure 5.7 as an example). Some options might be a photograph of a landscape or person important to you, a candle, a flower, a special geometric image called a yantra or a mandala (see figure 5.8).

If you choose to use a candle for gazing meditation, select one that doesn't flicker. Candles made with ghee (clarified butter) produce a very pure flame. You can make these yourself, as shown in figure 5.9(a), by cooking butter until it separates and then pouring the nondairy part off the top, or you can purchase ghee at your local health food store. A cotton ball can be floated in the ghee to make a wick as shown in figure 5.9(b).

Sanskrit Gem

So means I am, and *hum* means that.

Sanskrit Gem

Trataka means to look.

To practice: Sit in a comfortable position, and set the lit candle or other object at eye level. Pause, close your eyes, and become aware of your breath. Then open your eyes and focus intently on the flame or chosen object, trying not to blink or look away. When your mind wanders, focus again on the flame or object. When your eyes get tired or watery, close them and visualize the flame or object, perhaps on the back side of the forehead. When you can no longer see the image internally, look at it once again in the outer world. Start this practice very slowly at first; as it becomes easier, add more repetitions.

Sanskrit Gem

Yan means to support, and *trana* means freedom.

Sanskrit Gem

Mandala means circle, center, completion.

Group Meditation

The purpose of group meditation is not only to further your practice but also to create a sense of community. The benefit of group meditation is that it inspires personal practice and connects you to like-minded individuals, or a *sangha*. Meditating in a group can be very supportive and growth enhancing. There are many approaches to such a practice. An option I recommend is one of the ten-day retreats offered by S.N. Goenka at locations all over the world. Goenka's method, taught to him by Sayagyi U Ba Khin, is carefully designed.[3] Other retreats offering meditation may be located through your local yoga studio.

Figure 5.8. Sample mandala for meditation

Whatever method of meditation you choose, make a commitment to practice at a specified time and place, and for a certain duration. Having such a routine will encourage you to continue practicing. Also establish a ritual to perform that will set a positive tone and intent for your meditation. The ritual can be as simple as turning off your cell phone and shutting down your computer, or it can be an act that will enhance your meditation, like lighting a candle or incense, smiling at the birds outside your window, or draping a special shawl over your shoulders.

ASANA PRACTICE AS MEDITATION

Asana practice can be an act of meditation if you use your mind to continually come back to the breath and the present moment. This is likely to be effective whether you stay in poses for some time, continually move

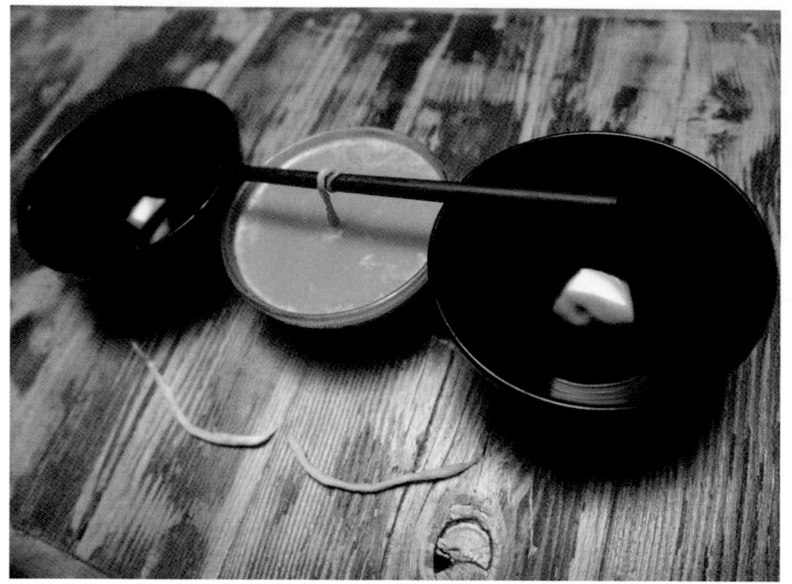

Figure 5.9(a). Making a ghee candle

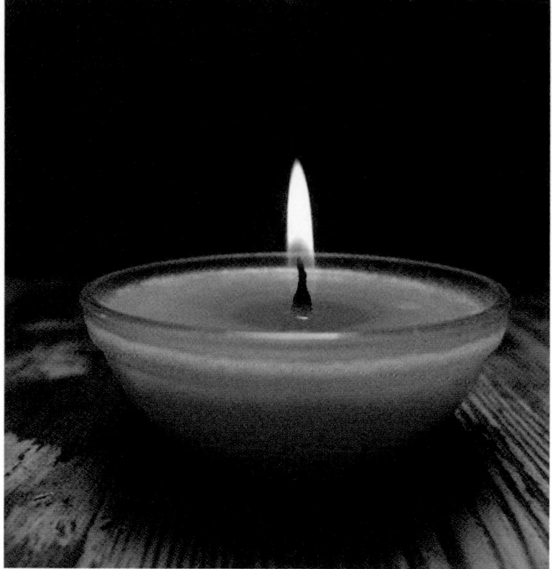

Figure 5.9(b). The pure flame of ghee

with the breath in vinyasa, or combine the two approaches. The idea is to continually return to your experience in the present, withdrawing sensory input from the outer world as you go inside, focusing on your gaze, and observing your thoughts without becoming distracted by the past or future.

In classes where you remain in a pose for a time, you may notice that your mind and body go through distinct phases. At first your body may make you aware of sensations, after which you may choose to either deepen your concentration to see if the sensations subside or back off of the pose altogether. In either case, eventually your mind will react to the pose. Then the work of meditation is to acknowledge the thought (perhaps even thank your mind for sharing it) and return to the sensations of the moment, knowing that at any time you can purposefully change the pose in a nonreactive way.

Vinyasa classes, which follow the same sequence each time, may help you to avoid being distracted by what happens next and thus permit you to more deeply connect to the breath and experience the quiet mind of yoga. Ashtanga and bikram yoga are popular examples of this type of practice; for a sample asana flow involving the primary sequence of Ashtanga, see figure 5.10. One student reports that only while practicing Ashtanga yoga, which requires a lot of vigorous movement, does her mind finally quiet down, allowing her to find peace.

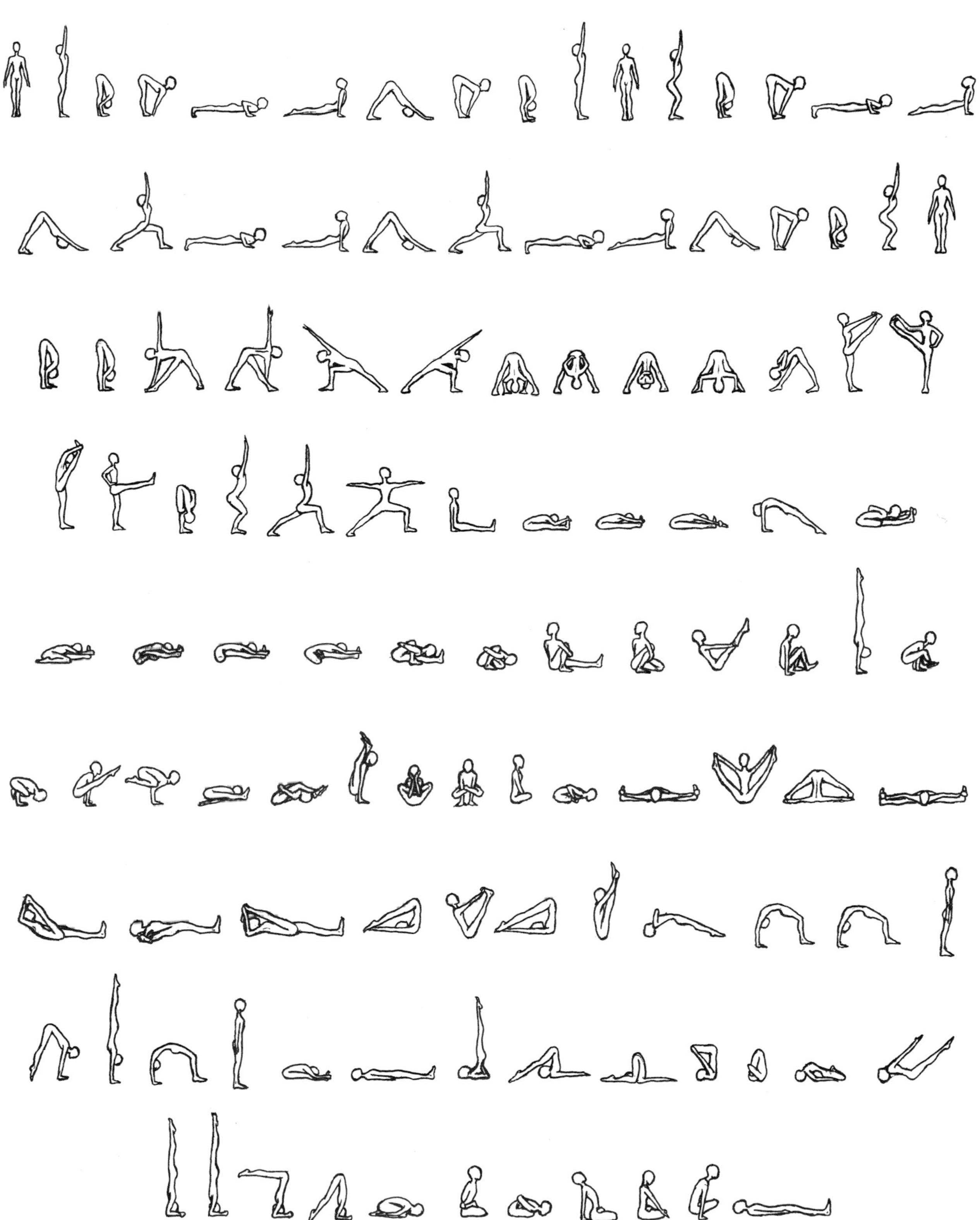

Figure 5.10. Ashtanga Primary Series

Create a ritual to perform before sitting each day, then meditate for a specified time, such as fifteen minutes, for forty days. Rituals can include lighting a candle, burning incense, placing a beautiful flower in front of you, or reading a short passage from an inspirational book. The rituals of one student are clearing the area where she will sit, lighting a candle, and reading from the Yoga Sutras; then, after five or ten minutes, determining an intention for her meditation, such as dedicating it to some individual, group, or cause; and finally setting a timer for twenty minutes.

Practice a meditation called *Neti neti,* here meaning I am not this and I am not that (see introduction). The purpose of this exercise is to remember that you are more than your thoughts or emotions. When a thought arises or you feel an emotion, say to yourself, "*Neti neti,*" before returning your focus to your breath. As you practice this, you will have a sense of freedom and may even briefly experience *samadhi.*

Draw your own mandala as a meditative practice. This exercise quiets the mind and assists in moving toward *samadhi* through an artistic medium. First, assemble materials such as paper, markers, paints, or pens, and on the paper draw or trace a circle. Then connect to your breath and, inside the circle, draw images from your life and dreams. If you are a visual person, you may find this practice especially nourishing and enjoyable.

The Web offers numerous interactive options for meditation. For example, at http://www.swamij.com/trataka3.htm you can set a timer and gaze online.

CHAPTER SIX

Poses for Freedom

This chapter addresses the facet people associate most with yoga—the asanas, or poses. In our practice of the third limb of yoga, asana, we bring to the mat knowledge from the other limbs of how to conduct ourselves as individuals and in relation to others; how to control the breath and withdraw our senses; and how to focus with increasingly greater concentration in meditation (see figure 6.1 for a visual reminder of the path). By bringing all the limbs to pose practice, we are able to have a full experience of yoga, encompassing physical, mental, emotional, and spiritual aspects, ultimately leading to peace and liberation.

This section begins with suggestions for finding the right yoga class for you and discusses the overall benefits of this limb. It also focuses on the importance of setting an intention before practice and presents enough anatomy to help you approach the poses intelligently. Because poses are supported by core strength, strategies for developing abdominal core strength are given, including specific poses accessible for all levels. Then key poses are discussed in detail with instructions and benefits, keeping in mind the Golden Rule of Practice: Find your breath, follow your breath to the place of sensation, and listen intently to your experience.

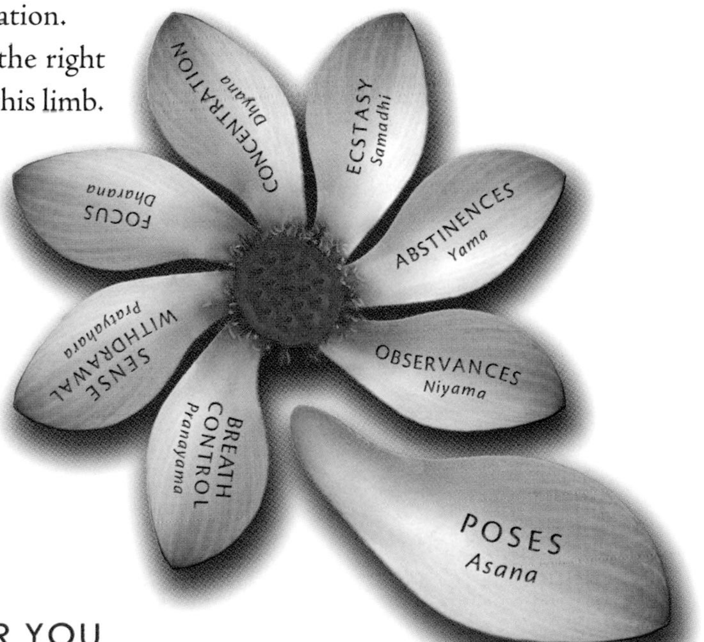

Sanskrit Gem

***Asana* means to sit, pose.**

Figure 6.1. The third limb of Ashtanga yoga, *asana*

FINDING THE YOGA CLASS FOR YOU

There are many styles of yoga with individual alignment recommendations and numerous books describing asanas (see bibliography). In this book, poses are presented with alignment principles based on the study and practice of a variety of approaches. And because there are so many, it is worthwhile researching and evaluating those best suited to your interests and abilities.

To assess the type of practice or teacher likely to benefit you the most, consider the following questions before and after attending a class:

- Is the teacher attentive and willing to provide individual consideration?
- Are the instructions clear and helpful?
- Do you feel better when you leave class, more expansive and alive, or do you feel like you are somehow flawed?
- Are you learning the poses, as well as something more about yoga and life?
- Do you look forward to going to class?
- Do you feel a sense of community inside the studio?
- Are the students treated with respect?
- Does the teacher practice and model the *yamas* and *niyamas*?
- Are you encouraged to ask questions?
- Are you permitted to find your own edge regardless of what others are doing?
- Are there aspects of the teaching that you emulate?

If you answer any questions negatively, give other environments and teachers a try. You may find that the teachers most beneficial to you are those at yoga conferences or workshops, on DVDs, or in books.

When you find a class and teacher that is right for you, look for yoga events outside of the regular asana classes. Often yoga studios offer *satsangs*, or community gatherings, for group study. Being with other students who are searching for meaning and growth through yoga, as well as minimizing interaction with people who are not, is an enormous support on your path, as the *Hatha Yoga Pradipika* emphasized hundreds of years ago: "The yogi succeeds by six qualifications: cheerfulness, perseverance, courage, true knowledge, firm belief in the words of the guru [which could be your inner guru], and by abandoning unsuitable company."[1] Such a yoga community, or yoga *kula*, will sustain you, though you may not choose to connect with others in this way due to your personal lifestyle.

Sanskrit Gem

Satsang **means gathering of like-minded individuals.**

Sanskrit Gem

Kula **means community of the heart.**

THE BLESSINGS OF PRACTICE

The more we practice on the mat with enthusiasm and dedication, the more likely we are to find relaxation, peace, equilibrium, and equanimity, or *samatvam*, in our daily lives, regardless of the turmoil around us. The potential physical benefits of yoga are practically limitless, depending on individual constitution and dedication over time. They begin with building strength, flexibility, balance, and endurance and continue with various forms of healing, including reduced stress, lower blood pressure, increased heart and lung capacity, body metabolism regulation, and improved sleep.

The mental and emotional benefits from yoga include a more relaxed and balanced approach to life due to increased detachment from thoughts and emotions impacting you during daily events, both from external situations and from negative self-talk. Yoga practice can teach you to notice when your thoughts veer toward self-defeating ideas and how to return to your yoga experience. For example, as you practice the poses you may experience negative self-talk in which you find fault with your poses in comparison with those of others in class, resulting in upset and feelings of inadequacy. But as you become aware of and detach from such thoughts through yoga techniques, your emotions are altered and you feel a greater sense of relaxation and well-being.

On the other hand, when you quiet your mind through practicing poses you may experience deep and difficult feelings that were previously repressed. You can also benefit from the emergence of these previously buried emotions as long as you watch them arise, tune in to their implications, keep breathing, remain focused on your pose, and allow the emotions to eventually pass. An appropriate response from a teacher upon noticing the eruption of difficult feelings in a student is simply to offer a tissue, express support, and then move on with the classwork. Yoga class isn't a therapy session, but it often becomes a safe and supportive environment for the release of emotions.

Once we are able to work with thoughts and feelings that surface, we move beyond the body, mind, and emotions and enter a spiritual world where we experience ourselves as part of a greater whole. This may feel as if a tight string that held you in tension and separateness has been released, resulting in a love for yoga, your classmates, your teacher, and all beings everywhere. Such moments may be fleeting at first, but the more you practice yoga by bringing all the limbs to the mat, the more often you will experience this state of freedom, or *samadhi*.

SETTING SANKALPA, INTENTION

Sanskrit Gem

Sankalpa **means intention, determination, purpose.**

Before beginning yoga practice, setting *sankalpa*, or intention, can help in achieving our goals. Without intention, yoga poses are merely movements of the body, lacking deeper meaning. By setting an intention, we create the backdrop for inner awakening. Indeed, intention has been referred to as a "call to awakening," which is the purpose of yoga.[2] The beloved poem of yoga, the Bhagavad Gita, encourages aspirants to set an intention to find the true self. A famous yogi, Swami Satyananda Saraswati of the renowned Bihar School of Yoga, said: "When *sankalpa* becomes the driving force, everything you do in life becomes successful."[3]

To set intention before beginning yoga practice, whenever you step onto the mat ask yourself why you have come to this practice and how you are feeling. Then set an intention for your own benefit and the benefit of others everywhere. You might want to use the *yamas* or *niyamas* or another ancient text as a basis for your intention—focusing, for example, on the concept of truth, self-study, or contentment. Once your intention is set, it works subconsciously as you go about the poses, although you might also recall it intermittently and reinforce it. Because intention is a powerful tool for manifesting outcomes, after setting an intention you are likely to intuit a solution for manifesting your intention or receive a vision linked to one.

JUST ENOUGH ANATOMY

While knowing the name of every muscle in the body is not necessary for practicing or teaching yoga, it is helpful to learn just enough anatomy—the main bones, joints, and muscles—to understand the physical implications of poses, easily follow directions, and ultimately give directions as teachers.[4] Also, comprehending basic anatomy helps us become more aware of our body's layers (*koshas*) and energy centers (chakras), so we can perceive our body as a refined organism.

First, we need to know the main bones of the body. As a student, you might hear both the common and anatomical names of bones—such as thighbone or femur, and sitting or sitz bones, or ischial tuberosities. As a teacher, you may want to say both names so students learn more about their physical structure. In addition, students should be made aware of the vast variation in the shape and size of human bones; for example, some individuals have an extra cervical spine or differently shaped femur heads. This is important to know because sometimes when students can't do the form of a pose demonstrated by a teacher, it is not because they lack flexibility, balance, or strength but simply due to the fact that their bones are shaped differently.

The spine, called the vertebral column, is central to all movements in yoga. According to yogis, we are as young as our spine is flexible. The spine is made up of approximately thirty-three bones, called vertebrae, divided into five regions: cervical (seven bones), thoracic (twelve bones), lumbar (five bones), sacrum (three to five fused bones), and coccyx (four fused bones) as shown in figure 6.2. The thoracic region is where the ribs are connected to the spine, with the cervical region above and the lumbar below, and the sacrum and coccyx below that. Each area has its own natural curve. The thoracic spine and sacrum form C-shaped curves with midpoints facing behind, called kyphosis if the shape is excessive. The cervical and lumbar regions curve in the opposite direction, putting sway into the neck and low back, called lordosis if exaggerated.

The main principle underlying spinal movement in yoga is elongation before movement. The basic movements of the back are extension (straightening the spine, bending backward), flexion (bending the spine or torso forward), lateral bending (bending the spine to the side), and rotation (twisting the spine). But before moving in any of these directions it is essential to elongate the spine. Because the vertebral column protects the

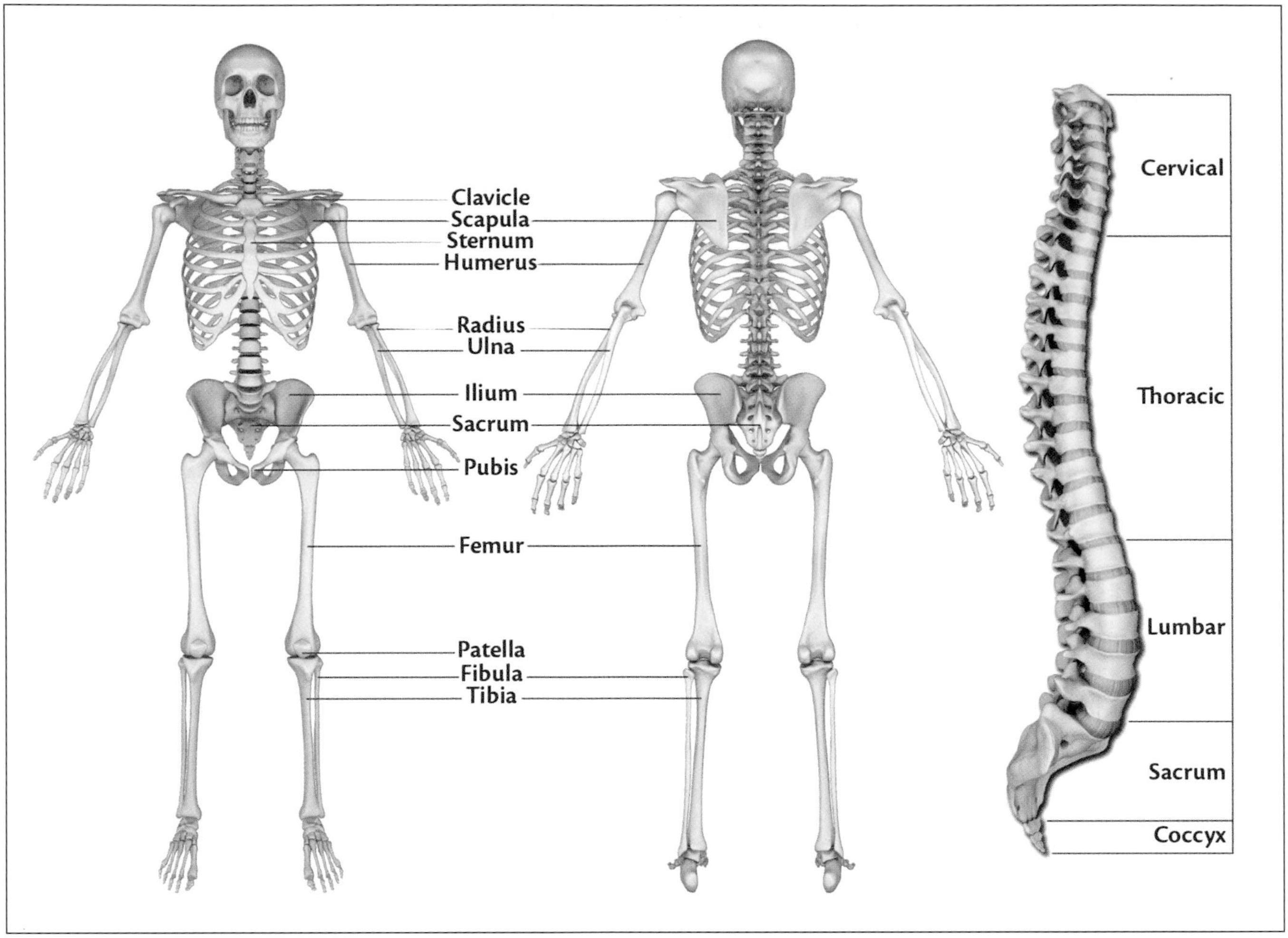

Clavicle
Scapula
Sternum
Humerus
Radius
Ulna
Ilium
Sacrum
Pubis
Femur
Patella
Fibula
Tibia
Cervical
Thoracic
Lumbar
Sacrum
Coccyx

Figure 6.2. Bones of the body: frontal view, posterior view, spine

"Sitting bones"
Ischial tuberosities

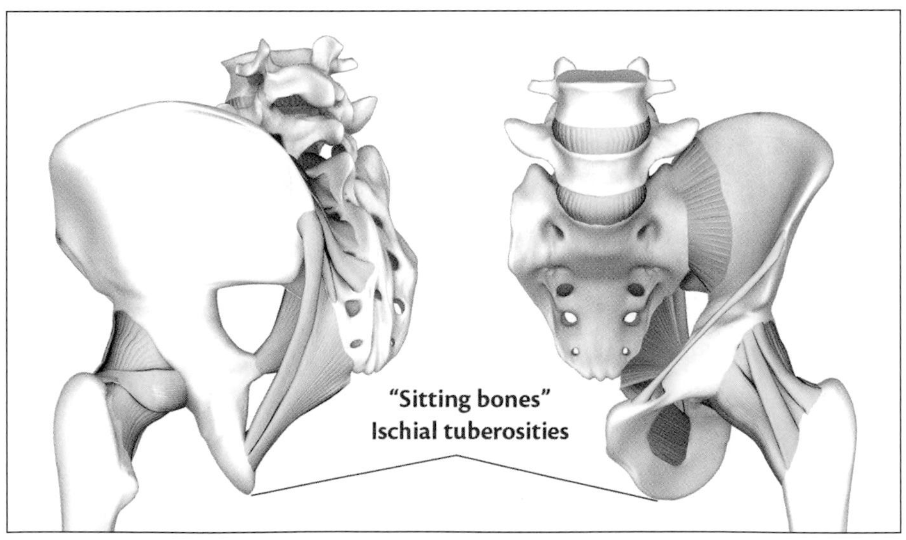

Figure 6.3. The sitting bones

spinal cord and the spinal nerves as they exit it and proceed to the body's muscles, joints, organs, and other vital tissues, keeping the spine elongated and flexible allows for proper neurological functioning.

The sitting bones also are important in yoga poses (see figure 6.3). Finding these bones while sitting is crucial to properly aligning the body and avoiding physical problems. Improper sitting, bad posture, weak core strength, or weak or inflexible muscles can cause us to put body weight in places not meant to hold it, such as the sacrum, resulting in numerous problems, including back pain, sciatica, chest collapse, tight middle-back, and tight shoulders.

Second, people practicing yoga also need to know the main joints of the body and how they function. A significant point to remember is that the body is composed of joints designed to move the bones but not to bear weight. Often, we rely on joints to bear too much weight—for example, by leaning on our wrists or overextending our knees. It is important to build strength around the joints equally so they move without torque and with equal support.

The largest joint in the body is the hip (figure 6.4). Notice how the head of the femur bone fits in the socket (acetabulum), and the bumps on the femur bone known as the lesser and greater trochanter. The greater trochanter can be located by rubbing the side of the femur. The lesser trochanter is the smaller knob on the inside of the femur, an attachment point for an important muscle group—the psoas (pronounced "so-az")—that connects the legs to the trunk and spine.

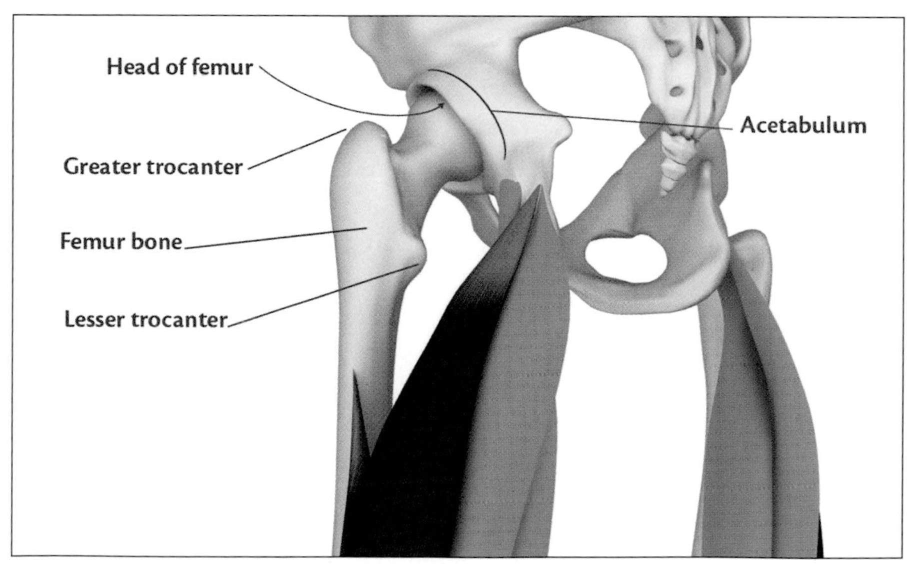

Figure 6.4. Hip joint

The hip joint is surrounded and supported by many muscles that move the bones. Appreciating how complicated and layered these hip joint muscles are (see figure 6.5 for an example) can make us realize the need for many approaches to opening the hips, which is a goal for most yoga

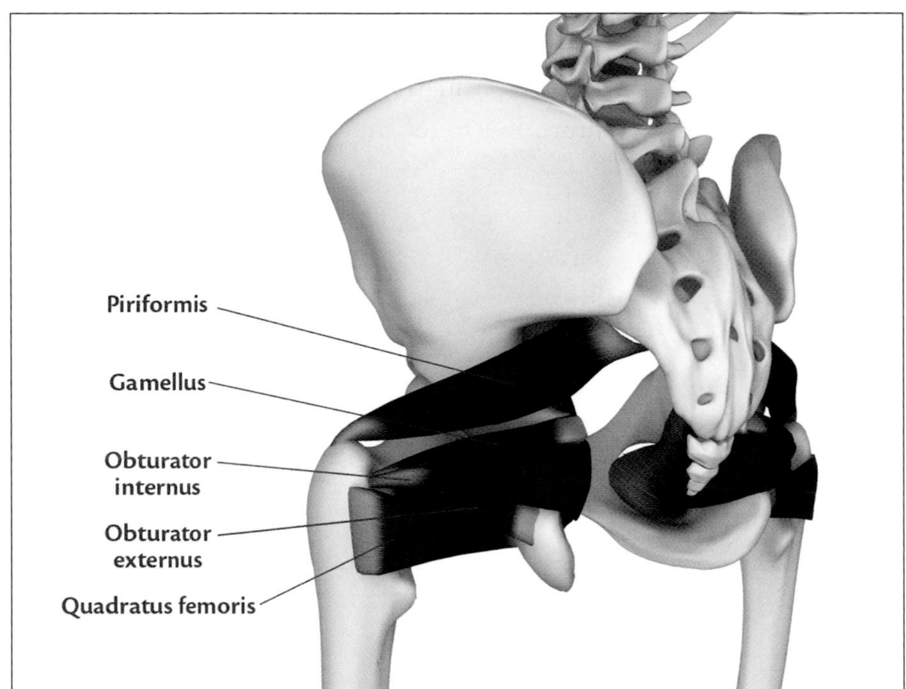

Figure 6.5. External rotators of hips

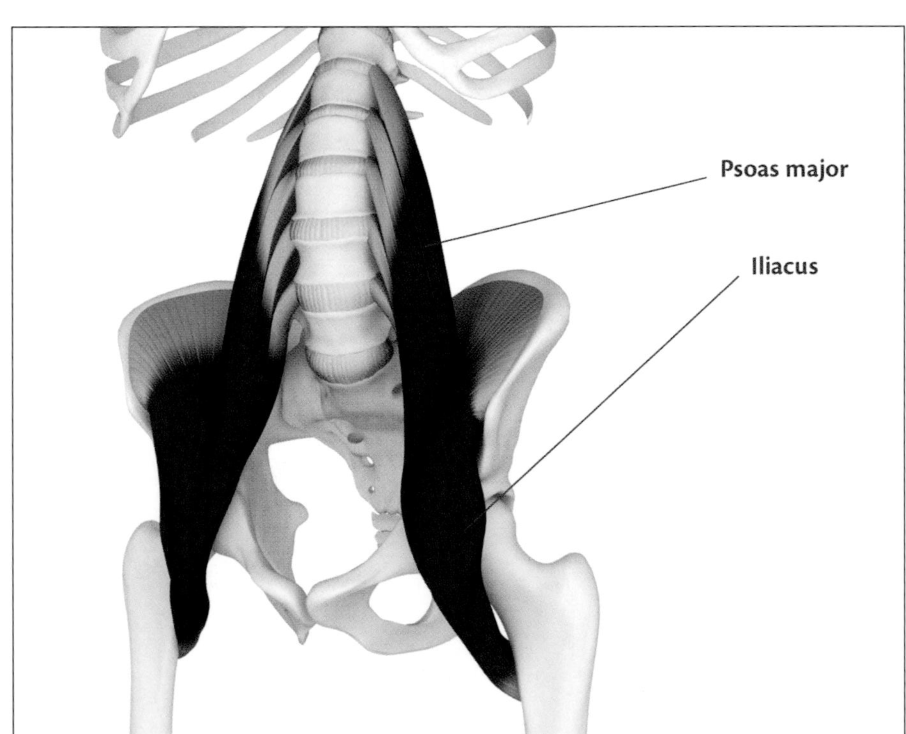

Figure 6.6. Psoas muscle group

students since many are stiff in the hips. Some students, on the other hand, suffer from overflexibility in this joint and require strengthening. For this group, the work is to build abdominal core strength, as discussed in the next section, coupled with pulling all muscles in to support the hip joint.

Third, it is useful for yoga practitioners to learn the principal muscles of the body, which can be layered and complex. For instance, the psoas, a significant muscle group connecting the legs to the trunk and spine, is often shortened in our culture, due to too much sitting. The psoas muscle group consists of the psoas major and the iliacus (see figure 6.6). These short and tight psoas muscles frequently lead to low back pain. Strengthening and lengthening the psoas, through yoga, can help us maintain a straight posture throughout our lives.

The primary muscles of the front legs, the quadriceps, include four muscle groups (see figure 6.7), and the back leg hamstrings involve three (see figure 6.8). These large muscle groups are composed of a number of distinct muscles with different attachments to the bones. Therefore, working to lengthen and strengthen muscles requires practicing multiple poses.

Figure 6.7.
The four quadricep muscles

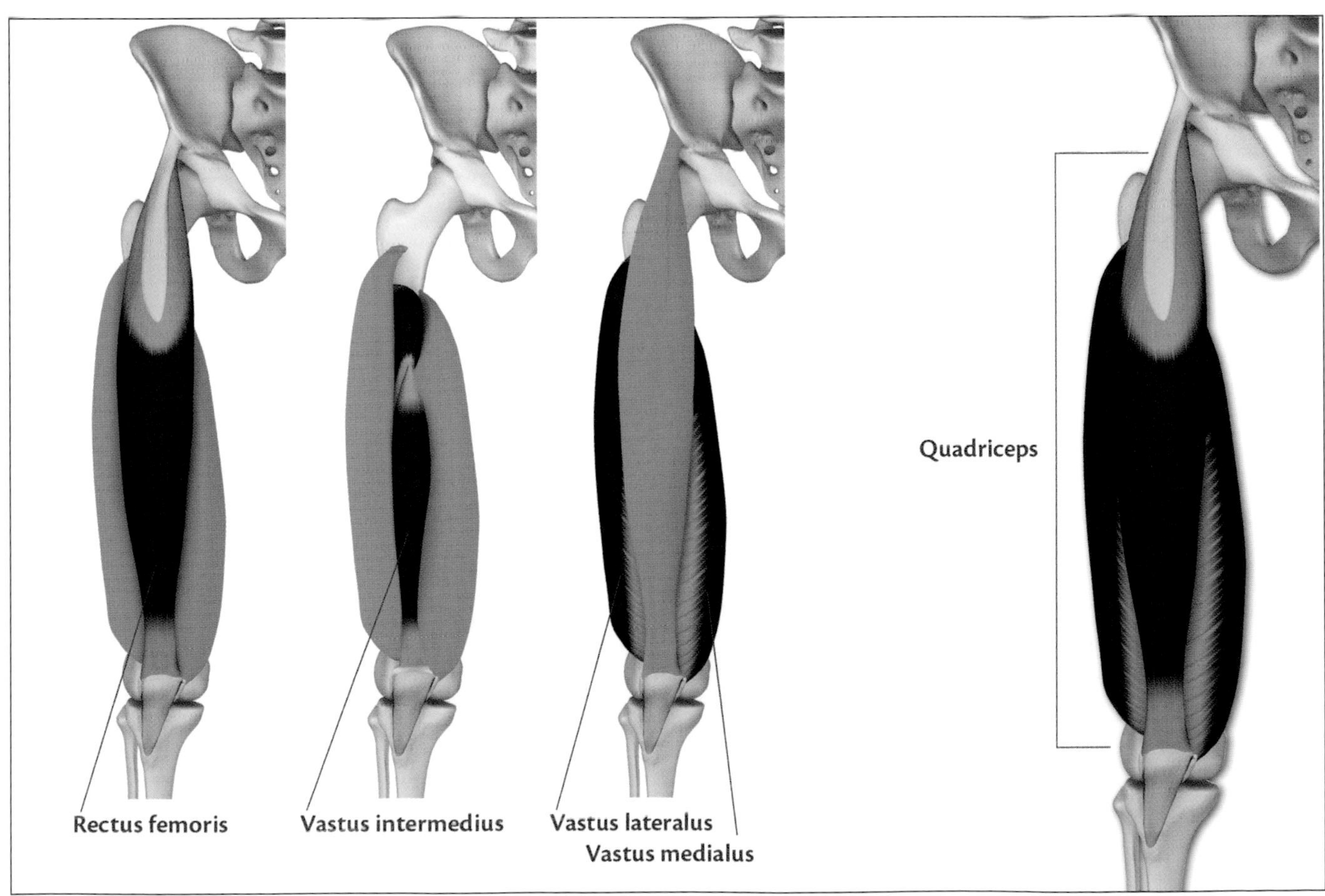

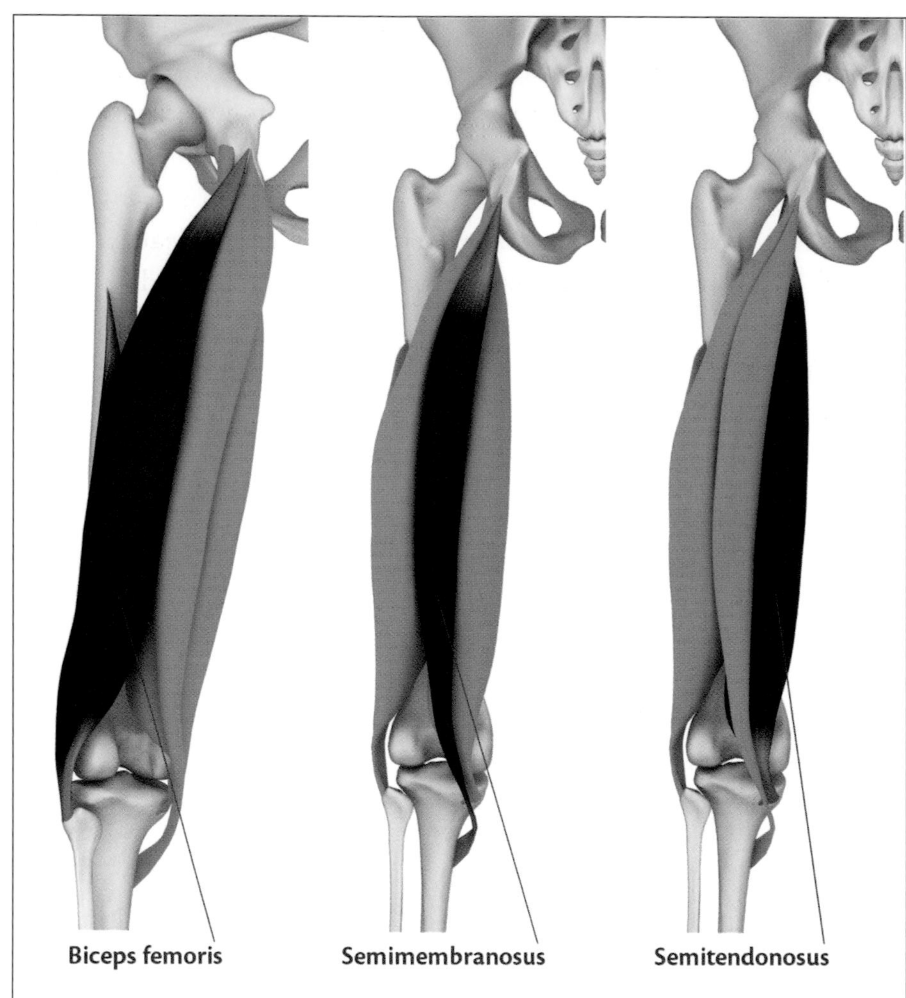

Figure 6.8.
The three hamstring muscles

Abdominal muscles, which include the side muscles, the obliques, are also layered and complex (see figure 6.9). Highly effective postures can strengthen this core group as well. Seeing how these muscles are layered and wrap the body allows us to experience them working in the poses and helps us understand why different poses are necessary to strengthen various aspects of the body's core.

Yogis additionally describe three diaphragms of the body: the pelvic floor, or perineum, between the anus and the genitals; the literal diaphragm, which moves as our lungs expand and contract (see figure 4.5); and the soft palate. The movement of these dome-shaped muscles ranges from the overt up-and-down movement of the literal diaphragm to the less obvious lift of the perineum and the even more subtle expansion of the soft palate.

The functioning of the diaphragms informs our understanding of breath practice. For example, the literal diaphragm is related to the three-part yogic breath (see chapter 4, "Breath, *Bandhas,* and Mudras: The Subtle Realm"). The lift of the perineum, also known as the *mula bandha,* is a powerful conduit for finding strength and support in the body. And relaxing the soft palate can relax the entire head, resulting in a sensation of softness streaming from the crown chakra down to the root chakra.

More anatomy is introduced later in this chapter, where relevant to specific poses. Additional discussions can be found in chapter 9, "Yoga Therapy Training and Yoga As a Profession."

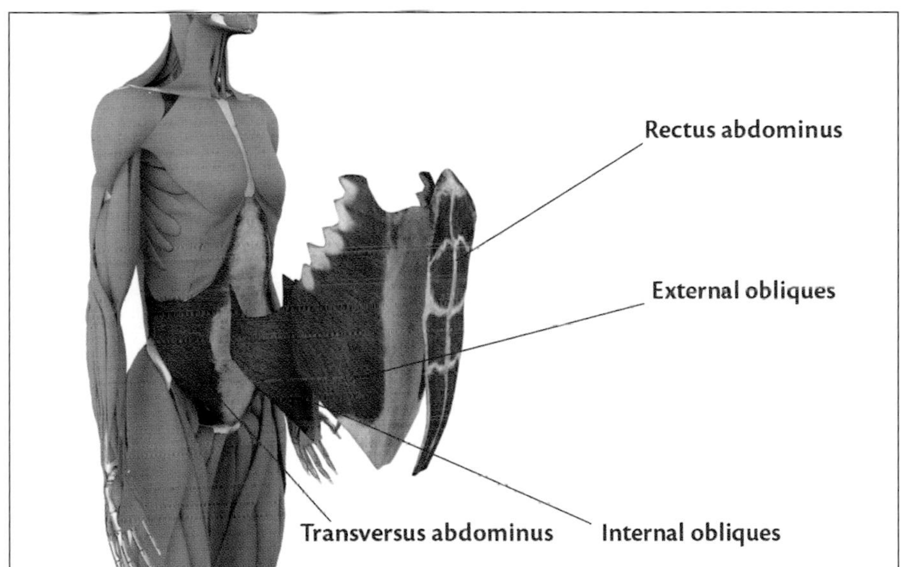

Figure 6.9. Abdominal muscles

POWER FROM CORE STRENGTH

Developing physical core strength allows us to perform many activities and tasks in life with ease and without injury, such as taking a long hike or carrying heavy luggage. Core strength supports mental, emotional, and spiritual strength and thus provides a foundation for attaining our goals, not just in asana or meditation practice but also in our daily lives. For example, there is evidence that young adults who participate in athletics are more likely to engage in healthy behaviors and exhibit higher self-esteem.[5] There is no doubt that when we have both physical and inner strength we feel different about ourselves—more alive and self-assured, as well as less vulnerable to stress and insecurities off the mat.

We build core strength by integrating the four components of breath, *bandhas*, skeleton, and muscles; and the benefit is increased physical strength, self-assuredness, and clarity about our identity and purpose. From that foundation, our interactions with others are marked by insight and calmness. For example, we may feel clear and grounded, rather than anxious, when we refuse to do something that we have habitually done in the past but doesn't serve us, or when we create boundaries around our time or relationships.

In working to develop core strength, it is crucial to realize that of the four components to be integrated, breath is the key to finding energy, while the *bandhas* provide the energetic lift in the body as we move the skeleton into alignment so the muscles are more easily engaged. Knowing that the main muscles of the abdomen attach at the pubis bone at one end and the ribs at the other end (see figure 6.9) reminds us that moving the lower rib cage toward the pubis bone and then contracting the muscles allows for far more efficiency than letting them move apart. Additionally, whenever we are working with core strength, it is important to remember to keep the rest of the body neutral or even relaxed so, for example, you don't find yourself clenching your jaw or straining your neck and shoulder as you work.

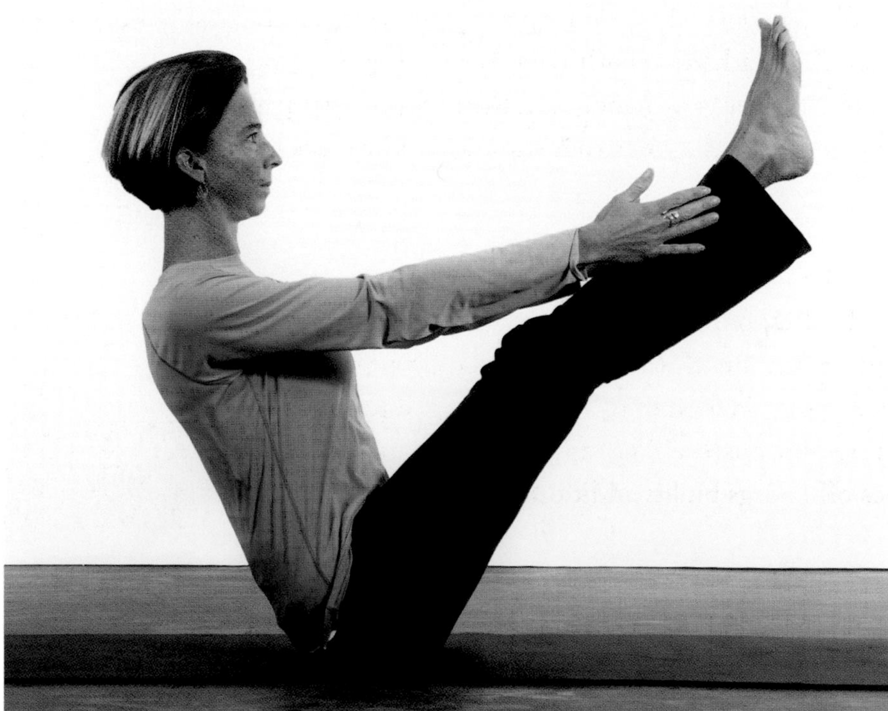

Figure 6.10.
Boat Pose—Navasana

Classical Core Strength Poses

Although all asanas can be used to develop core strength, the following classical yoga poses are particularly effective in doing so for individuals who already have a certain degree of strength.

Boat Pose—Navasana

Practice Boat Pose (figure 6.10) with bent knees, making sure there is no strain in your lower back. If you feel strain, hold your knees or shift to neo-asana poses (see page 132). As you lift your legs, engage your core in such a way that you experience the lifting from underneath, not as pulling up. Eventually, lift your sternum up; if you let it come down a bit initially, you may be better able to feel the abdominal muscles working.

Handstand Pose—Adho Mukha Vrksasana

All inversions can build core strength, especially handstand (figure 6.11). First place your hands on the floor about a hand length from the wall, move your shoulders over your hands, and then lift one leg up as you move your hips over your shoulders. Then kick up.

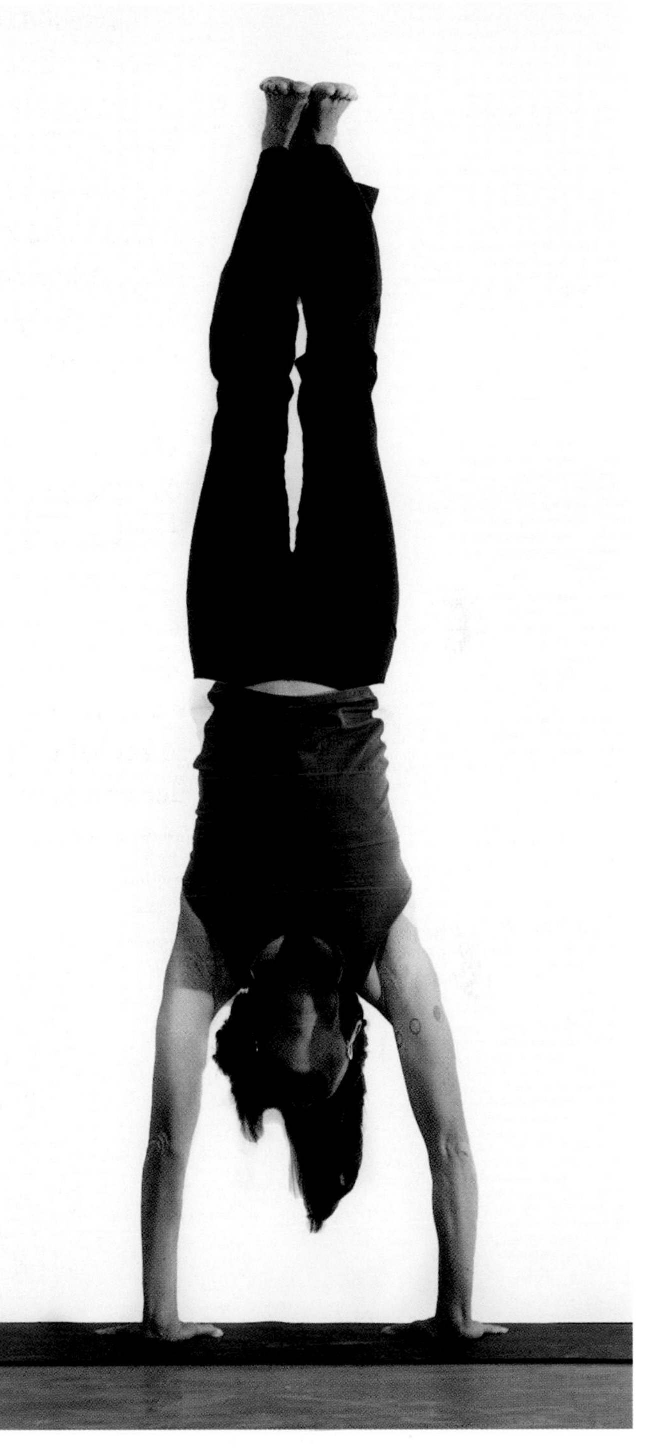

Figure 6.11. Handstand—Adho Mukha Vrksasana

Fierce Pose—Utkatasana

In this pose (figure 6.12), it is necessary to engage abdominal muscles to prevent arching of the back. Back paraspinal muscles are also engaged to maintain an upright posture. Demand on the quadriceps muscles of the legs builds additional leg strength.

Plank Pose—Plankasana

This pose (figure 6.13) is often a bridge to other poses. Electromagnetic tests performed by a physiotherapist and yoga teacher in Oregon have

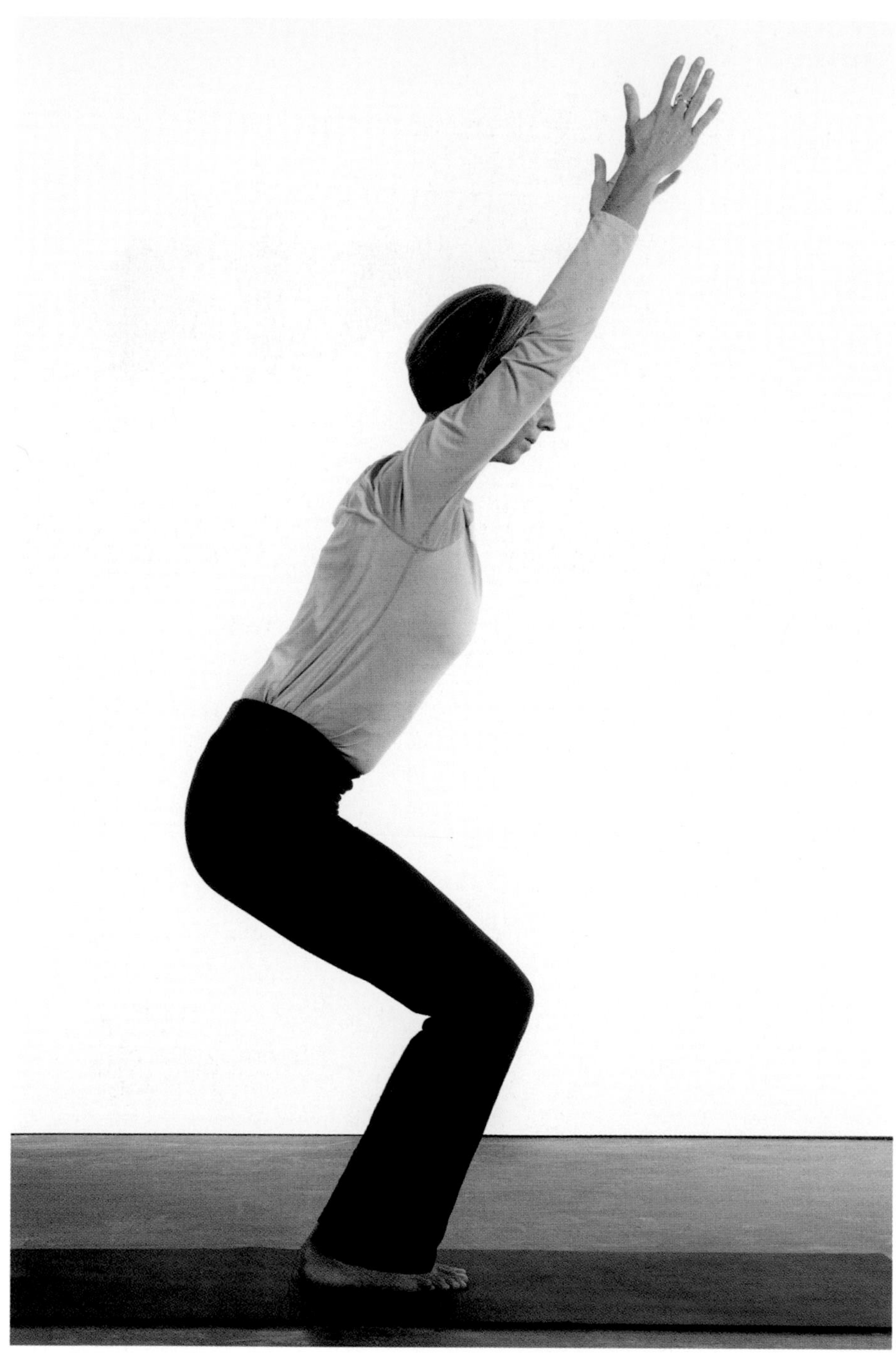

Figure 6.12. Fierce Pose—Utkatasana

shown that this asana engages all four layers of the abdominals more fully than any other abdominal exercise. Work with the pose by isometrically moving your hands down toward your feet and then toward each other, noticing how the work in the abdominal area changes with each action.

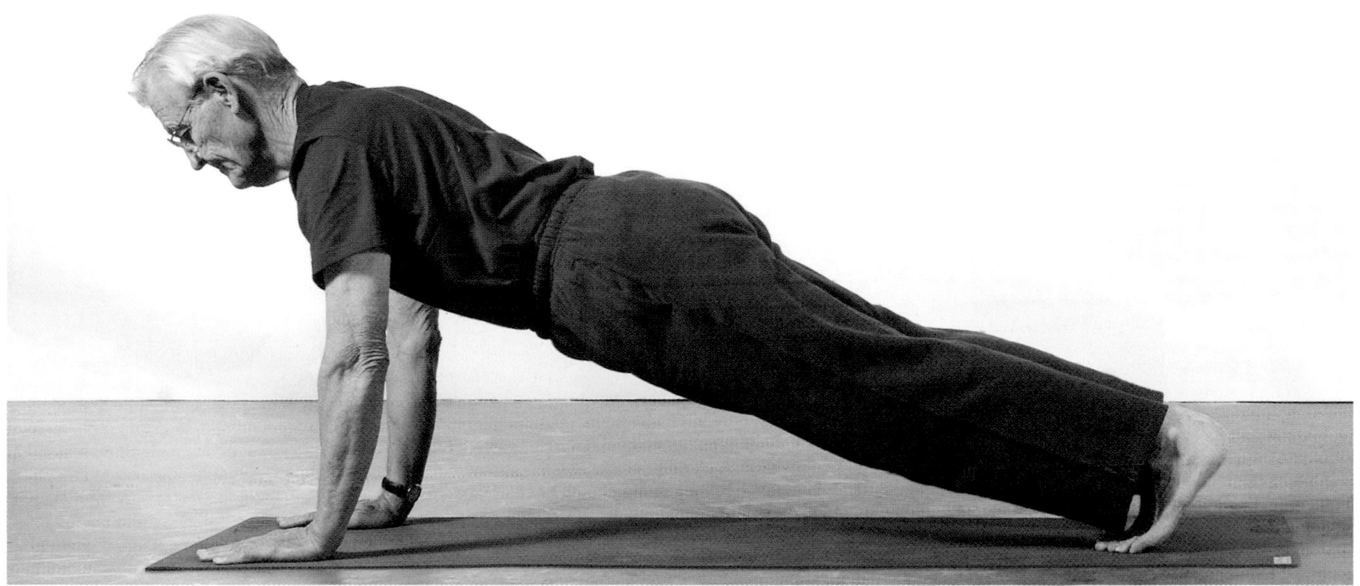

Figure 6.13. Plank Pose—Plankasana

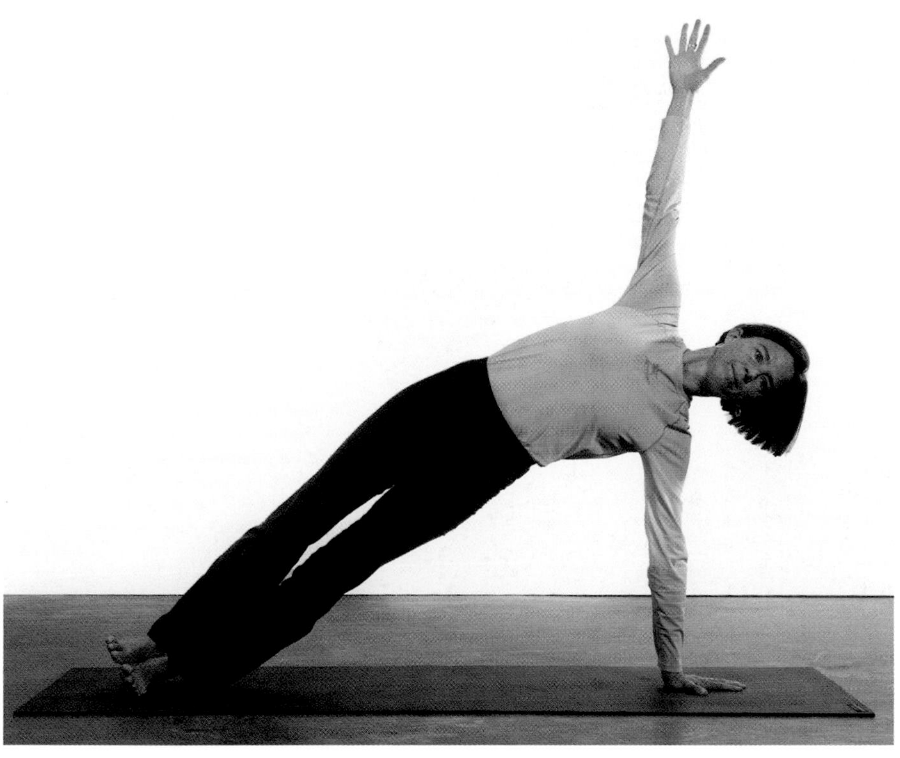

Figure 6.14. Side Plank Pose—Vasisthasana

Side Plank Pose—Vasisthasana

This pose (figure 6.14) engages all four abdominal layers, as well as gluteus medius (buttock), quadriceps (front thigh), and triceps (underarm) muscles.

Neo-Asana Poses for Core Strength

Neo-asana poses are modifications of classical poses that allow beginning students to build core strength in a safe manner and to practice with intensity but not pain. If the classical yoga poses discussed above are too difficult for you and cause feelings of strain, begin instead with the following neo-asana poses.

Lying Release with Leg Lift Variations

Keep your shoulders relaxed and on your back. Inhale and lift your knees up. Move your knees close to your chest. Then move your knees away from your chest so that your thighs are straight up and down. Notice how your low back has arched slightly, with your sitting bones moving down. Exhale and engage *mula bandha* and *uddiyana bandha,* pulling your belly toward the floor, almost feeling like your belly is riding under your rib cage. With your hand on your lower ribs, move your rib cage down a bit in order to access the muscular action. Continue breathing and engaging the *bandhas,* moving the skeleton (rib cage) down, and strongly contracting the abdominals.

Then try moving your legs in these variations:

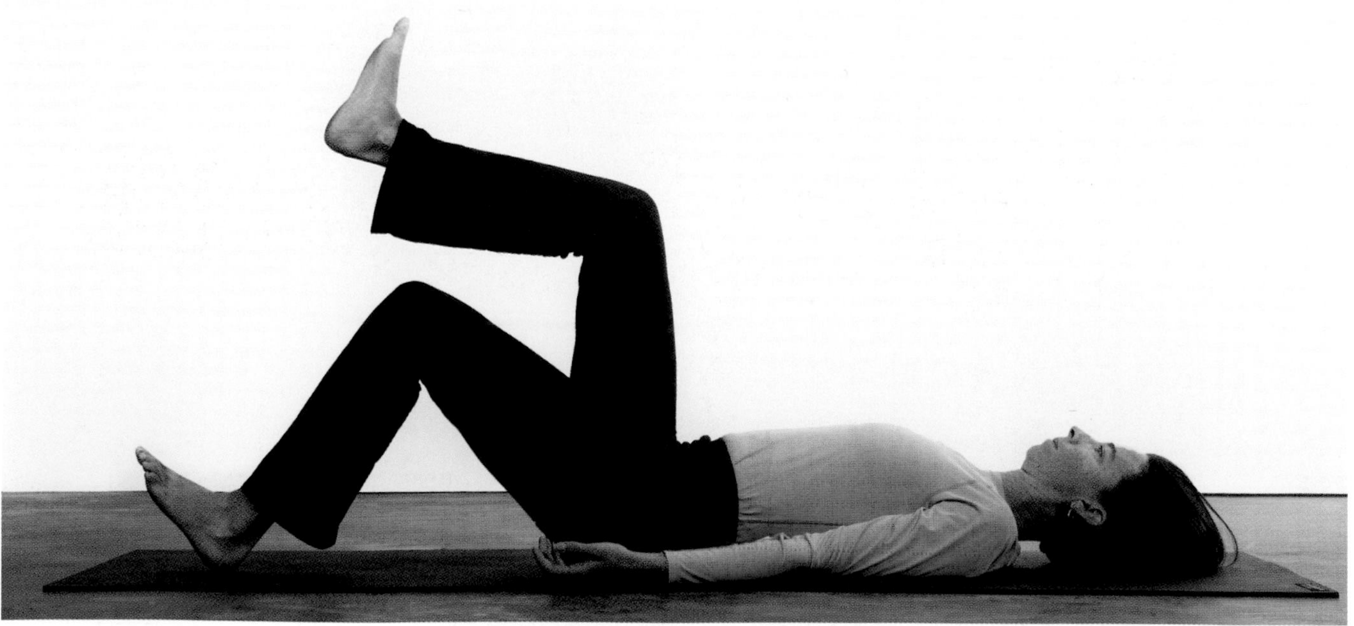

Figure 6.15. Lying Release with Leg Lift Variations

- With knees bent and feet flexed, touch one foot to the floor at a time (figure 6.15). Rest after ten cycles, then do another round with the foot pointed, touching toes to the floor one foot at a time.
- With one leg straight up, move the other, keeping the bent knee away from your torso. Move your knee slowly and see how you work more and more to keep the core engaged and low back on the floor.
- With both knees bent, move them toward the floor together, first with flexed feet, then with pointed feet.

In all these variations, be sure to move slowly and keep your mind focused on the river of energy moving up between your legs. If thoughts arise, simply acknowledge them and return to your practice. Should you be unable to engage the core, then it is time to rest.

Cat/Cow with Leg Lifts

Come to all fours on the floor and begin to practice Cat/Cow Pose (figure 9.3, page 255): Inhale, let your spine sink down and head lift in line with it, then exhale, tuck your tailbone, and round your back like a mad Halloween cat. Go back and forth between these positions slowly, and

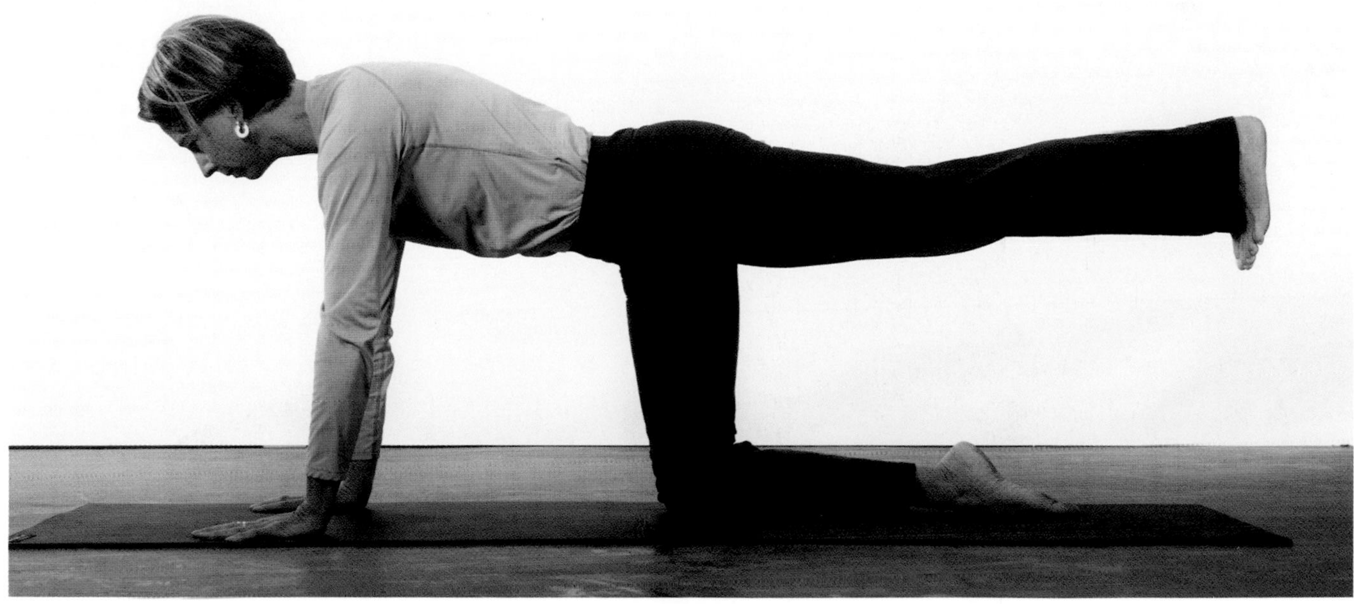

Figure 6.16. Cat/Cow with Leg Lifts

with your breath work to find *mula bandha* in this way: On the inhale isometrically move your thighs away from each other and feel a slight stretch of the *mula bandha*. Then as you exhale lift up from that spot and pull the abdominal muscles up and under for the Cat Pose. Hold the exhale a bit longer and see if you can find *mula bandha* again and *uddiyana bandha* as the skeleton and muscles all work together. Continue practicing Cat/Cow Pose, focusing on core strength, then come to neutral and rest in Child's Pose (figure 6.48, page 170).

Come again to all fours and inhale. Then exhale and bring one leg with bent knee toward your chest, inhale, and extend your leg out behind you. Hold it there as you continue to breathe and engage the core. Bring the opposite hand around to the back waist to see if it is dipping down at all. Work to lift your belly button up so that your back waist is flat as shown in figure 6.16. Continue holding and breathing for about ten breaths, then release, pause, and rest in Child's Pose (figure 6.48, page 170). Repeat with the other leg.

Sandbag Navasana Variations

With your knees bent, put a sandbag on your feet and position yourself with hands on knees. Let your lower rib cage move down so that you can find your core. Next, release your hands from your legs and see if you

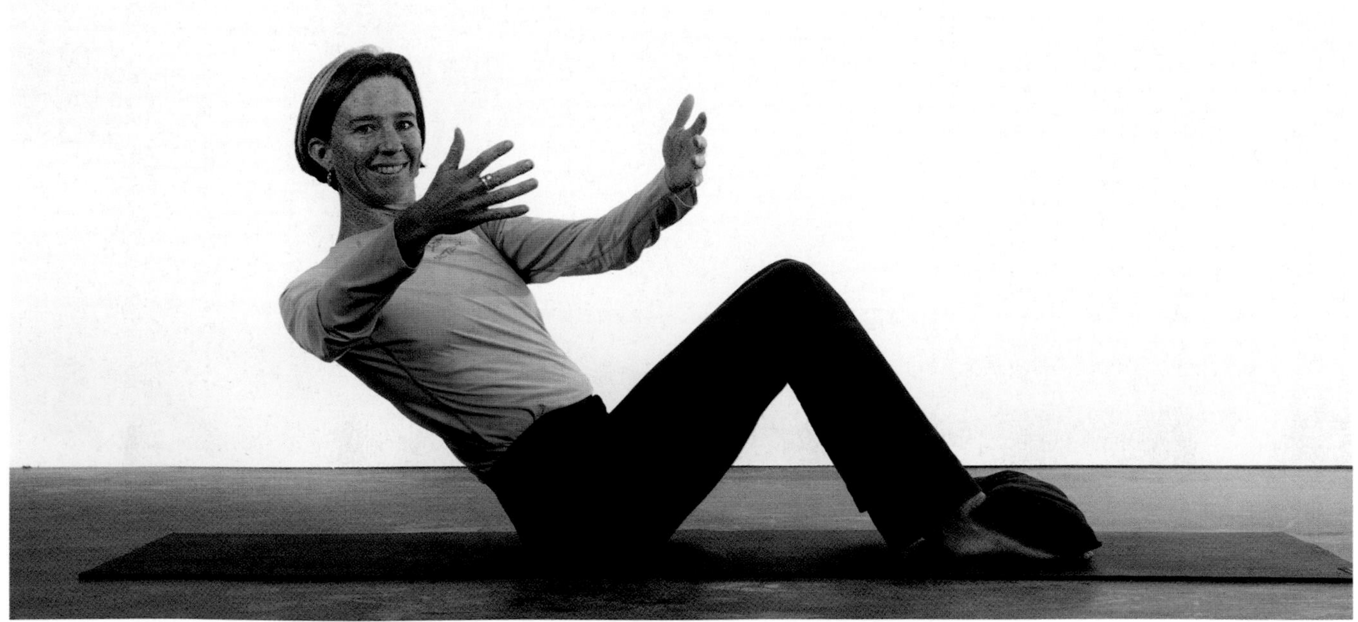

Figure 6.17. Sandbag Navasana Variations

can maintain the position of your spine. If you feel any stress in your back, keep your hands on your legs. If not, inhale, bring your arms up, and hold while breathing, keeping your mind focused on your core. Then bring your arms to your sides and inhale. Turn to one side and practice five breaths on each exhale; turn a bit farther, inhale to center, and exhale to the other side for five breaths in the same manner. Rest and fold forward, with your head on your knees.

Return to upright with arms straight out to your sides. Inhale, then exhale and reach to one side, stay there, and pulse by inhaling and reaching to the side for five breaths. Inhale to the other side and repeat for five breaths (see figure 6.17). Rest.

Return to upright, engage all four elements of core strength, and slowly lower yourself toward the ground, hovering wherever you can maintain strength without tension in your neck, shoulders, jaw, or eyes. Relax your jaw, and smile as you practice. Then rest.

Always follow core work with a counterpose, which moves the body in the opposite direction, to release and relax the muscles and train them to become responsive and flexible. For example, practice **Easy Wide Leg Bent Knee Twist** slowly focusing on the breath (see figure 6.18). Lying on

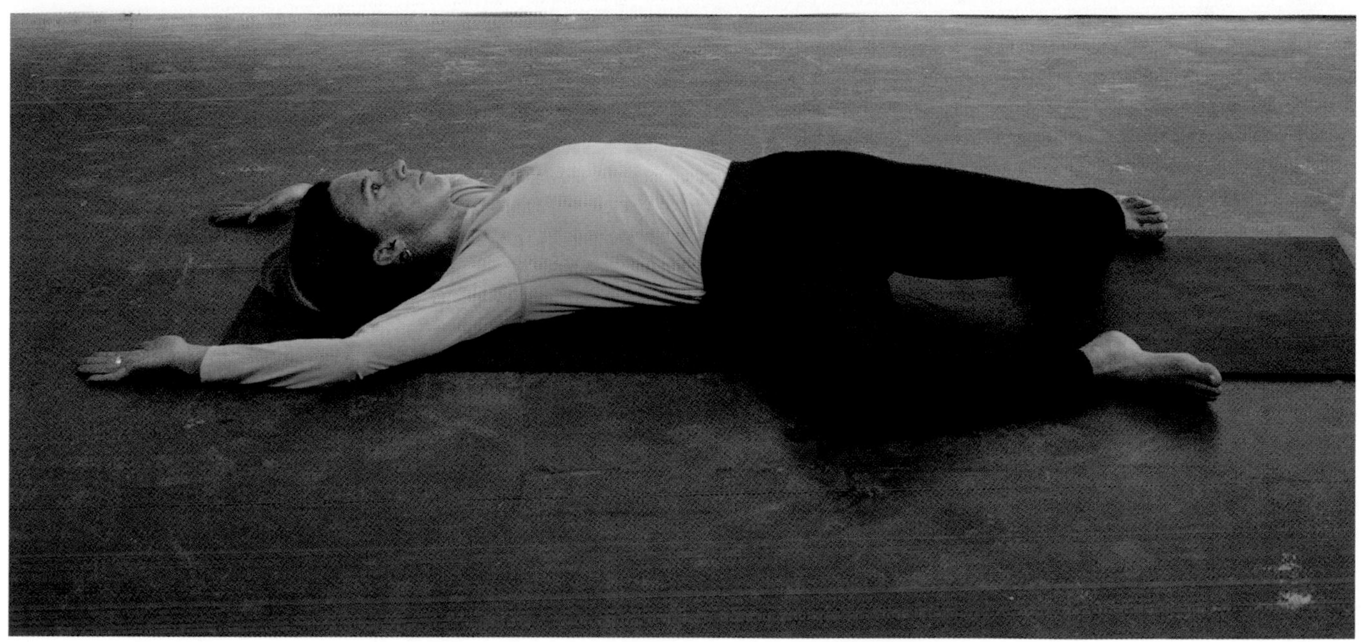

Figure 6.18. Easy Wide Leg Bent Knee Twist

your back, inhale with knees bent upright. Exhale and let your knees go to one side, keeping your legs wide and rolling on the side of the feet. While on this side, gently pulse your top knee toward the floor and away from your chest, feeling the stretch of the area that was just worked. After ten breaths, inhale, bring your knees back up to center, and exhale, allowing them to go to the other side, then repeat the same actions. After ten breaths return to center and hug your knees gently to your chest, drawing small circles with them in both directions. Then rest in any variation of Corpse Pose (figure 6.63 on page 185), noticing the sense of activation and warmth in your core.

THE THIRD LIMB: ASANAS, POSES

The practice of asanas is called hatha yoga, meaning balance of oppositional forces. There is never a movement spent in one direction without attention given to balancing the force in some way. Yoga poses involve working with such oppositional forces as stability and freedom, and edges. In every pose there is a minimum edge and a maximum edge. The minimum edge is the first place you find sensation, and the maximum edge is the place of most sensation before feeling pain. Many people are able to push to the maximum edge, bypassing the minimum edge. It may be useful, however, to play with the minimum edge first, to explore sensations. As you move deeper into a pose, you can then discover how far to go before reaching the maximum edge. And since your edges can change over time depending on your condition and perspective, strive to come to the mat each time with a fresh approach, releasing the results of previous practices and anticipating working with the poses anew in the present.

The Yoga Sutras provide relatively little detail concerning asanas except that poses must be steady and comfortable:

> Yoga pose is a steady and comfortable position.
> *Sthira-sukham asanam.* [6]

Fortunately, we can apply the Golden Rule of Practice to all poses for all levels of practice: Find your breath, follow your breath to the place of sensation, and listen intently to your experience by playing your edges. The first step is to breathe consciously, feeling the sensation of breath moving along your spine, as practiced in *pranayama* (see chapter 4). The second step is to take your breath and awareness to a place in your body where you feel something, such as intensity or soreness. In yoga, we say where the mind goes *prana* goes, so we take our breath by way of our consciousness to whatever we are feeling. Finally, the third step is to listen very carefully to messages you are receiving from your body. You may want to work intensely and with great focus (*tapas*) and discipline, but you don't want to experience pain. If you are working intensely, you can always back off, but if you push yourself too hard and experience pain you may have no control over the result. The distinction between states of intensity and pain is at the heart of yoga practice, and it is crucial to recognize the difference. On the other hand, at times you may want to deliberately practice gently because you need a more restorative and relaxing experience. In that case, find your breath, follow it to the sensation, and then play your edges at an easier place.

It is important to remember that each pose balances the oppositional forces of stability and freedom. If there is too much stability in a pose, you lose freedom; and with too much freedom you lose stability. You want to have a pose with a strong foundation that can support the openness and expansion available. Finding the correct balance between stability and freedom that allows for both is not only a focus of yoga but also a metaphor of life. For example, we've all experienced going too far in something, perhaps in drinking, eating, or working, and also staying too grounded and thus unable to spontaneously enjoy things. Balancing these two concepts on the mat can build confidence in maintaining balance off the mat.

There are many yoga poses from which to choose—some texts say 8,400,000,[7] while others claim 20,000. Regarding this variety, one ancient text states: "Asanas are as many as there are numbers of varieties of creatures in the world. According to Lord Shiva the total number of yoga asanas is 8,400,000. Out of that, however, only 84 are important for the good and welfare of man."[8]

One reason to practice a variety of poses is that it's helpful to know a range of them so that you can build strength, flexibility, balance, and endurance in your whole body. Also, as you practice your body will become accustomed to the same poses, and you will need a new challenge. If you can create a pose in your body without effort or concentration, it actually isn't yoga but just a body shape. It's the process of attaining the poses that makes it yoga. Consequently, poses of greater difficulty are needed as you progress along the path.

Some yoga schools have a preset series of poses that are done each time in the same way in the same order, while other schools use a variety of poses. We will discuss these different strategies more in chapter 8, "Teaching Yoga." Here we will study groups of poses: 1) Standing, 2) Balance, 3) Backbends, 4) Inversions, 5) Seated, 6) Twisting, and 7) Finishing. For each group of poses, the benefits, key principles, key anatomy, and instructions are outlined. For each pose the names are given (English, Sanskrit transliteration, and Sanskrit Devanagari), together with information about the pose and instructions for practicing it. The transliteration includes special marks, called diacriticals, to indicate the precise sound. Sanskrit sounds are defined by where you create the sound in your mouth. For example, when you say "t," your tongue is behind your teeth; when you see a dot under a letter, your tongue should flip to the roof of your mouth instead; a short accent mark above an *s* indicates a "sh" sound; a line over an *a* denotes a long *a* sound; and a dot over a consonant signifies a nasal sound, like "m." Additional illustrations show students with varying degrees of flexibility demonstrating the poses to indicate the range of body types usually found in yoga classes from quite flexible to less flexible and more stable.

Practice these poses over time, observing how you experience them both physically and on other levels—emotionally, mentally, and spiritually. As a guide, suggestions are made about experiencing the poses beyond the physical level, but for every individual this will be different. As you become proficient in some poses, add more poses to your repertoire.

Props illustrated in some versions of poses are meant to make them more accessible to people who lack flexibility or are physically injured or sick. If the props don't help or if you have an aversion to using props, choose poses without props. Props were first championed by the well-known yogi B.K.S. Iyengar from Pune, India, who brought yoga to America. He claimed that yoga was his salvation after experiencing many illnesses and problems in his early life. He found that for Americans, who often lack flexibility, the use of props made yoga more accessible (see more information about his teachings in chapter 1).

Indeed, the way Americans use their bodies is quite different from how people in India do. In America, as soon as babies are born they are put in carriages, car seats, and bouncing chairs. As adults they also spend considerably more time sitting. By contrast, in India squatting rather than sitting is common and considered comfortable. As a result of this difference, Americans generally have less flexible joints, especially hip joints, and thus may find props helpful in attaining comfortable and steady poses.

Poses are presented here first as individual postures with specific descriptions of alignments so you can comprehend the components and learn how to work with them. Ultimately, the poses can be linked together into a flowing movement by following the breath and holding them for as few as five breaths or substantially more. Examples of the classic sequences known as Sun Salutations and Moon Salutations are given after the discussion of individual poses.

Before entering poses, remember to set an intention to give them purpose. Similarly, exit poses using consciousness and intention.

Each pose that follows, demonstrated by three yogis of differing ages and abilities (see figure 6.19), is just right as illustrated; one model's demonstration is not better or closer to "real" yoga than another's. Ultimately, the perfect pose is the one that is done with awareness and enthusiasm, not to match an external picture.

Standing Poses

Benefits: Standing poses provide a sense of being grounded and connected to the world, as well as open to possibilities due to the upward lift of the trunk. These are good poses to do when you feel confused or overwhelmed. Therapeutic aspects include strengthening the legs and arches of the feet, strengthening and elongating the spine, and building core abdominal strength.

Standing poses may allow you to simultaneously practice the other limbs of yoga—for example, cultivating the *niyama* known as *santosha* (contentment) or dharana, focusing attention on the third eye. Such practices done as standing poses may result in a feeling of relaxation throughout the body.

Key Principles: Often new students imagine that they will begin yoga practice seated on the floor in cross-legged, or Lotus, position as they have seen in images of yogis meditating. Actually, since seated poses require more flexibility, it is helpful for most students to begin with standing poses and then move to seated poses. It is best to start standing poses with the Mountain Pose, which is symmetrical, and then add asymmetrical poses to build flexibility and balance.

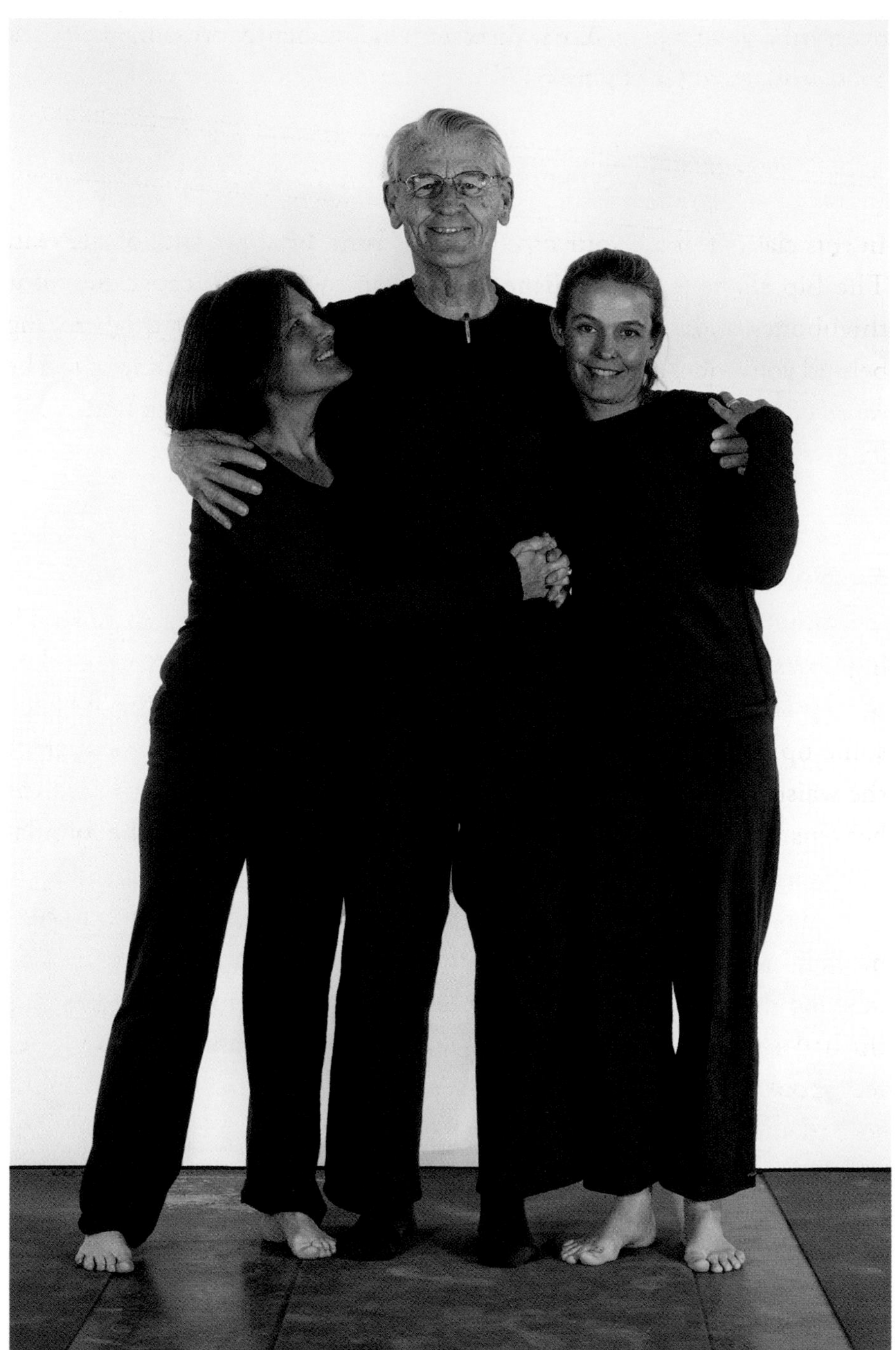

Figure 6.19.
The three models hugging

Key Anatomy: For standing poses, it is important to know which way your hip points are facing and how to tilt the hips, using core strength. Locate the hip points or the anterior superior iliac spine. Notice that you can rotate or tilt your hips either forward, in an anterior tilt, or backward, in a posterior tilt. Use of a block can help you determine if you are overtilting your hips in either direction, inadvertently pressing the block back or forward (see figure 6.20).

HIPS FACING FRONT OR SHORT END OF THE MAT

In this class of poses your hips face the front, or short end, of the mat. The hip shape is accomplished by moving your legs, especially your thighbones. Generally the leg in back will have the inner thigh rolling behind you, and the leg in front will have the inner thigh rolling out. The revolved poses are more challenging, so be sure to use props to find stability or choose the more stable pose shape.

Mountain Pose—Tadasana

tāḍāsana
Mountain Pose

About the pose: Tadasana is home base, the pose to which all standing poses relate. Establishing the foundation is critical so that the roots of your legs go deep into the earth to support the flight of your torso and spine up toward the sky. We allow gravity to penetrate the pose from the waist down and use breath to expand from the waist up toward the heavens. As one yogi says, "Nobody can go to heaven unless the foundation is firm."[9]

Instructions: Begin with your feet creating the "four continents of connection," which are the main points of contact with the gravity of the earth in standing poses. To find them, begin by lifting your toes and pressing the ball mount of your big toe, little toe, inner heel, and outer heel. Your feet should point straight forward, which means that the line between the second and third toe should point forward regardless of the outer shape of the foot. As you find the foot connection, notice the relative strength of your legs, inner versus outer, front versus the back. If your arches are dropping, press down more strongly with the ball mount of your big toe and roll your ankles slightly out as shown in figure 6.21. Release your toes downward, but keep the energy in your feet.

To find the strength and power of your legs, begin by rolling your inner legs toward the wall behind you as you press the top of your thighbones back (your buttocks will stick out slightly) and feel the space between your sitting bones. Press your inner thighs away from each other; strongly tuck your tailbone, lifting from between your legs and low belly; then press your shins in.

Two extremes of the way we hold our legs are sometimes called the Marilyn Monroe and John Wayne stances (see figure 6.20, left and center, respectively). In yoga, strength comes from the middle way, using neither extreme, though you might have fun noticing how people in the supermarket or mall use Marilyn Monroe or John Wayne stances.

Once you have the foundation set in your legs, elongate your torso and spine evenly in the front and back. Put your hands on your hips and slide them to your rib cage; imagining a light in your rib cage, shine it directly into your pelvic bowl, neither in front nor behind. You can maintain the two planes of the body (front and back) even if you keep noticing where your lower ribs are in relation to your pelvic bowl. Lifting energetically between your legs, raise the abdominal muscles up and back slightly.

Once you have elongated your spine, set the foundation of your shoulders. They may have lifted while you were working to elongate the spine, creating a long side body. If so, move the head of your arm bones back, lift your sternum or breastbone (the scapulas or shoulder blades will move along your back), then broaden your entire upper chest, front and back

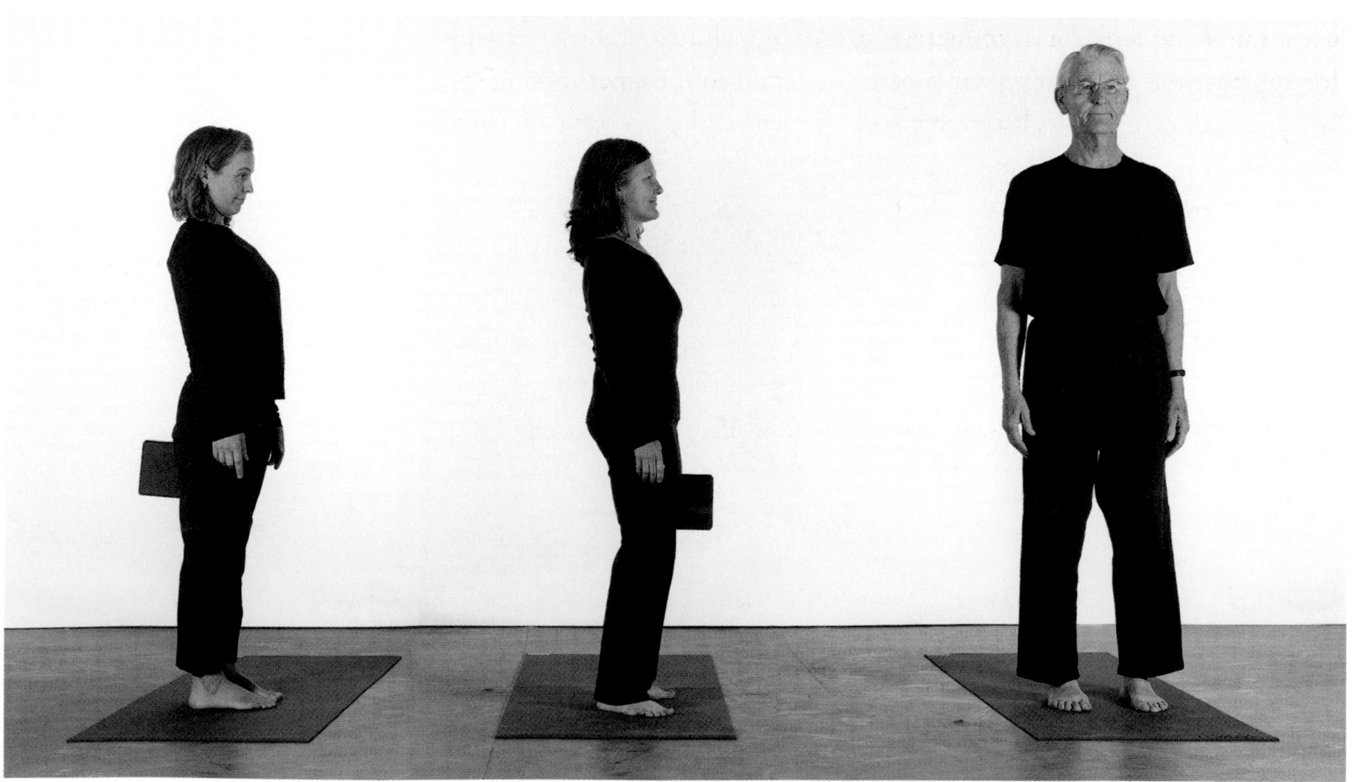

Figure 6.20. Mountain Pose—Tadasana:
Overarching lumbar spine (left); overtucking tailbone (center); steady pose (right)

planes, as your shoulder blades drop down your back. Resist the temptation to overwork your shoulders by pulling them down your back. Remember to keep the relationship between your rib cage and pelvic bowl, and use the lift of the core to prevent your low back from crunching.

Once your shoulders are in place, your head may not feel comfortable on your spine. The best way to realign it is to find your breath. Breathing from the bottom of your spine, watch the breath move through the center core of your body to your throat, and see if your soft palate is aligned over your throat. As noted earlier, to find your soft palate place the tip of your tongue behind your upper teeth and slide your tongue back along the roof of your mouth until it becomes soft. Now as you breathe, try to align your soft palate over your throat by moving it forward and backward—which also moves your head forward and backward—until your breath flows easily from the base of your spine through your torso, throat, soft palate, and into your head.

Relax your arms. You may want to shake them and roll your upper arms slightly back so your palms face your body. Find your breath, and move your body to feel the sense of simultaneous groundedness and flight.

Experience the pose completely from the inside out. You may want to use a mirror to look for asymmetries externally while looking internally for contractions and using your breath for expansion. Remembering the Golden Rule of Practice, listen to your experience. Shake everything out, relax, and then begin again.

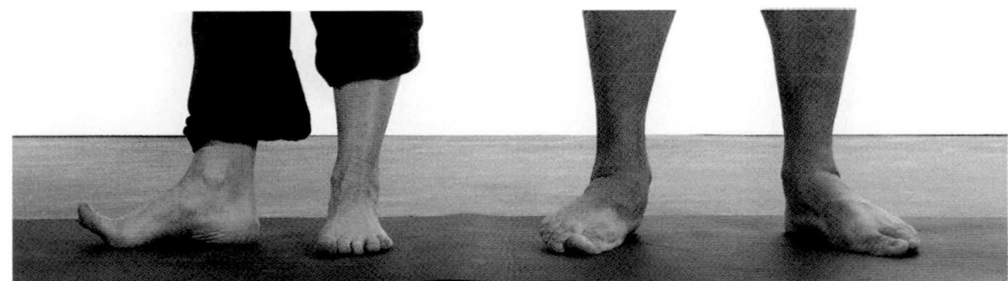

Figure 6.21. Mountain Pose—Tadasana: Arches steady (left); arches dropping (right)

Upward Facing Arms Pose—Urdhva Hastasana

About the pose: This simple pose of lifting your arms up can be a meditation pose in which you receive the energy of the earth with your legs and the energy of the heavens with your arms. Holding this pose for even a few minutes can be surprisingly strenuous. Often, tight shoulders restrict movement, so be sure to use the modifications provided if you experience pain.

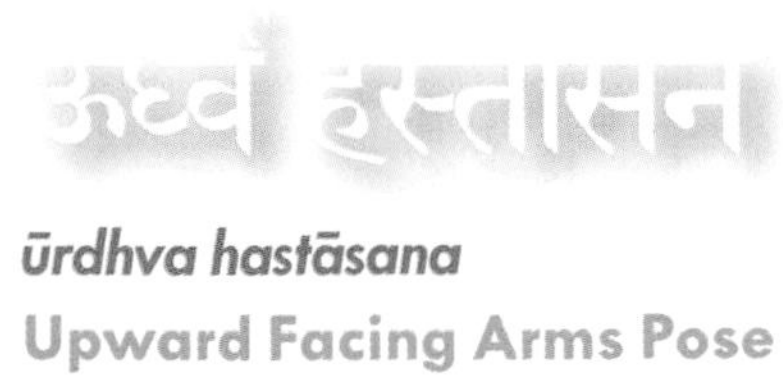

ūrdhva hastāsana
Upward Facing Arms Pose

Instructions: Standing in Mountain Pose, press down with your feet as you inhale and lift your arms forward, pause and suck your armpits back, and exhale. Then inhale and continue raising your arms, rolling the creases of the elbow back as shown in figure 6.22. If your shoulders are tight, bend your arms and move to a wider V shape. Be sure to support your spine with your core strength by lifting between your legs and feeling an inner rise up your body. If you have more flexibility, you can move your arms back slowly with hands facing back as shown in figure 6.22.

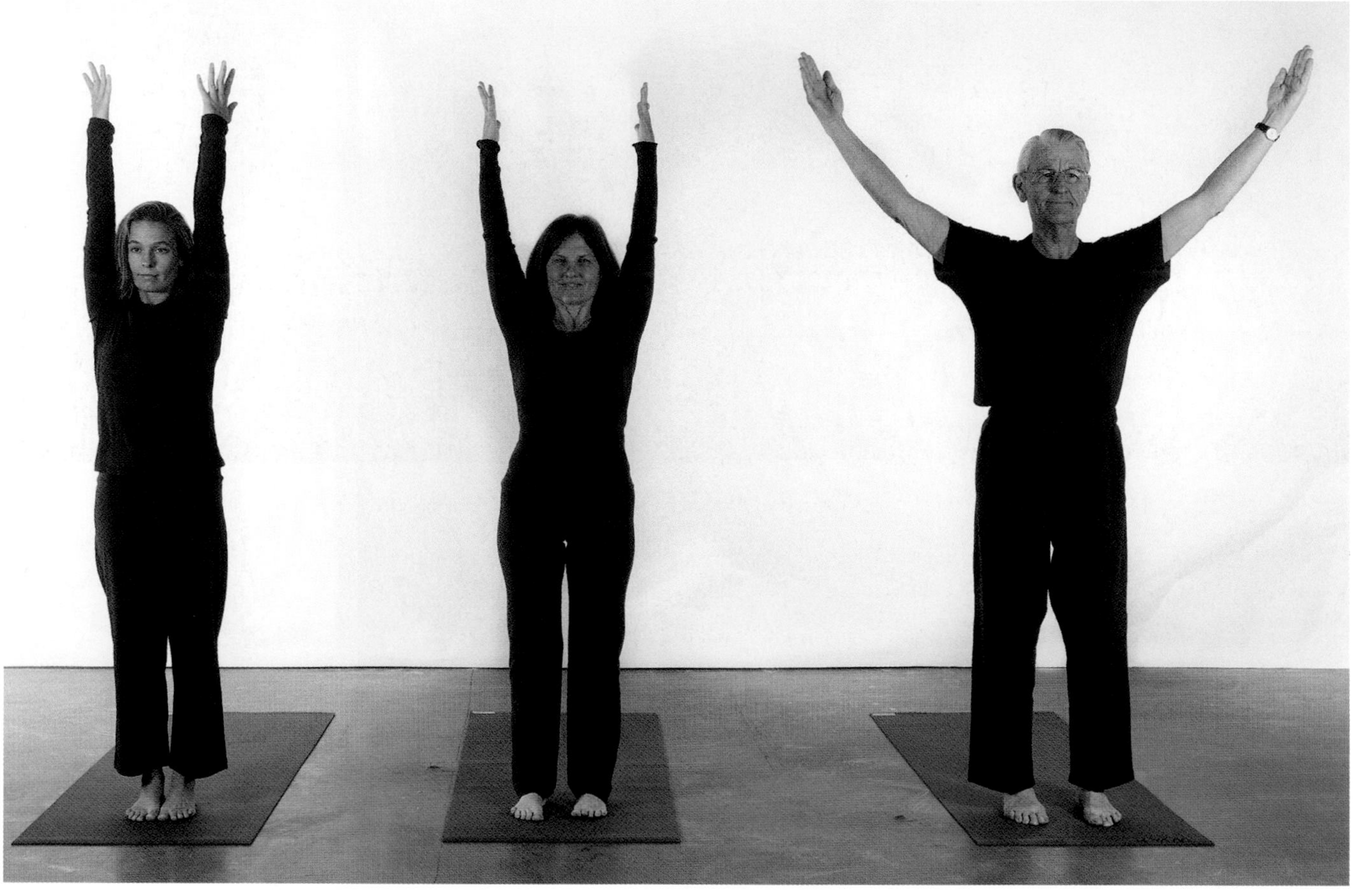

Figure 6.22. Upward Facing Arms Pose—Urdhva Hastasana

Standing Forward Fold Pose—Uttanasana

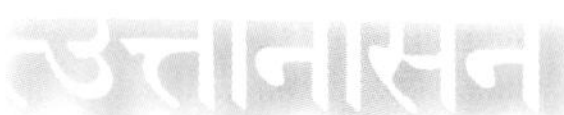

uttānāsana
Standing Forward Fold Pose

About the pose: Folding over often makes beginning students feel inflexible. Most people have some shortness in their hamstrings because of their lifestyle, so be sure to use modifications when necessary. Never compromise your spine just to get your hands or fingers somewhere. Remember what the yogis say: "Long spine, long life."

Instructions: From Upward Facing Arms Pose, inhale and lengthen your spine, then exhale and slowly begin to fold forward as shown in figure 6.23. If there is any tightness in your back, bend your knees as you fold and then rest your hands on blocks or a chair, making sure your shoulders are on your back as shown in the variations in figure 6.23.

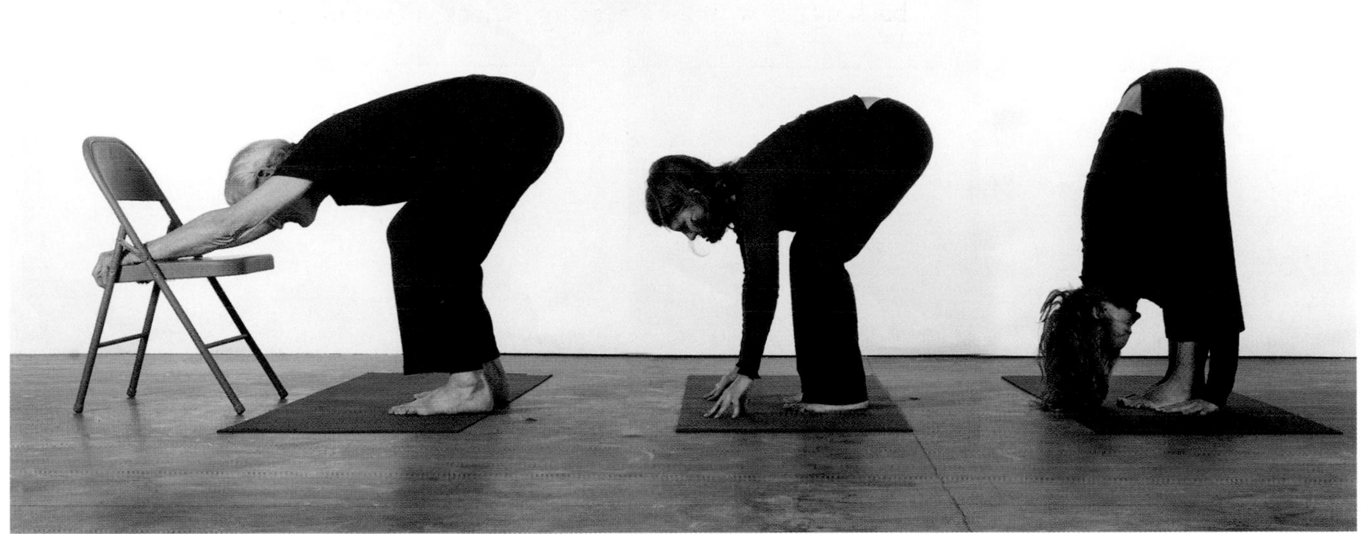

Figure 6.23. Standing Forward Fold Pose—Uttanasana

Warrior I Pose—Virabhradrasana I

About the pose: Warrior I Pose is not about warfare but about supporting yourself as you focus on your divine purpose and follow your unique path with confidence and power despite distractions from the external world. One yogi tells about practicing this pose in the parking lot before going into a divorce proceeding. Another describes doing this pose in a bathroom before entering a difficult meeting. The therapeutic aspects of the pose include strengthening the legs and feet, lengthening the spine, and cultivating the breath.

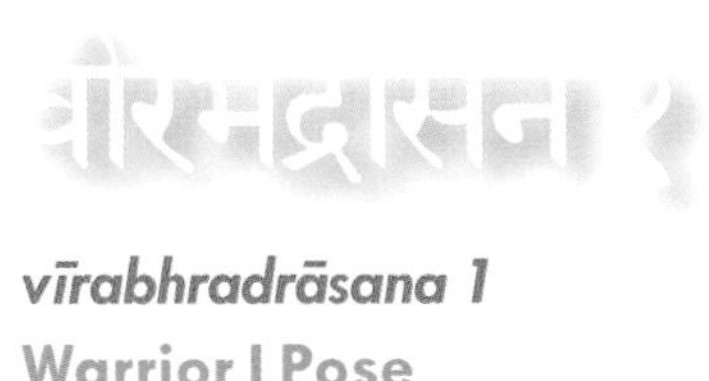

vīrabhadrāsana 1
Warrior I Pose

Instructions: Begin in Standing Forward Fold Pose and step back with one leg, keeping your front foot facing straight forward with your knee bent and moving toward the little toe side of your foot as shown in figure 6.24. On the leg that is forward, move the flesh of your buttock down from the back of the waist and then move your knee toward the outer side of the foot. Strongly press all four points of connection of the foot, especially the ball mount of your big toe.

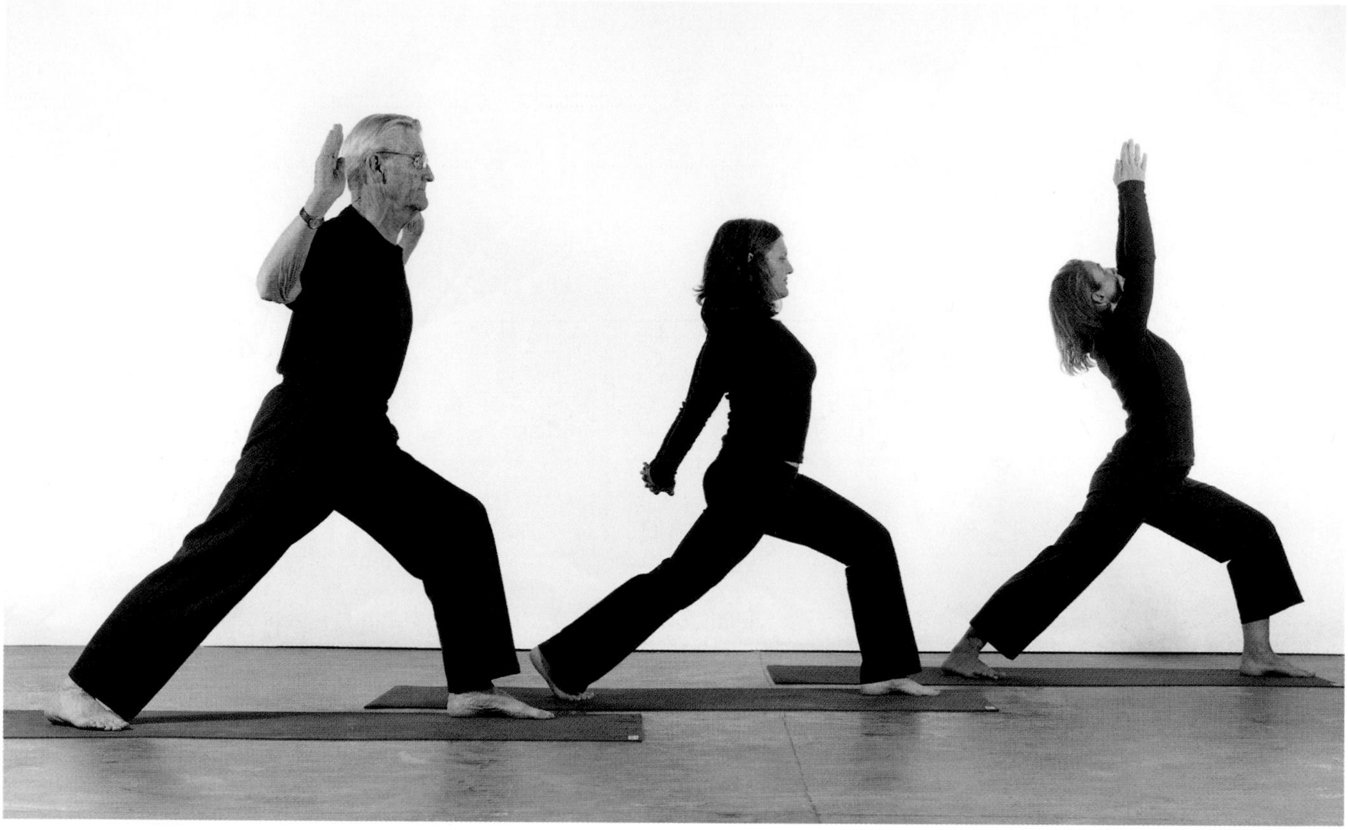

Figure 6.24. Warrior I Pose—Virabhradrasana I (Notice feet and arm variations.)

Inhale as you rise up, keeping your back inner thigh moving back and into the top of your thighbone, bringing your hips forward. Be sure to support your low back by using your abdominal core to lift your root up and tuck your tailbone. Then add opening of your shoulders and perhaps a bit of a backbend, although that is really a flourish once the legs and core are set. Try lifting your back heel to bring your hip forward as shown in figure 6.24. Your torso remains elongated as your breath moves freely along the center channel of your body. You can shorten the pose for more stability or lengthen it for more freedom, depending on what you need. Repeat on the second side.

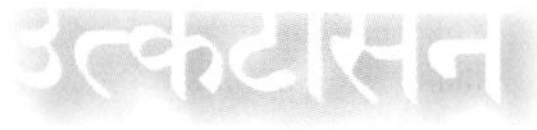

utkaṭāsana
Fierce Pose

Fierce Pose—Utkatasana

About the pose: Fierce Pose is well named as it requires a lot of energy and stamina. Being fierce can be useful in life while attempting to discover your true nature.

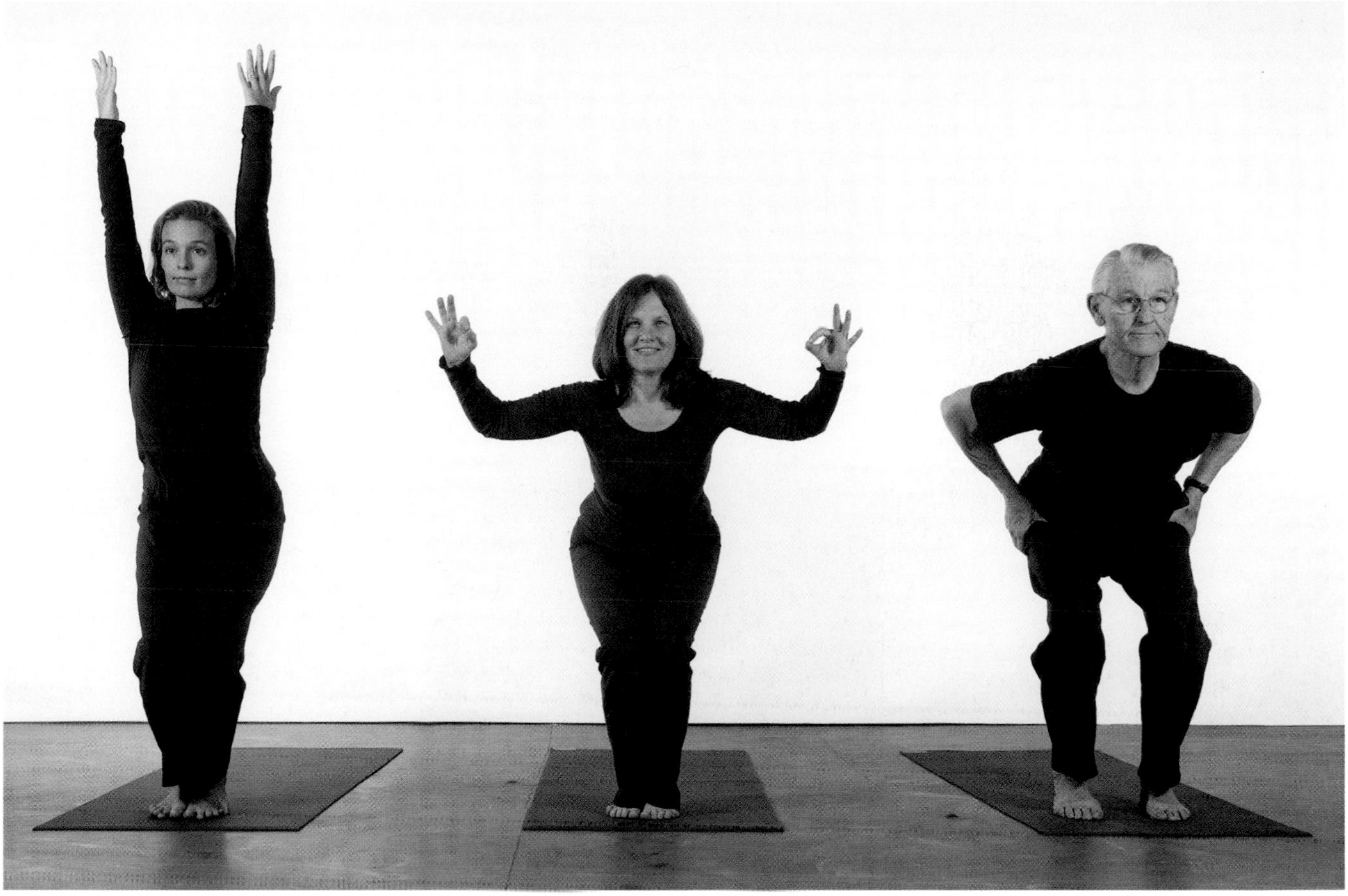

Figure 6.25. Fierce Pose—Utkatasana (Arm variations help keep shoulders relaxed.)

Instructions: From Mountain Pose, bring your big toes together and heels slightly apart. Inhale to prepare, then exhale and sink down and touch the floor. Sit way back, letting your hips move behind you. Lift your core up and then your torso and arms (see figure 6.25). If your shoulders are tight, move your arms down to your hips or bend your elbows. You can also rise up higher and move your arms back.

Revolved Fierce Pose—Parivrtta Utkatasana

About the pose: Revolved Fierce Pose is even stronger than Fierce Pose. You can feel a massage of the viscera and a revolving of the spine.

Instructions: Begin in Fierce Pose, then bring your hands to *anjali* mudra and inhale. Elongate your spine and exhale. Twist to one side and hook your elbow, keeping your knees level (see figure 6.26). You can also begin with your legs apart and put an elbow between them for more

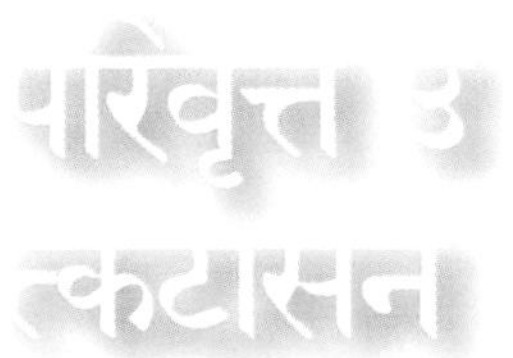

parivṛtta utkatāsana
Revolved Fierce Pose

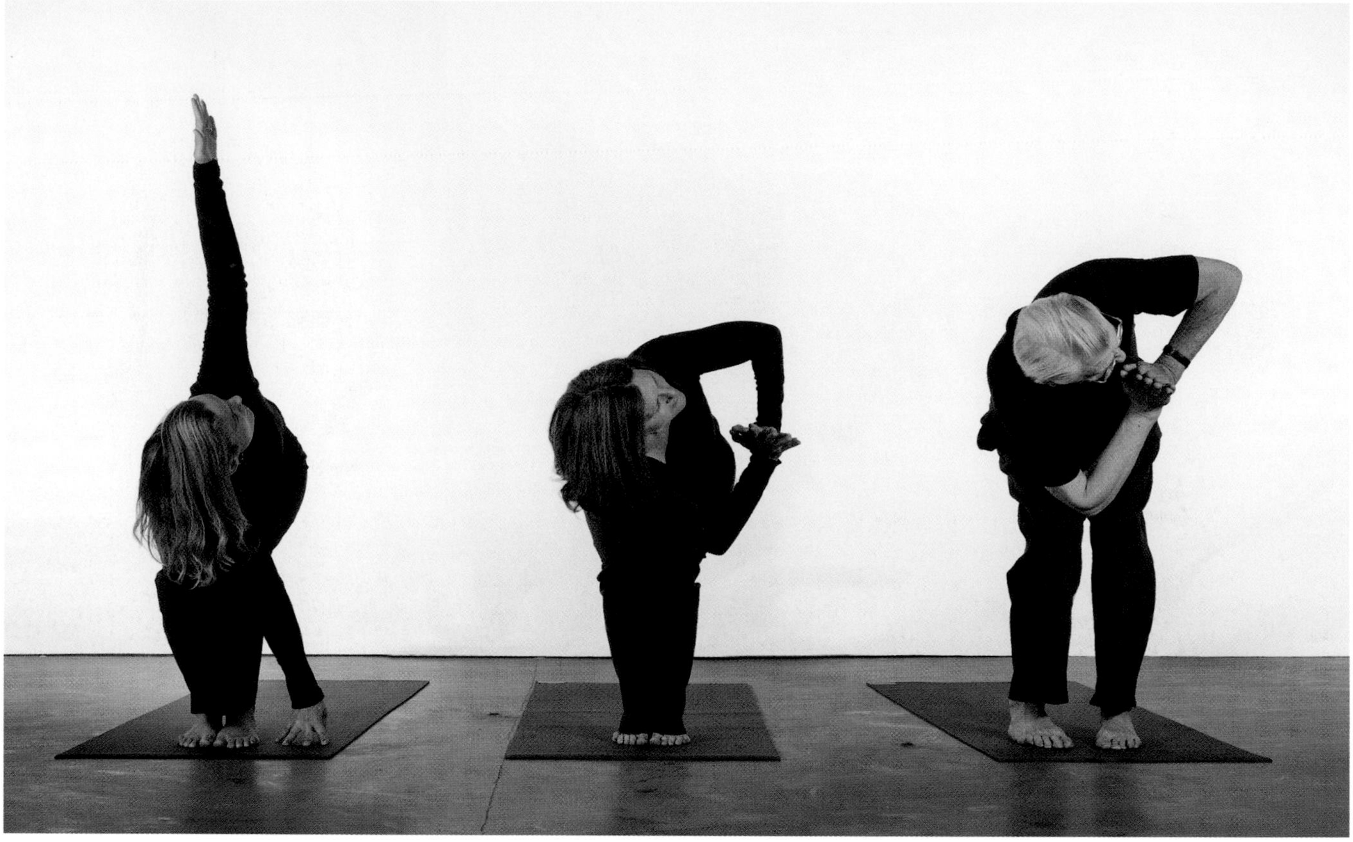

Figure 6.26. Revolved Fierce Pose—Parivrtta Utkatasana

stability. Or you can reach both arms out, letting them take any number of shapes once your legs are set. Repeat on the second side.

Side Stretched Out Pose—Parsvotanasana

About the pose: The leg action in this pose is straightforward, but keeping your hips facing forward can be challenging.

Instructions: Start in Mountain Pose and step back with one leg. Engage your leg muscles as you draw the inner edge of your back thigh back, rotating your front outer hip back so your hips are square with the front of the mat. Inhale and bring your arms out to the side. Exhale and bring them behind you as you roll your shoulders back and lightly down. Either put your hands in Reverse Prayer Pose, grasp your wrists or elbows, or release your hands to blocks, as shown in figure 6.27. Inhale and lift your sternum, lengthening your spine. Exhale and fold your trunk over your front leg, pulling your outer hip back from your front leg as you breathe.

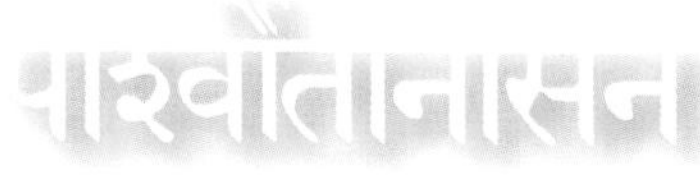

pārśvotānāsana

Side Stretched Out Pose

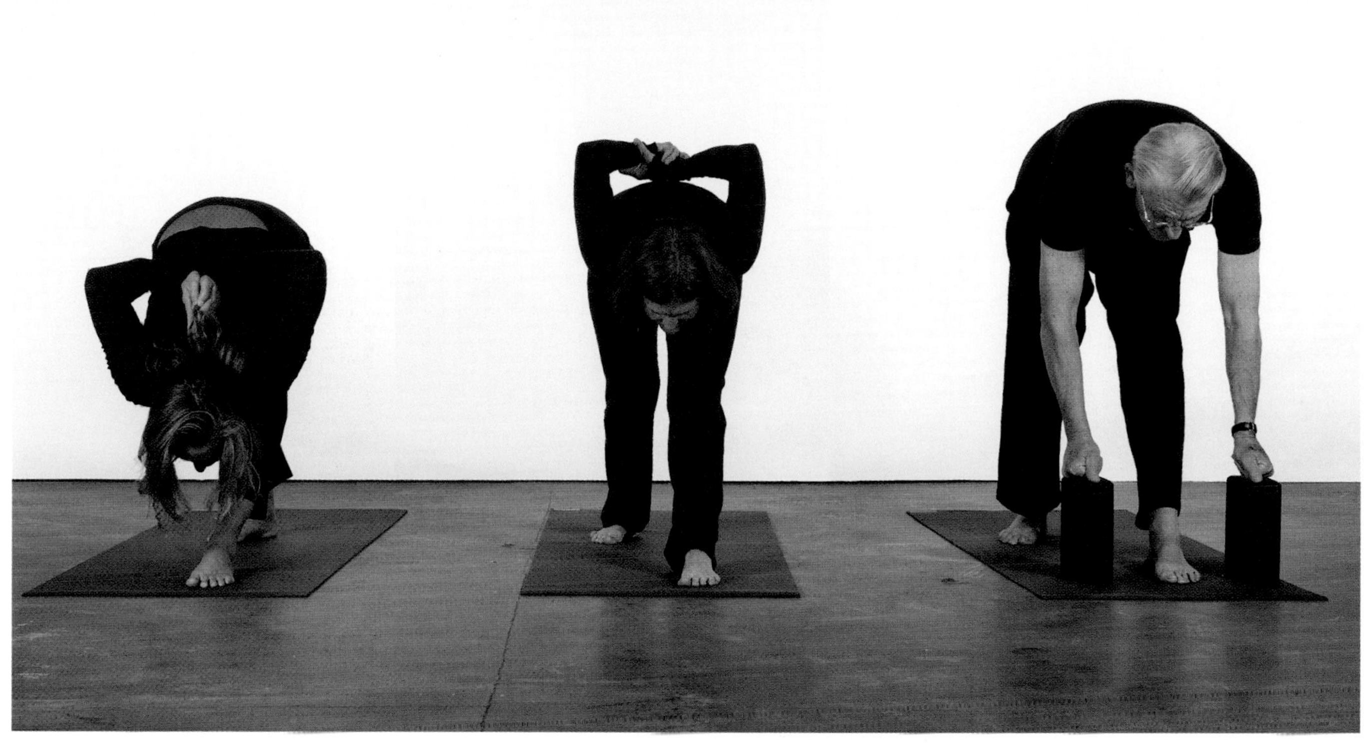

Figure 6.27. Side Stretched Out Pose—Parsvotanasana

If your back is rounded, try bending your front leg and then straightening it, slowing with the exhale. If your back is still rounded, come up farther and hold level to the ground. Repeat on the second side.

Revolved Triangle Pose—Parivrtta Trikonasana

About the pose: This pose provides a wonderful stretch and twist for the spine and massage for the digestive organs. It is also excellent to counteract confusion. It requires a surprising amount of balance and intense focus.

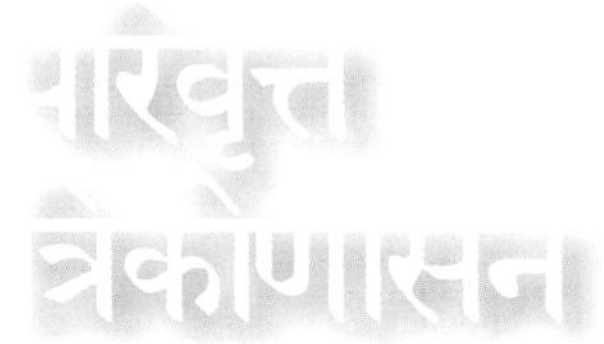

paṛivrtta trikoṇāsana
Revolved Triangle Pose

Instructions: Start with Side Stretched Out Pose and pause before folding over. Next, instead of putting your arms behind your body, lift up the arm that is on the same side as the back leg and reach forward, then down, either inside or outside the front arch, slowly lifting the other arm toward the heavens (see figure 6.28). For more stability, put your hand inside the arch of your front foot on a block (or two) and keep your upper arm at your hip, rolling your shoulder back. Repeat on the second side.

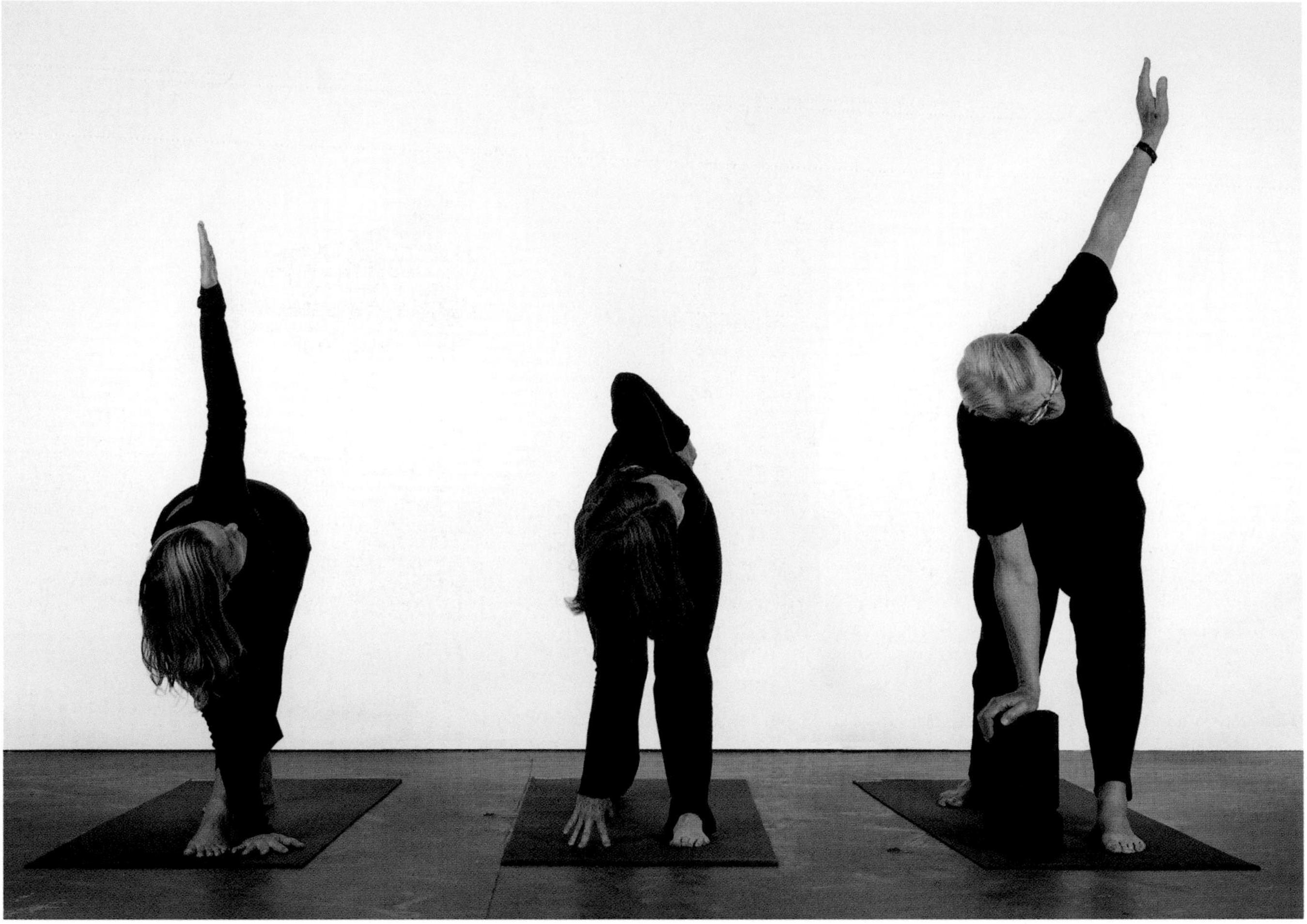

Figure 6.28. Revolved Triangle Pose—Parivrtta Trikonasana

Revolved Side Angle Pose—Parivrtta Parsvakonasana

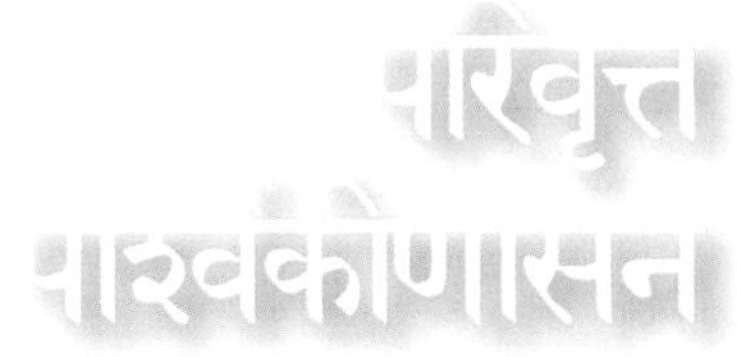

parivṛtta pārśvakoṇāsana
Revolved Side Angle Pose

About the pose: This pose gives you a sense of squeezing to center and can feel like you are flushing your digestive organs. Poses with this amount of twist help you enjoy your meal after yoga class. By staying on your knees, you can work at twisting and breathing into your belly, and by lifting your leg and even dropping your heel you can work more on stability, balance, and flexibility.

Instructions: Begin this pose on your hands and knees. Bring one leg forward, and put your foot solidly on the floor, with all four points of connection on the mat. Lift your torso and inhale, raising the opposite arm while lengthening your spine. Then exhale and hook your elbow over your bent knee, putting your hands together in *anjali* mudra or extending your legs. If you feel steady, you can tuck your back toes under and lift your back leg. If you are still steady, you can bring your heel to the

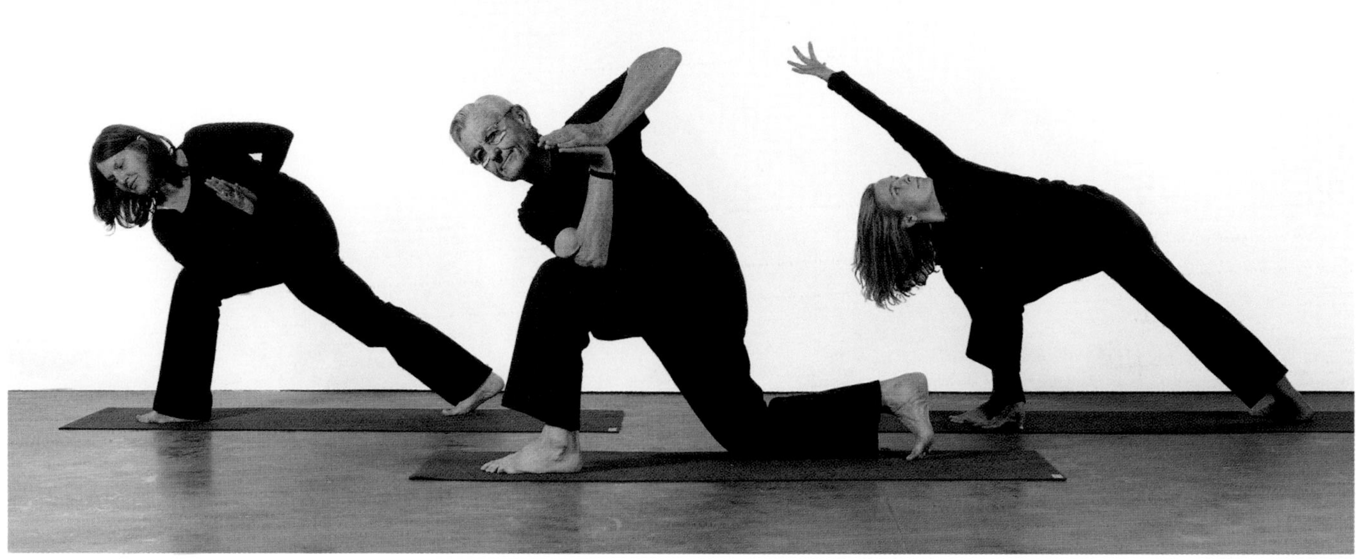

Figure 6.29. Revolved Side Angle Pose—Parivrtta Parsvakonasana

ground, with your toes angling toward the short end of the mat as shown in figure 6.29. Repeat on the second side.

HIPS FACING SIDE OR LONG END OF THE MAT

In this group of poses the leg action sets the hips facing the long end of the mat.

Triangle Pose—Uttitha Trikonasana

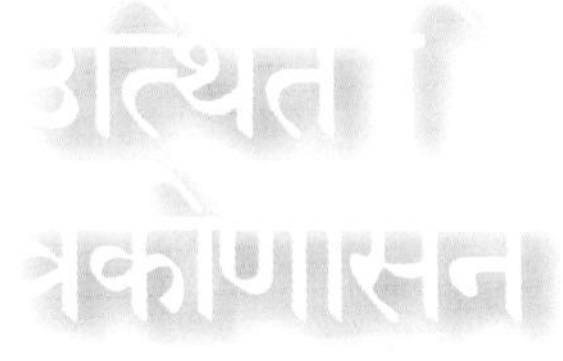

uttitha trikoṇāsana
Triangle Pose

About the pose: This pose relieves stress and tension and opens the heart. It's an excellent pose to do after sitting at a computer for a long time. Therapeutic aspects include lengthening and strengthening leg muscles, opening shoulders, and elongating and twisting the spine.

Instructions: Step wide to face the long side of the mat, then turn one leg forward with your feet either aligned heel to heel or heel to arch of the back foot. Inhale, bring your arms up, exhale, reach out and then down (see figure 6.30). Engaging all your leg muscles enthusiastically, rotate your front leg outward so that your knee moves toward the little toe side of the foot. Hold that position without hyperextending your knee. Oppositionally, move the top of your back thigh into the top of your hip socket (toward the wall behind you) and then roll your thigh out from the

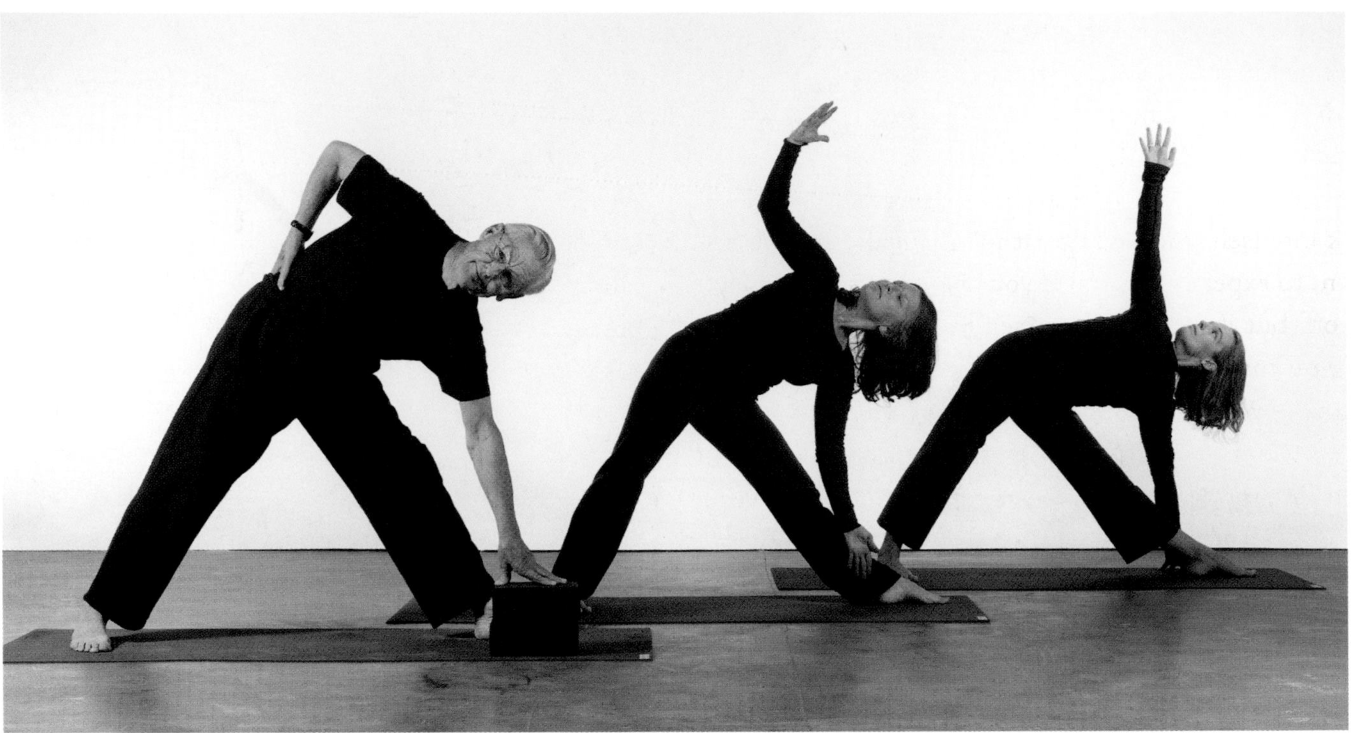

Figure 6.30. Triangle Pose—Uttitha Trikonasana

midline. Breathe up from the core of your body, using the abdominal lift to support your low back. You may use props to keep your spine lengthened (see figure 6.30). The pose can be narrower or wider, depending on what allows you to fully explore your body. Repeat on the second side.

Warrior II Pose—Virabhradrasana II

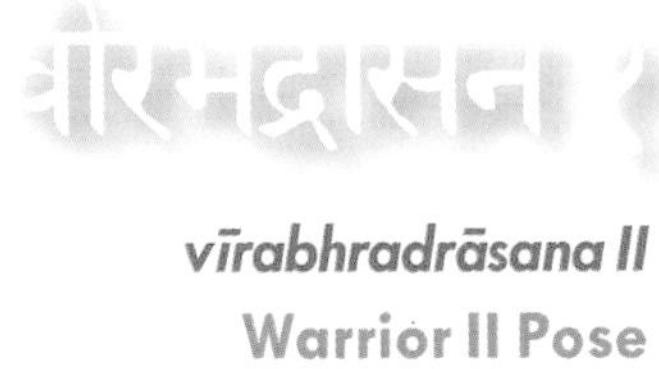

vīrabhradrāsana II
Warrior II Pose

About the pose: This strong pose can be seen as representing the clarity of your path, with the torso being the present moment, the back arm the past, and the front arm the future. In this pose your torso tends to bend forward, reflecting the fact that we often lean toward the future. Your gaze can be directed toward your front middle finger as you contemplate the warrior's strength required to stay true to your purpose in the face of many external distractions.

Instructions: Step wide to the long side of the mat and turn the front foot out to the short end of the mat. Then bend your knee, moving it toward the little toe side of your front foot, and, keeping your back leg straight and strong, inhale and raise your arms as shown in figure 6.31. Inhale and

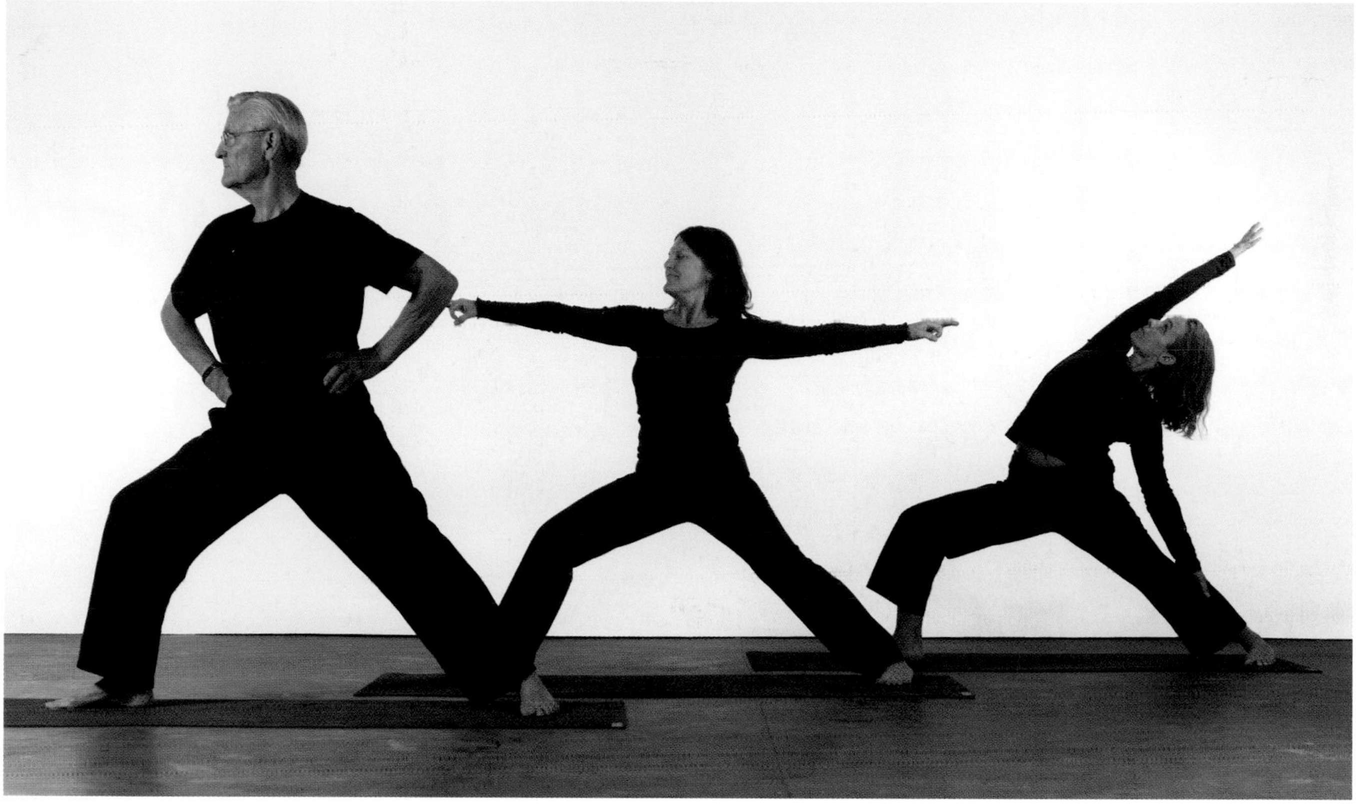

Figure 6.31. Warrior II Pose—Virabhradrasana

lengthen your spine, tucking your tailbone and stretching the crown of your head toward the heavens. You can also put your arms on your waist or reverse the arms for Reverse Warrior II Pose. Repeat on the second side.

Side Angle Pose—Parsvakonasana

About the pose: This pose, which requires considerable strength and focus, is excellent for steadying your mind and body. If you hold it for a number of breaths, or even minutes, you will build body heat and awareness. This pose seems to reach toward infinity as the energy pattern runs up your back leg and your outstretched arm.

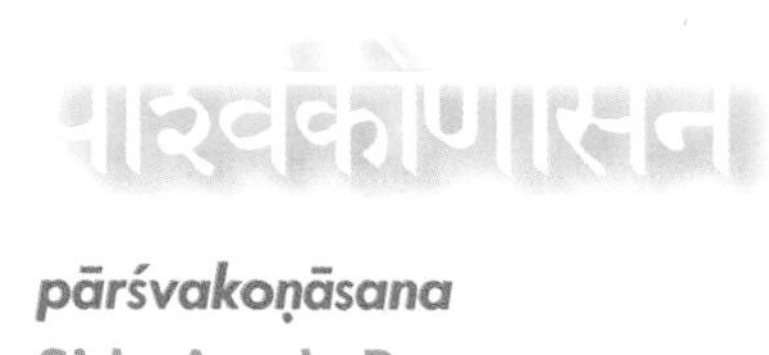

pārśvakoṇāsana
Side Angle Pose

Instructions: Come to Warrior II Pose and reach your front arm forward, putting your elbow on your knee and keeping your back leg from moving forward, as shown in figure 6.32. Inhale and lengthen your spine; exhale and twist around your center core as you spiral up toward heaven. For a greater challenge, release your hand outside or inside your leg. Repeat on the second side.

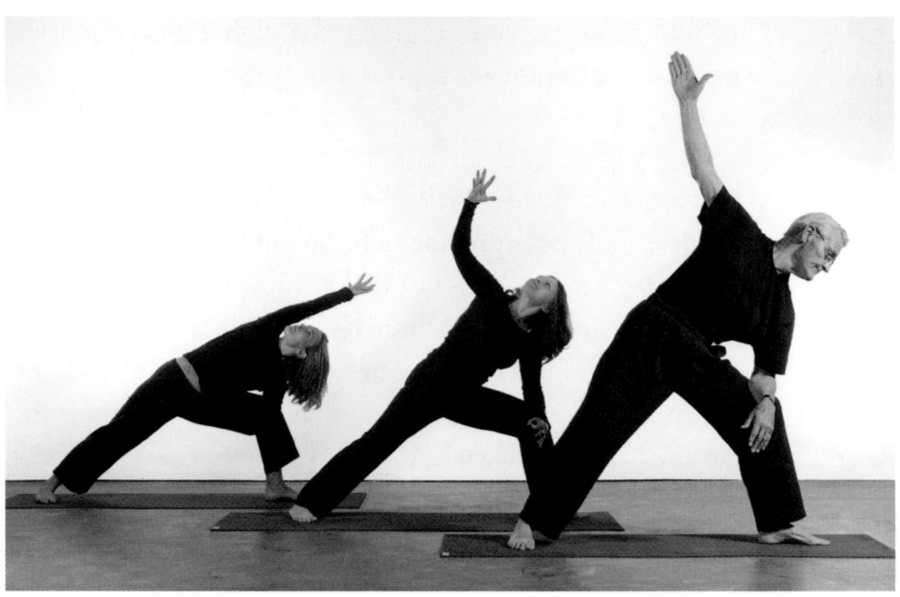

Figure 6.32. Side Angle Pose—Parsvakonasana

Pyramid Pose—Prasarita Padottanasana

प्रसारित पादो-
त्तानासन

prasārita pādottānāsana
Pyramid Pose

About the pose: This pose feels good after and in between the other standing poses and is an excellent back leg stretch.

Instructions: Start with wide legs, feet slightly pigeon-toed, and press down with your legs as you exhale. Inhale with your hands at your waist as you lengthen your front spine, and exhale as you fold down toward the ground (see figure 6.33). You can use blocks and experiment with various

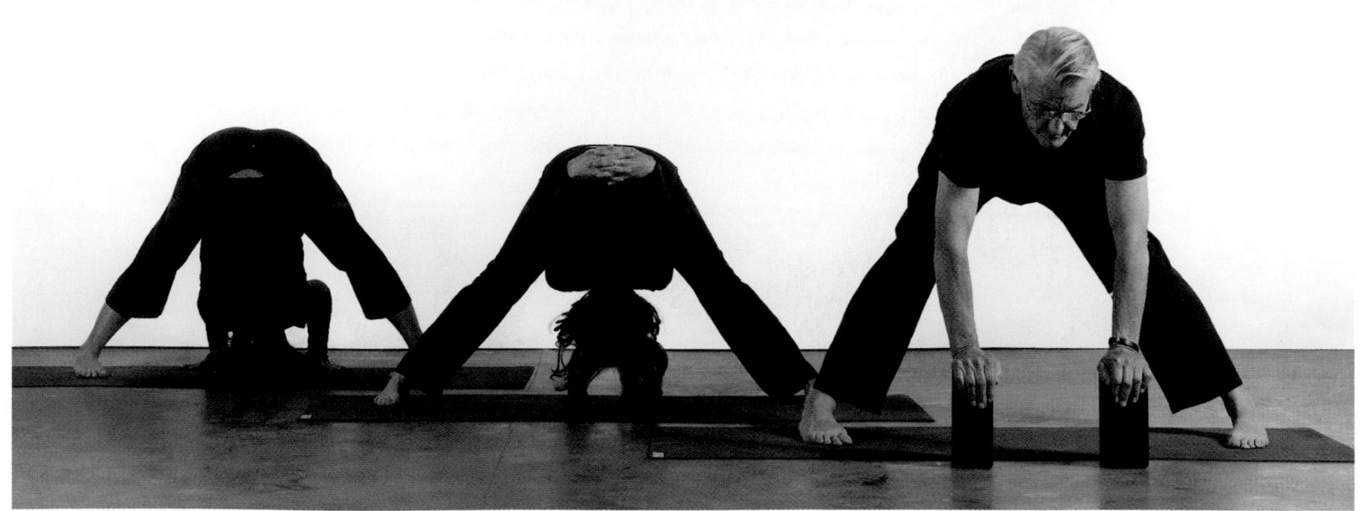

Figure 6.33. Pyramid Pose—Prasarita Padottanasana

arm shapes, including clasping your fingers and straightening your arms, making sure not to compromise your spine in the process.

Downward Facing Dog Pose—Adho Mukha Svanasana

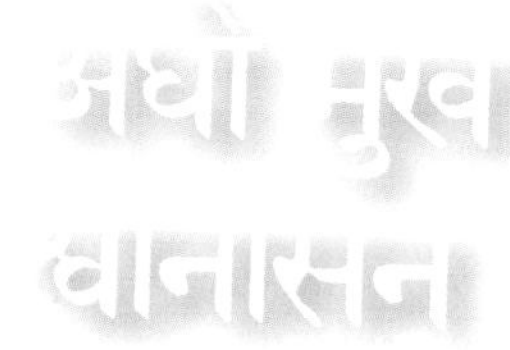

adho mukha śvānāsana
Downward Facing Dog Pose

About the pose: This pose provides a feeling of being supported by the earth, while also creating a sense of flight, allowing us to feel both bound and free. Dogs spontaneously do this pose, as do horses, cats, and other animals. Down Dog (as it is sometimes affectionately called) calms the heart and helps promote positive thoughts. It has been said that this is the only pose anyone really needs and that by practicing it repeatedly for about ten minutes the body will gain flexibility, grace, and energy. Downward Facing Dog encourages flexibility of the hips and shoulders, as well as tones and strengthens arms, legs, and the low back. It also improves digestion, supports reproductive organs, and releases tension from the body. Although this pose can seem difficult, as there is often too much weight on the arms caused by tight shoulders and hips, you can alleviate this using one of the modifications with bent knees given below.

Instructions: Begin on your hands and knees, hands under your shoulders, knees slightly behind your hips. Create a foundation by spreading your fingers, moving your weight off your wrists to your fingers, and keeping your arms straight. You can move your hands wider than your shoulder distance if your shoulders are tight. Move your armpits upward, underarms away from the floor, hips lifted up, with knees deeply bent, and breathe into your

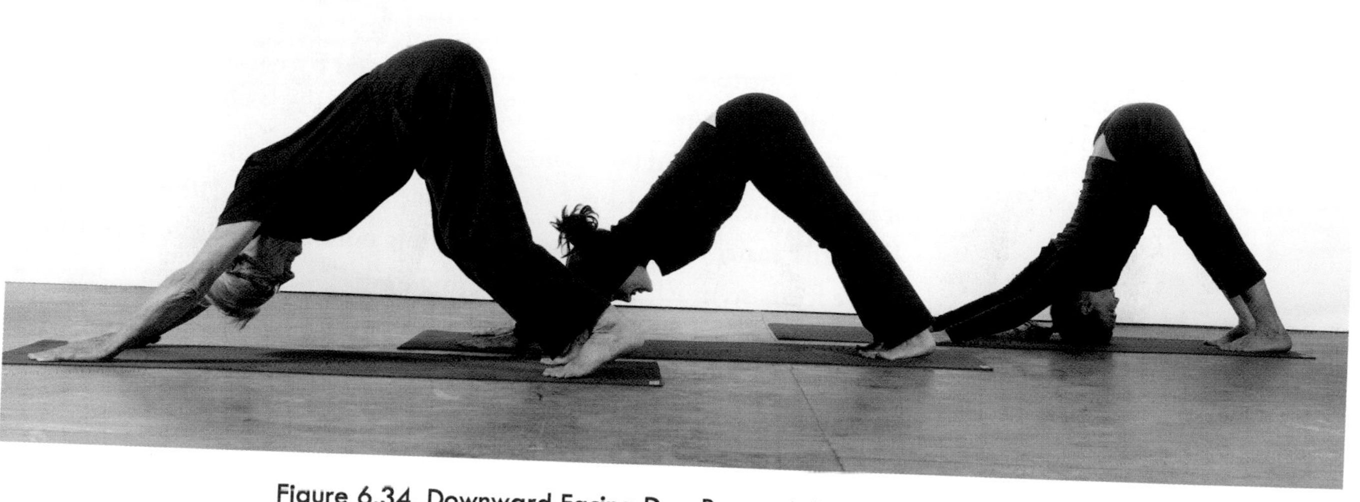

Figure 6.34. Downward Facing Dog Pose—Adho Mukha Svanasana

try other variations, including moving your arms toward the bent knee. Release when you are ready, and practice on the other leg.

Half Moon Pose—Ardha Chandrasana

अर्ध चन्द्रासन

ardha chandrāsana

Half Moon Pose

About the pose: This pose can feel like you are alive in an uplifting way and taking flight. The more you engage your leg muscles and breathe deeply, the more elevated and free you will feel.

Instructions: You can begin the pose by leaning against a wall and then work to move away from the wall. Standing in Mountain Pose, inhale and lift your arms. Then exhale, fold halfway, and bring one leg behind you. Put your hands on the floor or a block, one hand in front of and to the outside of your standing foot. Bend your standing knee and roll it toward the outside of your foot, feeling your buttock move down and your inner thigh roll out. In this pose, the hips are not level but are stacked (see figure 6.36). Keep a slight bend in your knee if you feel any pressure in your hip

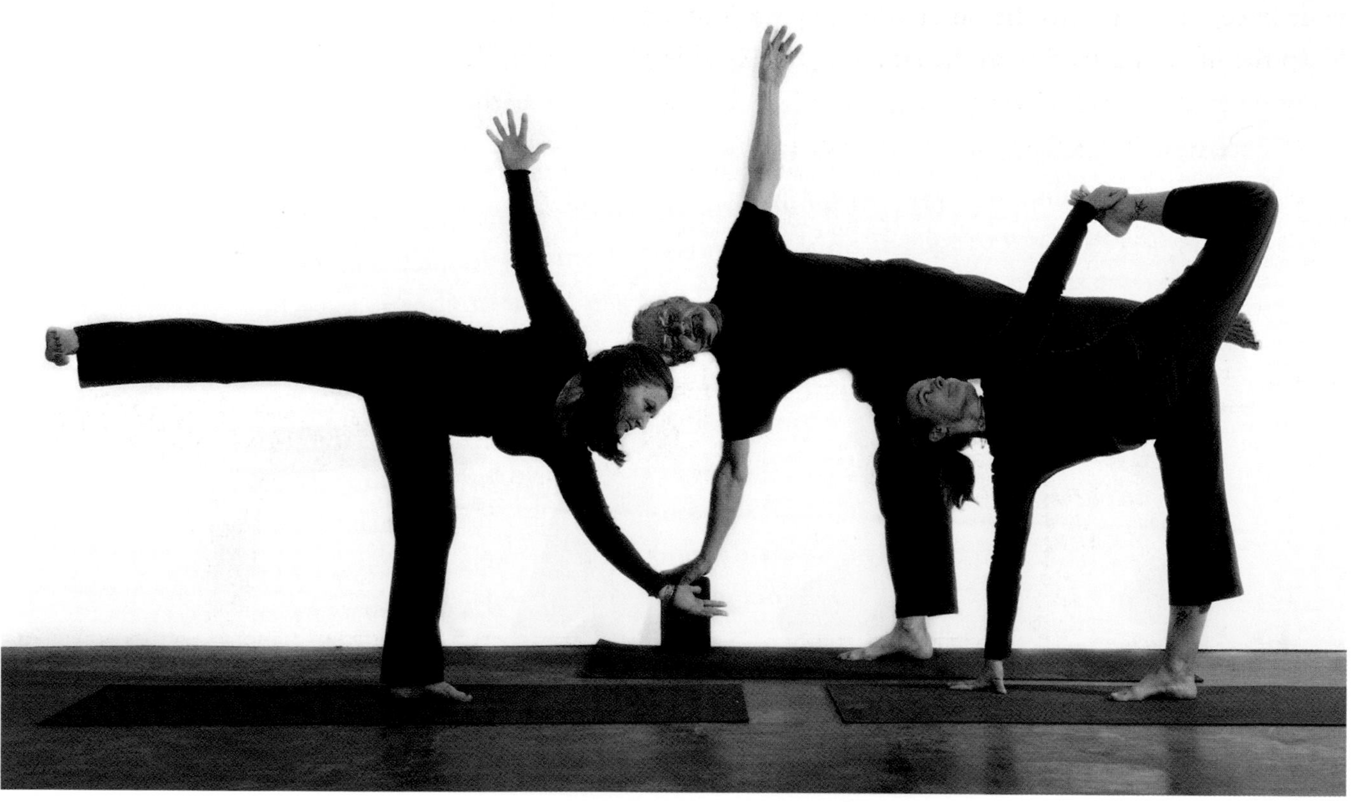

Figure 6.36. Half Moon Pose—Ardha Chandrasana

as you raise the other leg slowly up and back, flexing your foot. Initially move your lifted leg forward as you inhale, and as you exhale bring the leg back and up as you roll your heart toward the sky. Eventually, when the lifted leg is in the same plane as your torso, breathe and feel the sense of being grounded in the standing leg, yet taking flight. Slowly return to standing and repeat on the other side. Use a block and lean into a wall for greater stability.

Warrior III Pose—Virabhradrasana III

About the pose: Warrior III is about finding balance on your path and discovering how to be your unique self uninfluenced by the expectations of others. This involves focusing intently, *dhyana*, and maintaining that focus even if your body begins to feel unstable.

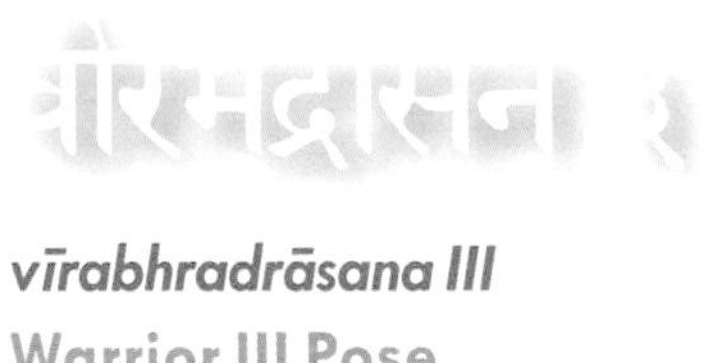

vīrabhradrāsana III
Warrior III Pose

Instructions: Standing in Mountain Pose (figure 6.21, page 142), focus on a single point. Inhale and lift your arms to Upward Facing Arms Pose (figure 6.22, page 144), then lift one leg behind you as you fold over, extending your arms as in figure 6.37. For greater stability, you can bend your knee, keeping it to the outer edge of your foot, and slowly stand. Keep the lifted hip level with the standing hip, working the core up for support. You may try different arm variations, including arms beside your torso, and *anjali* mudra. Repeat on the second side.

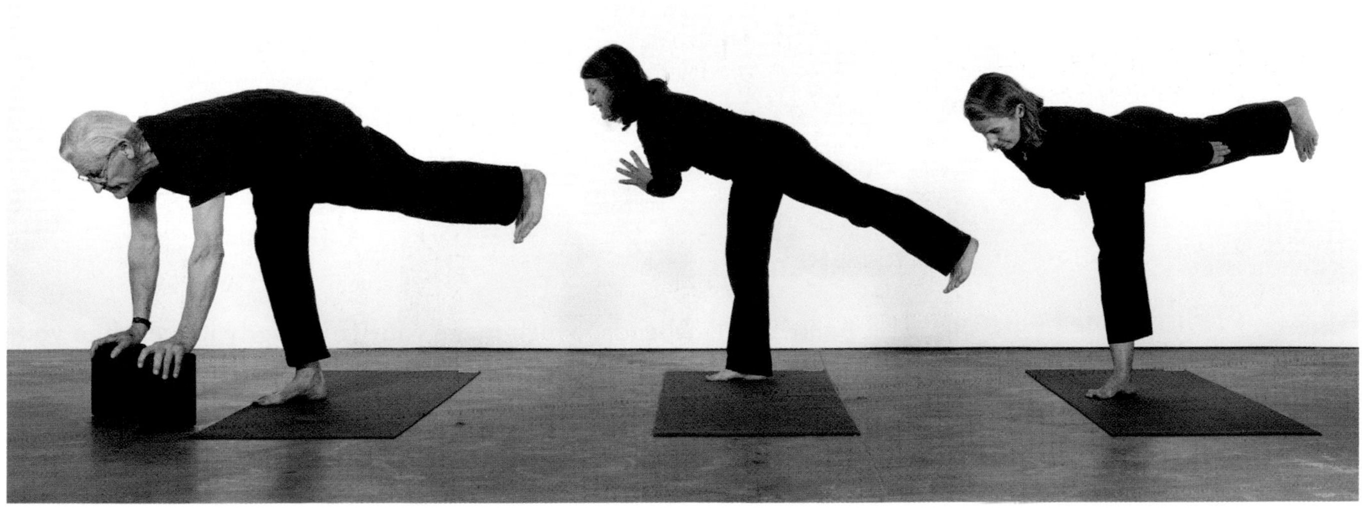

Figure 6.37. Warrior III Pose—Virabhradrasana III

Upward Facing Dog Pose—Urdhva Mukha Svanasana

About the pose: This is a tricky pose because it looks accessible, but if you don't have the strength to hold the pose and support your spine you can hurt your lower back. Also if you don't have enough strength in your arms and core you can sink into your shoulders, putting too much stress on your shoulder joints, and collapse forward. To determine whether you are ready to try Upward Facing Dog, do **Four Limb Staff Pose—Chaturanga Dandasana** (figure 6.42), which looks like a push-up with your elbows at your sides and shoulders above them. Begin in Plank Pose and move forward as you bend your elbows toward your body, using your legs strongly and lifting your core. If you can hold this pose steadily without dropping your hips, and with all the key alignment points, you can safely do Upward Facing Dog.

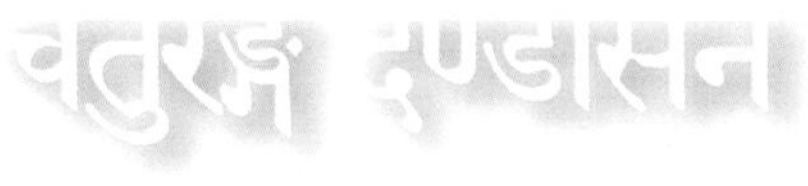

caturaṅga daṇḍāsana
Four Limb Staff Pose

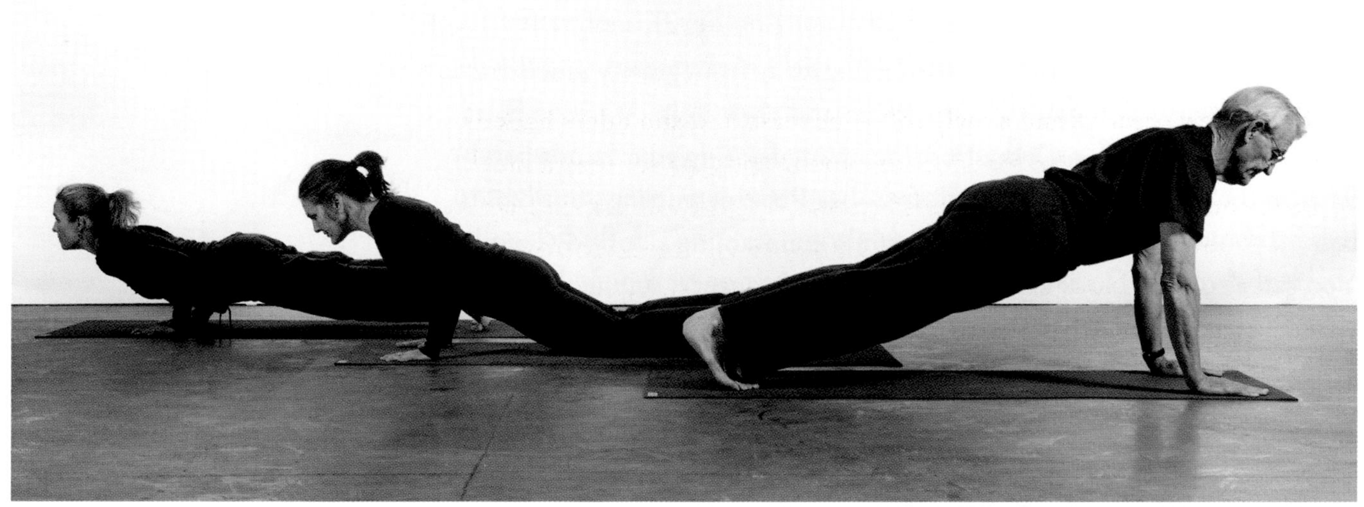

Figure 6.42. Four Limb Staff Pose—Chaturanga Dandasana

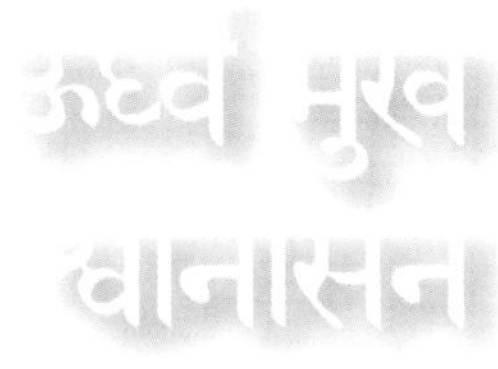

ūrdhva mukha śvānāsana
Upward Facing Dog Pose

Instructions: Start with Four Limb Staff Pose and then move to Up Dog (an affectionate nickname). Use a modification if you are not able to hold Four Limb Staff Pose. Begin in Plank Pose and hold steady, pressing your heels away, keeping your hips in line with your shoulders, and rolling your shoulder blades back. Slowly move forward as you bend your elbows toward your body, but do not let your shoulders drop below the height of your elbows, and keep your legs strong and your core engaged.

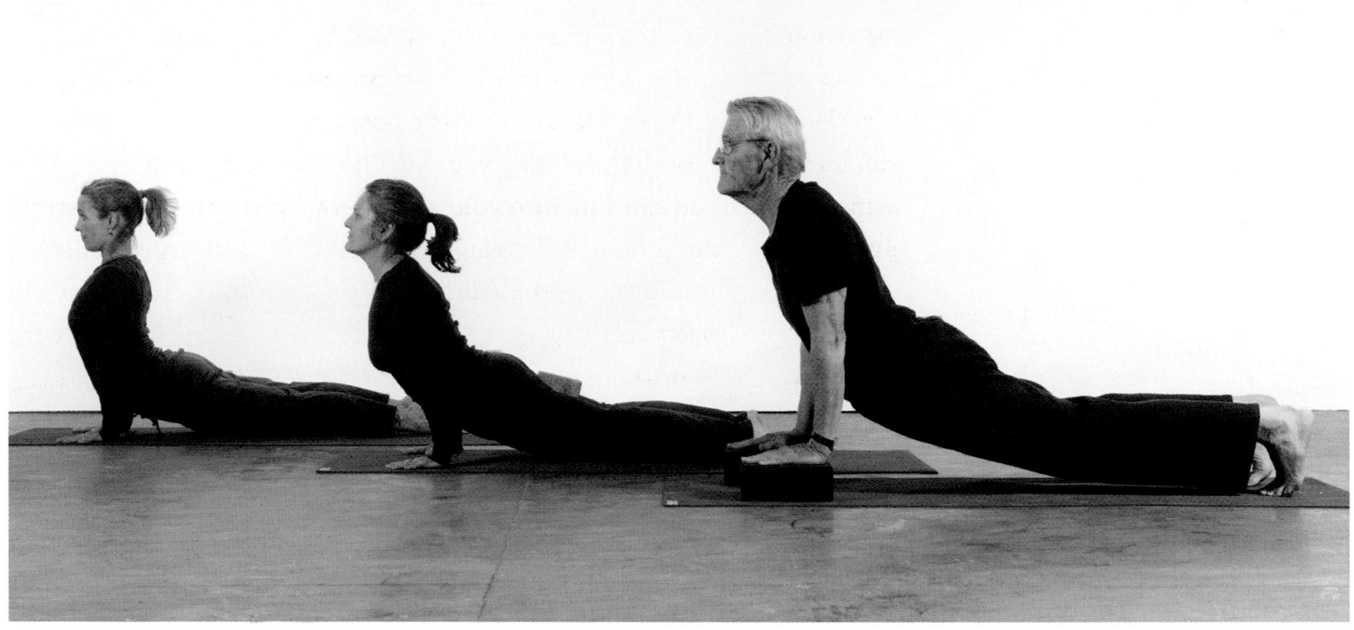

Figure 6.43. Upward Facing Dog Pose—Urdhva Mukha Svanasana

Hold for a few breaths, and slowly roll your torso and shoulders back as shown in figure 6.43. Use blocks under your hands, or squeeze a block between your legs and hold it to build strength. Or simply stay in Plank Pose, building strength there for a few breaths, then release down and do Cobra Pose as your backbend instead of Upward Facing Dog.

VERTICAL

For vertical backbends we use the same principles as for horizontal backbends: creating an inner spiral of the legs, tucking the tailbone, lengthening the side body, moving the heads of arm bones to the back body, moving the soft palate back, and lifting your chin slightly. Always watch the relationship between your back waist and core abdominal lift, and the opening of your sternum to prevent any crunching of your low back. If you feel sensation there, do less, lifting your core as you open your sternum forward. Vanda Scaravelli, the Italian yogi who was bent over "ready to die" when she found yoga in her forties, became known for her deep and beautiful backbends up until the end of her life as shown in figure 6.44.

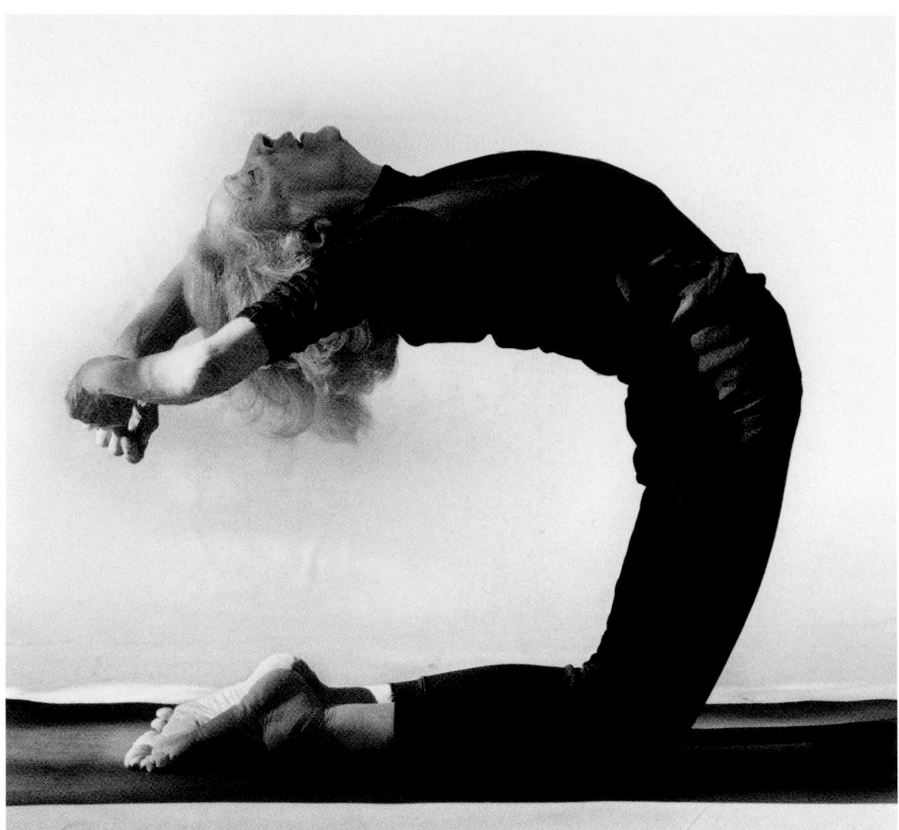

Figure 6.44.
Vanda Scaravelli in Camel Pose
while in her eighties

Camel Pose—Ustrasana

उष्ट्रासन

uṣṭrāsana
Camel Pose

About the pose: This pose, which looks like its name, is an excellent way to open and lift the sternum, symbolically lifting your heart's desires to the heavens. The challenge is to use the legs and not sink into the low back.

Instructions: Begin on your knees facing a wall, with two blocks on either side of your legs. Put your hands at your back waist, tuck your tailbone, and engage your core. Inhale and lengthen your spine, lifting your shoulders up. Exhale, roll your shoulders back, and begin to curl away from the wall, peeling your heart back while still pressing your hips to the wall (see figure 6.45).

You may want to keep your hands on your hips, lightly touch the blocks, or reach back for your heels. If you feel any sensation in your low back, move out of the pose, reengage your core, and then try again but not as deeply. If you have no discomfort in your low back, you can move away from the wall and reach toward your heels as you lengthen your spine. You can also use your arms and hands in other ways—for example, reaching

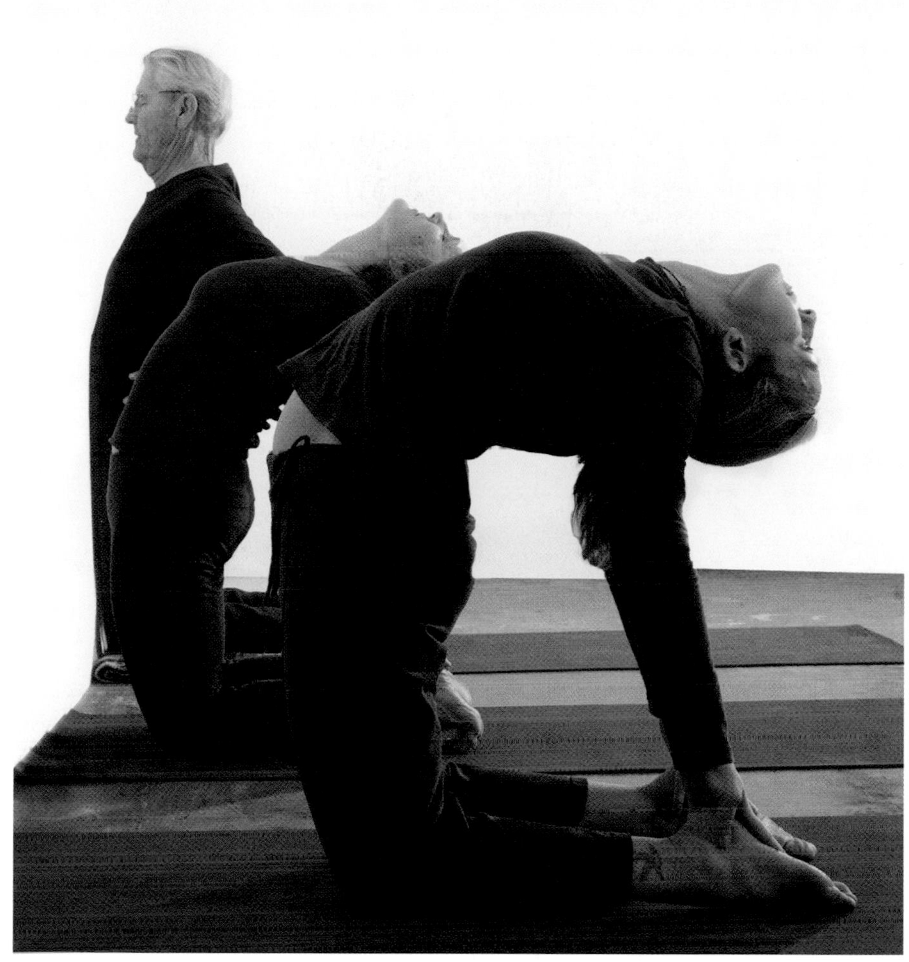

Figure 6.45.
Camel Pose—Ustrasana at wall

for your heels and lifting your heart upward, or interlacing your hands and reaching your heart upward (see figure 6.46).

Upward Bow Pose—Urdhva Danurasana

rdhva danurāsana
Upward Bow Pose

About the pose: This pose is the perfect antidote to stress in your shoulders and in your life. Exhilarating, it gives you a sense of boundless possibilities.

Instructions: Begin by lying on your back, with your knees bent over your ankles. Spiral your legs inward. Inhale and lift your arms to the sky. Exhale and seat your armpits down. Inhale and bend your elbows toward each other. Exhale and place your hands under your shoulders, with your fingers pointing toward your feet (see figure 6.47). Inhale and let your breath lengthen your spine and lift your belly slightly. Exhale and lift

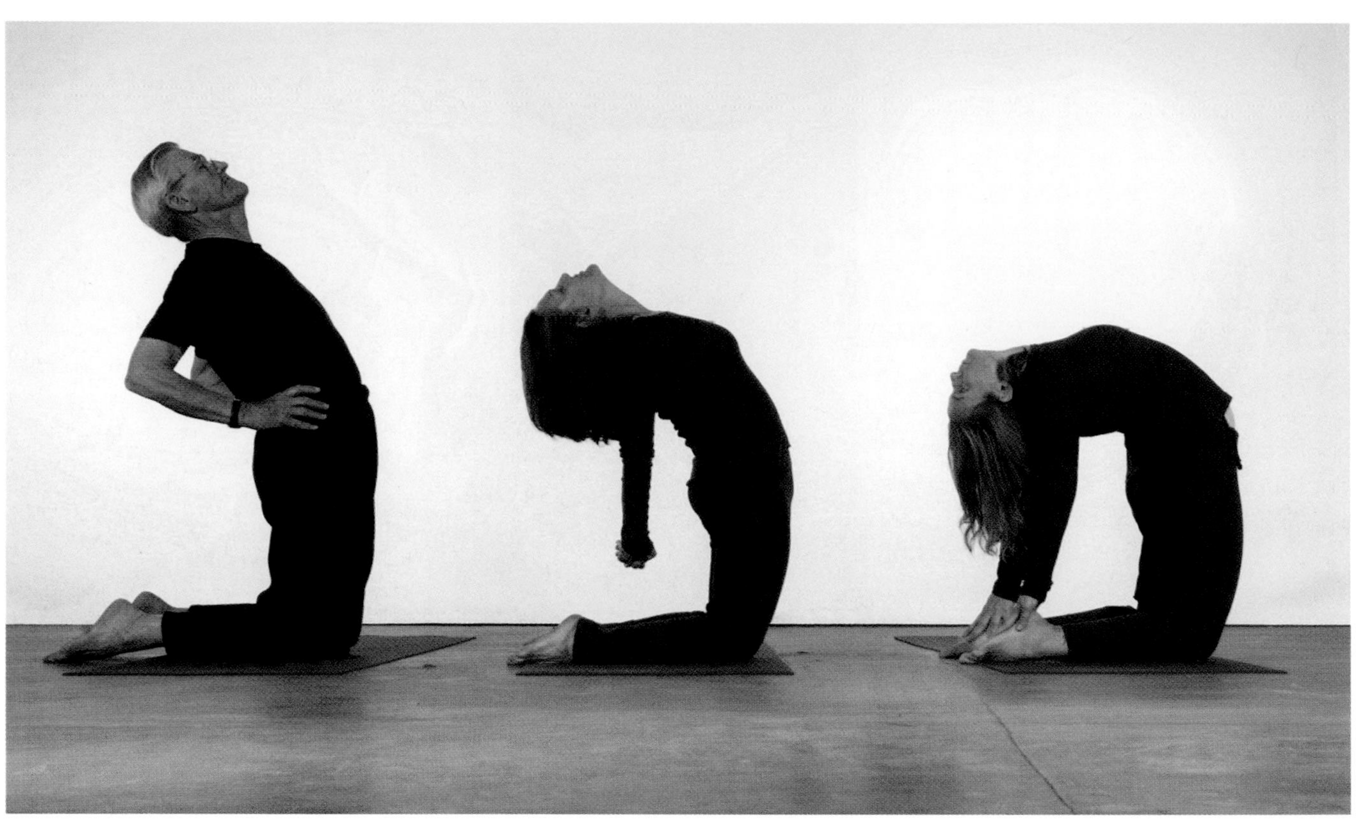

Figure 6.46. Camel Pose—Ustrasana

your core, pressing your back waist to the floor and your heels down. On the next inhale, keeping your tailbone tucked and your thighs spiraled inward, lift up to the top of your head. Pause, reaffirm that your elbows are moving toward each other, roll your head slightly so that your chin lifts, and inhale to continue lifting up to the full pose. Breathe deeply and play with using breath. For example, inhale and bend your elbows slightly; exhale and straighten your arms. For some students, props are very helpful when practicing this pose, including blocks or a blanket at the wall for the hands, a block between the legs, or a strap for the arms.

Another alternative is to practice Bridge Pose—Setubandha Sarvangasana, as shown in figure 6.47 (center). Interlacing your fingers under your hips, tuck your tailbone as you move your sternum toward your chin, being careful to watch for low back sensation (in which case, use abdominals more), and press the back of your head down so as not to overly flatten your neck.

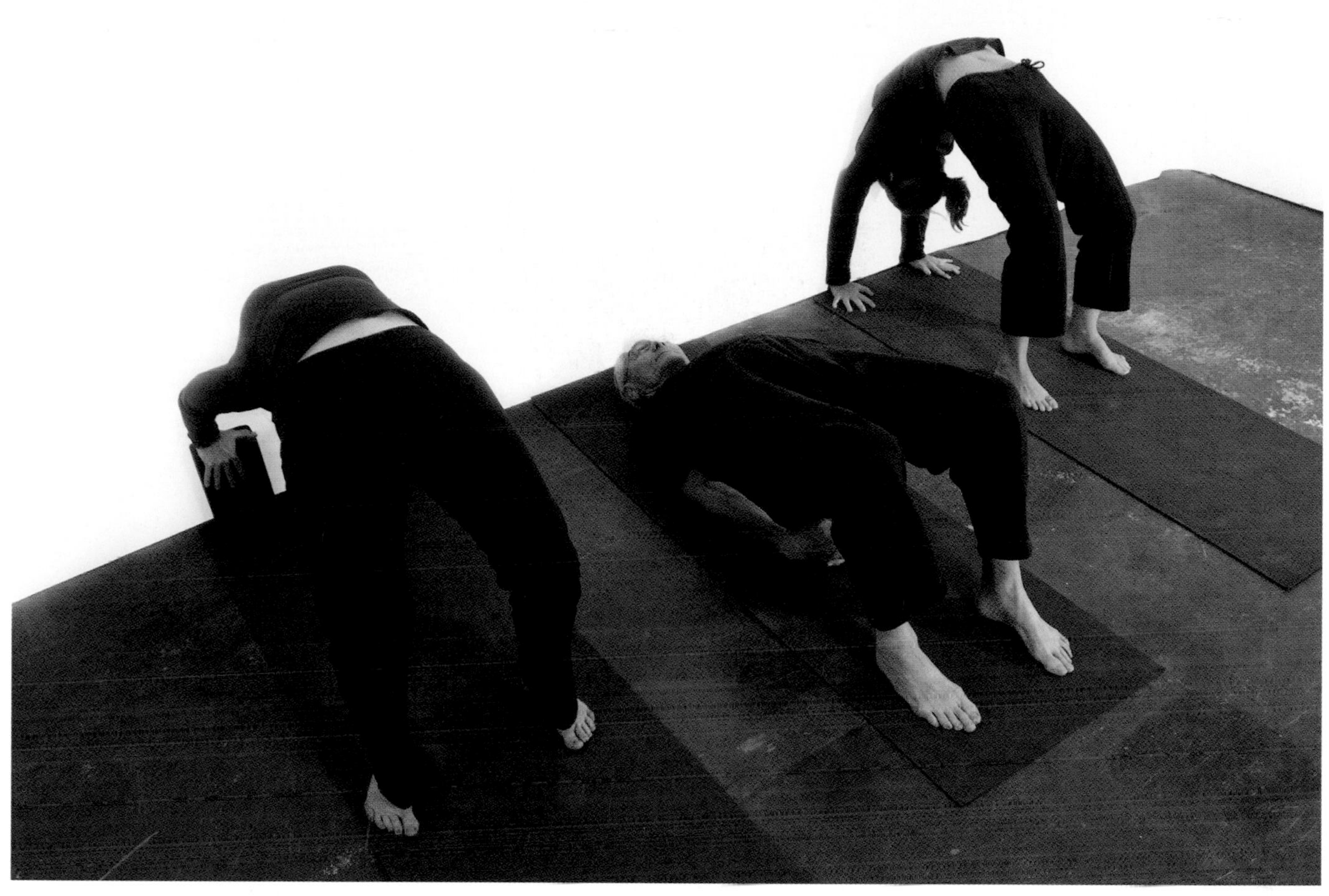

Figure 6.47. Upward Bow Pose—Urdhva Danurasana with blocks for support (left); Bridge Pose—Setubandha Sarvangasana (center); Upward Bow Pose—Urdhva Danurasana (right)

Inversions

Benefits: Inversions offer a way to get a different perspective when we feel overwhelmed or confused. They allow us to move the life energy in a new way in relation to gravity and thus reenergize the body, especially the four major systems—circulation/cardiovascular, lymphatic, nervous, and endocrine—as they change the pressure on all valves of the organs.[11] The *Hatha Yoga Pradipika* sings the praises of inversions:

> *While practicing this [the inversion Viparita karani], increase the duration gradually every day. After six months, wrinkles and gray hair disappear. He who practices this for a yama (three hours daily) conquers death.*[12]

Key Principles: Contraindications for practicing inversions are high blood pressure,[13] glaucoma, and dizziness. You may also have a fear about being upside down, in which case be sure to find a teacher for assistance. After a while, you may want to explore your edges, including fear. How much time you spend in inversions is critical. Begin with very short periods, gradually adding breaths, then minutes. After inversions, always rest with your head down in **Child's Pose—Balasana** (see figure 6.48) for a minimum of ten breaths, although longer is better.

Key Anatomy: When you are inverted, it is possible to forget about your legs, but in these poses the legs help us lift off whatever is supporting us to reach up toward the sky.

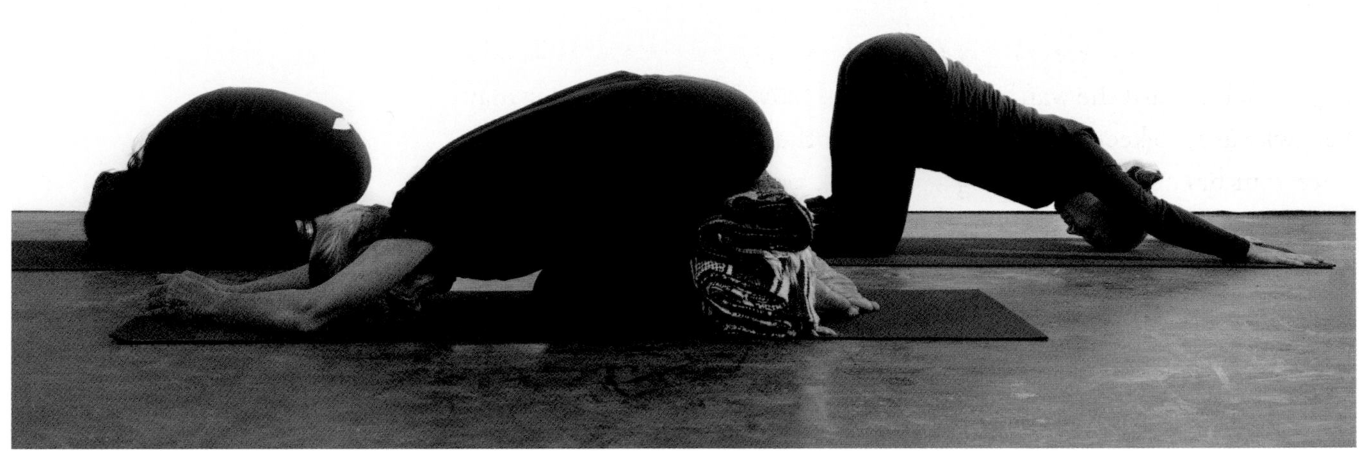

Figure 6.48. Child's Pose—Balasana

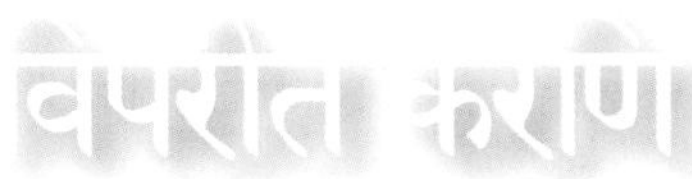

viparīta karani
Legs up the Wall Pose

Legs up the Wall Pose—Viparita Karani

About the pose: Begin practicing inversions with this rejuvenating and accessible one and gradually build toward others. Besides practicing this pose on the mat, Legs up the Wall Pose can be done upon arriving in a hotel room after a long day of work, or even with your legs on a couch.

Instructions: Sit sideways to a wall, knees bent. Swing your hips up, and put your feet on the wall. Lift your hips and bring them down on the floor, folded blankets, a bolster, or a block as shown on page 172 in figure 6.49 (left), with your tailbone either tucked or untucked. Allow your thighs to deepen in your hip sockets. You can put a sandbag on your feet for added weight, unless that is uncomfortable. Breathe deeply, allowing your shoulders to relax and spread out to your sides. Let your soft palate open, and lift your chin slightly, creating a seal at the throat. Variations include bending your knees, opening your legs, and a combination of the two.

Handstand Pose—Adho Mukha Vrksasana

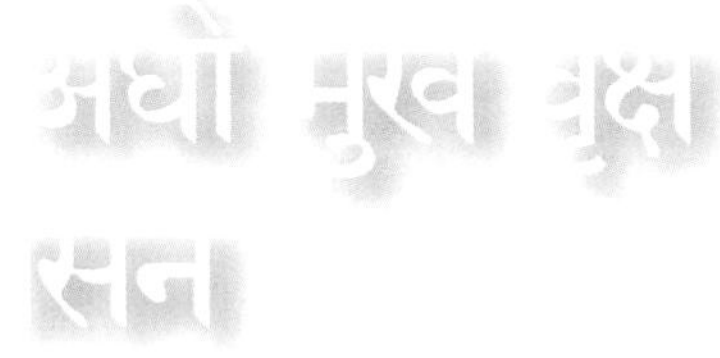

adho mukha vṛkṣāsana
Handstand Pose

About the pose: Handstand Pose, shown in figure 6.49 (center), is an excellent way to build overall strength and practice balancing upside down. It is a pose with no weight on the neck, shoulders, or head, so if you feel compromised in these areas it is a good choice for an inversion. You can work toward Handstand Pose by practicing Table Pose, illustrated in figure 6.49 (right). Once you can easily get up into Handstand, work the pose by staying for longer and longer periods of time.

Instructions: For **Table Pose**, begin in Downward Facing Dog (figure 6.34), with your feet at a wall. Then move your hands one hand's length back toward the wall. This shortened Downward Facing Dog may feel awkward, so keep your knees bent. Another way of finding where to place your hands includes sitting at the wall, extending your feet, putting your hands where your feet are, and then doing Downward Facing Dog. Whichever way you start, you may need to adjust the distance from the wall based on your body's flexibility. You may also want to initially start with your arms wider than shoulder width to account for tighter shoulders, working toward putting your hands under your shoulders.

Keep lifting your hips and sitting bones up toward the sky in Downward Facing Dog, engaging your core abdominal strength, and then one leg at a time walk up the wall to the height of your hips. Keep your knees bent slightly as you work to lengthen your spine and move your mid-spine toward the wall. Breathing deeply, keep lifting your hips up as you tuck your tailbone and use your legs strongly. When you are fatigued but not yet exhausted, walk your legs slowly down the wall and return to Child's Pose (figure 6.48).

For **Handstand Pose**, place your hands a hand's length from the wall. Inhale, roll your shoulders up toward your ears, and exhale as you feel your shoulders firmly on your back. Walk your legs forward so that your shoulders are directly over your hands. Bring one foot forward and donkey kick up so that eventually your legs touch the wall.

Once your legs are up, lift your hips up with core strength, tuck your tailbone, and move your lower rib cage toward your back body. Counting your breaths, feel the simultaneous lift off the earth and the pull of gravity. When you are finished, bend one leg and slowly return to Child's Pose (figure 6.48). Variations of Handstand include lifting your head to the wall, diamond-shaped legs, putting one leg on the wall, and Pumping Pose. Pumping Pose, which is basically lifting or pumping your body weight, involves inhaling as you bend your elbows and exhaling as you straighten them.

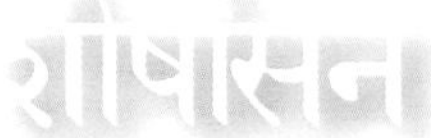

śīrṣāsana
Headstand Pose

Headstand Pose—Sirsasana

About the pose: Sometimes called the king of poses, Headstand is an inversion with many benefits, according to B.K.S. Iyengar:

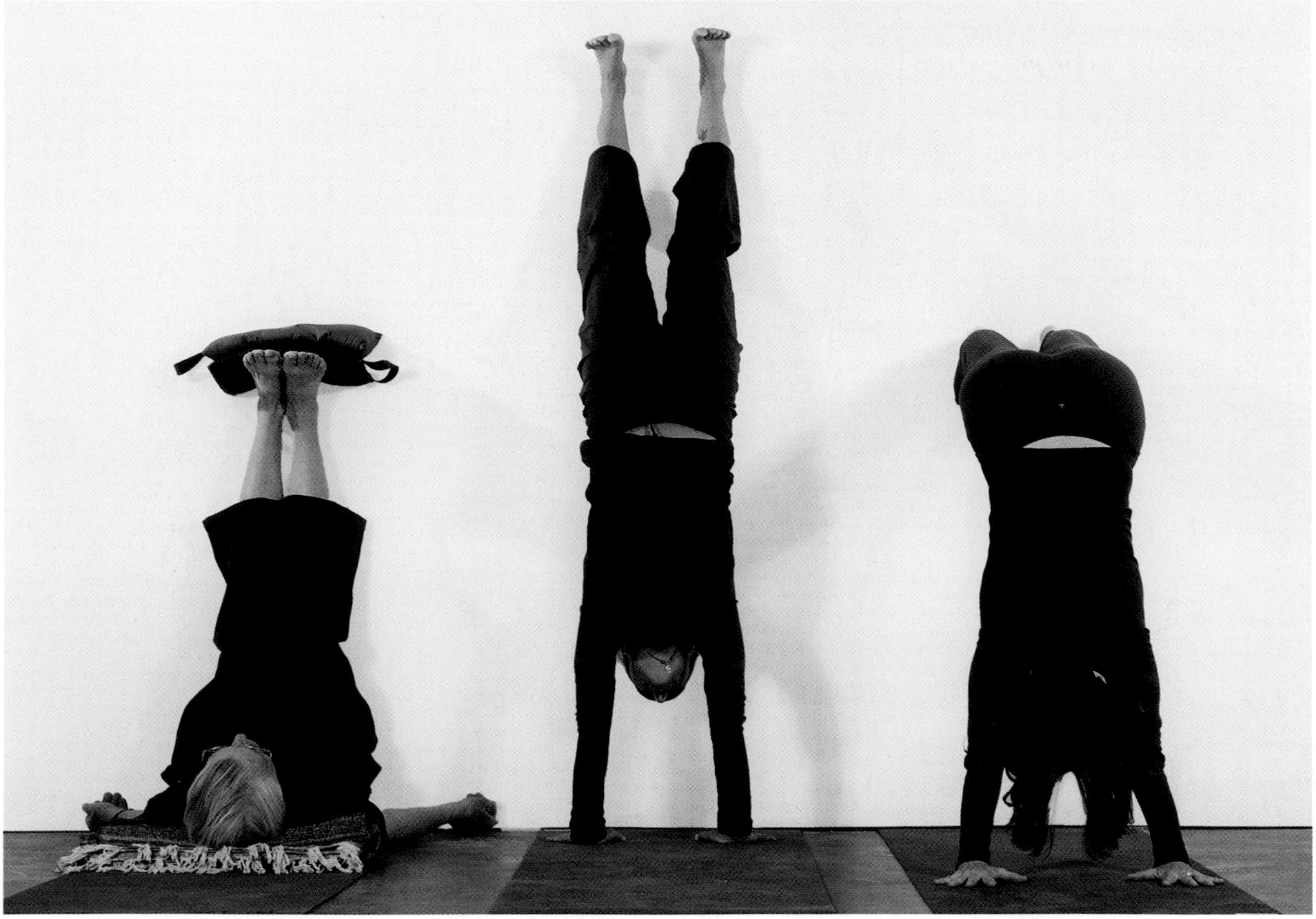

Figure 6.49. Legs up the Wall Pose—Viparita Karani (left); Handstand Pose—Adho Mukha Vrksasana (center); and Table Pose (right)

Regular and precise practice of Sirsasana develops the body, disciplines the mind and widens the horizons of the spirit. One becomes balanced and self-reliant in pain and pleasure, loss and gain, shame and fame and defeat and victory.[14]

For your first few decades of practicing yoga, in Headstand you'll want to be able to lift your head slightly off the ground with your arm and core strength. If you don't have that much power at the beginning, be sure to only stay in Headstand Pose for a few breaths and then rest in Child's Pose (figure 6.48). Advanced practitioners who have much strength and flexibility in the spine can try Headstand variations in which the entire weight of the body is on the head.

Instructions: Kneel down facing a wall. Put your nose on the floor and keep rolling your heel on the mat until you find your crown, a relatively flat spot on the top of your head. Then move your head in circles to discover the edges of your crown (see figure 6.50). Once you have found

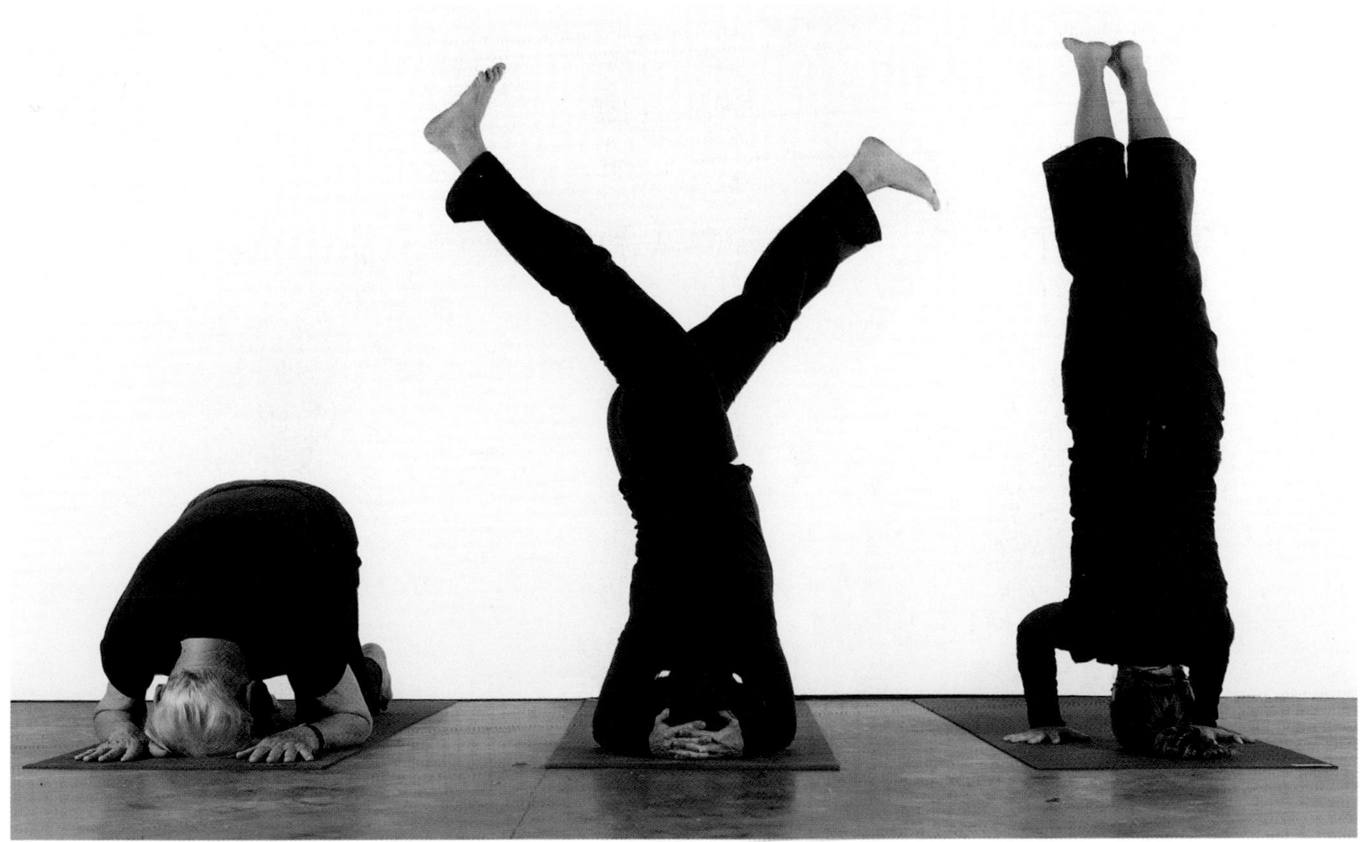

Figure 6.50. Headstand Pose—Sirsasana

your crown, you may move slightly toward your hairline if your neck is considerably flattened.

Next, create the shoulder and arm support for the pose. Interlace your pinkie fingers so they are stacked, and cup your head with your hands. Put your elbows directly under your shoulders (not wider than your shoulders), inhale, and lift your shoulders to your ears and then away from your ears, pressing down firmly with your forearms and hands to create a stabilizing foundation. Tuck your toes under and walk your feet closer to your head until your hips are almost over your shoulders. Then bring your legs over your head, either one leg at a time or both together. Slowly and carefully practice Headstand. Make sure your abdominal core is engaged, your lower ribs are moving toward your back body, and your inner thighs are moving behind you as you tuck your tailbone. With your arms, shoulders, and core supporting you away from the floor, there should be very little weight on your head. Now spread your toes, breathe deeply, and smile. Hold the pose for just five breaths at first, then slowly come down to Child's Pose (6.48). Work up to holding the pose longer as you become more comfortable with it. Variations can include lowering straight legs halfway down and then bringing them back up, or crossing the legs, or twisting them.

Shoulderstand Pose—Salamba Sarvangasana

About the pose: Shoulderstand Pose has many benefits, including contributing to the health of the thyroid and parathyroid glands and, according to some yogis, regulating body weight. Having heard that Shoulderstand regulates body weight, one of my teachers tested the theory. One summer when she was in her late fifties and had been practicing yoga for decades, she kept her daily yoga routine exactly the same except for eliminating Shoulderstand to see if she detected any difference in weight. By the end of the summer, she had gained twelve pounds and has since been convinced that Shoulderstand does indeed help regulate body weight.

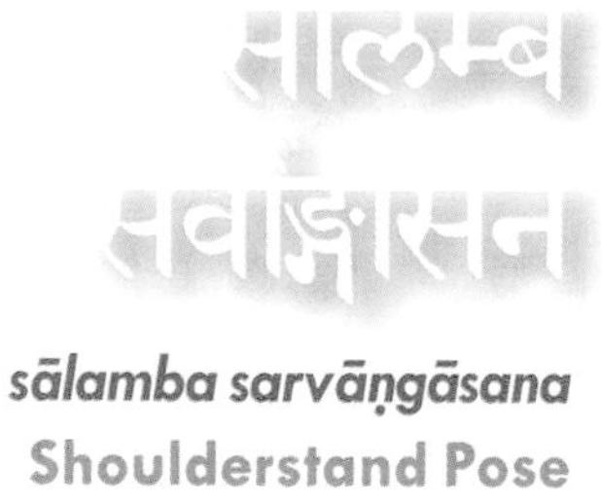

sālamba sarvāṇgāsana
Shoulderstand Pose

Despite its benefits, however, Shoulderstand Pose can be risky, especially for people who aren't able to fully rotate their shoulders as they may end up putting too much weight on their neck and feel pain or sustain injury. To avoid this outcome, you will want to remain aware of the condition of your neck and shoulders. If you use props and cannot tell whether your neck is being compressed, assume that it is and release to a modification such as the one demonstrated in figure 6.51.

Instructions: Begin by gaining awareness of your neck so you can assess its condition while practicing Shoulderstand. This you can do by bringing your chin to your chest and feeling the pointed bone, called C7 or cervical 7, at the bottom of the neck, which goes all the way up to the base of your skull. If while doing the pose you aren't able to tuck your shoulders under that bone, it may stick out toward the floor and take weight from your body. When practicing Shoulderstand, you want to remain sensitive to the neck, especially at the base on C7.

Lie sideways alongside a wall and swing your legs up the wall. Bend your knees, pressing your feet to the wall. Lift your hips up and reach your hands underneath, interlacing your fingers and strongly pulling your shoulders under. You want to feel that you have weight on the back of your head and sides of your arms but not on your neck. Then use your legs to keep lifting your hips over your shoulders, eventually lifting your legs straight up (see figure 6.51).

During this movement, if you feel the weight move to your neck, return your feet to the wall, bring your hips down, and change to Half Shoulderstand, untucking your tailbone and putting a block under your sacrum.

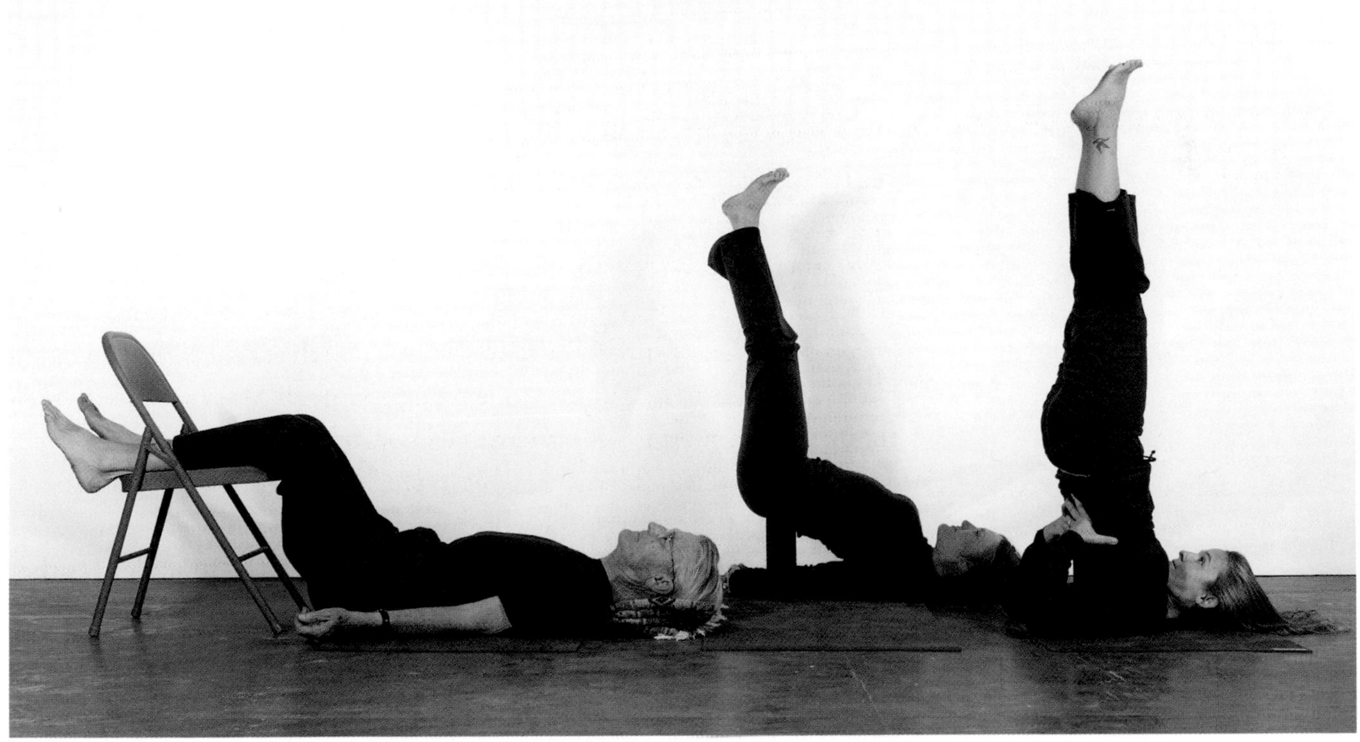

Figure 6.51. Shoulderstand Pose—Salamba Sarvangasana

Come out of the pose slowly and rest for at least twice the number of breaths you were up in the pose or for as long as it feels good to you, whichever is longer. After Shoulderstand practice **Fish Pose—Matsyendrasana** (figure 6.52), to move your chest in the opposite direction by lying down and then coming up on your elbows and reaching your heart up as your elbows move toward the center of your body. Then rest again.

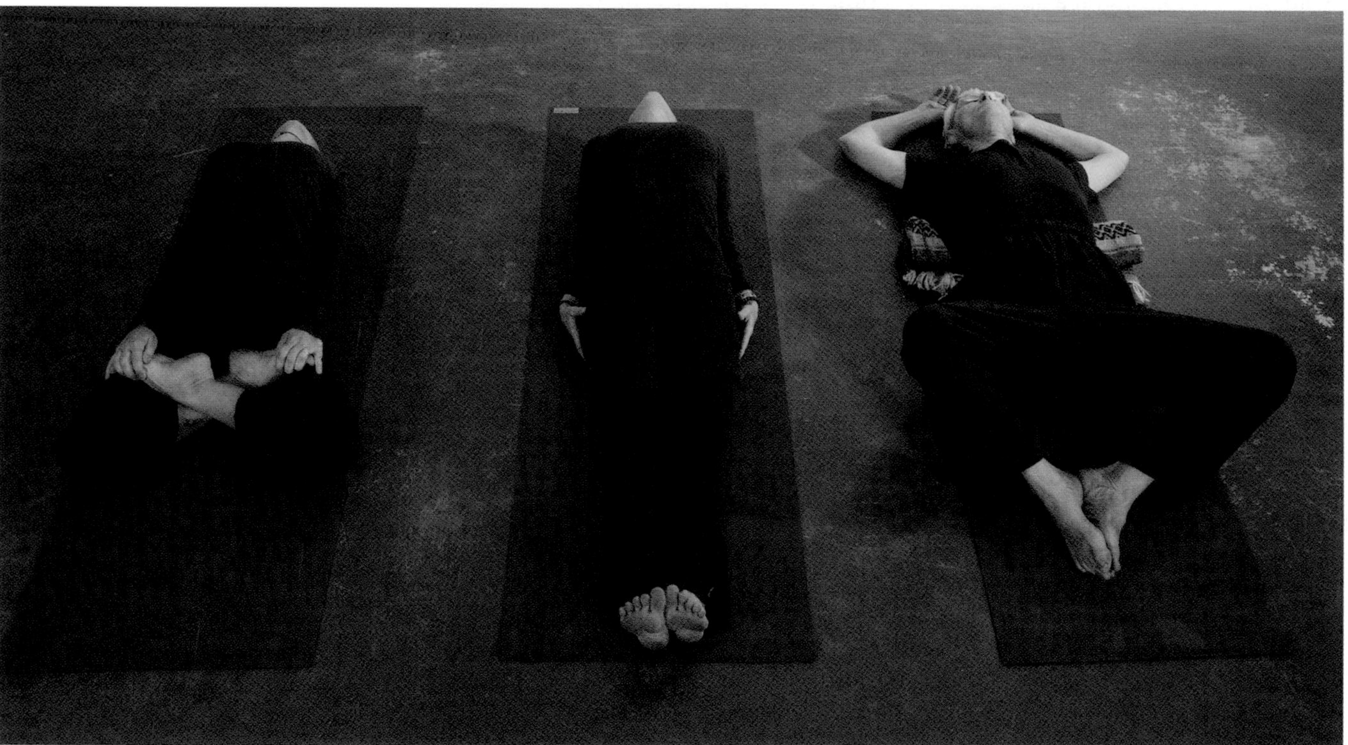

Figure 6.52. Fish Pose—Matsyendrasana

Seated Poses

Benefits: *Asana* means to sit, and all yoga poses prepare us for sitting and meditating. Therapeutic benefits of seated poses include lengthening the hamstrings and back body, opening the hips, and calming the central nervous system. Emotional and spiritual benefits include feeling more connected to nature and the world, and simultaneously to ourselves, as we are able to feel the lift of the spine and vibration in the central channel of energy.

Key Principles: Seated poses are often the most challenging, as they require considerable flexibility and length in the hamstrings. Whatever your level of yoga practice, be sure that you are working toward the primary goal of lengthening the spine and not only focusing on some secondary goal like touching your head to your knee as you practice Knee to Head Pose. You want to first lengthen the spine and then move it down toward the legs.

Key Anatomy: Instructions for most seated poses include moving to the front of the sitting bones, so it is important to understand what this entails in relationship to the skeleton and use props, if necessary. Often for the hip tops to tilt forward a lift is required, which may be produced by sitting on blankets, a sandbag, or a bolster or by bending the knees.

Seated Forward Fold Pose—Pascimottanasana

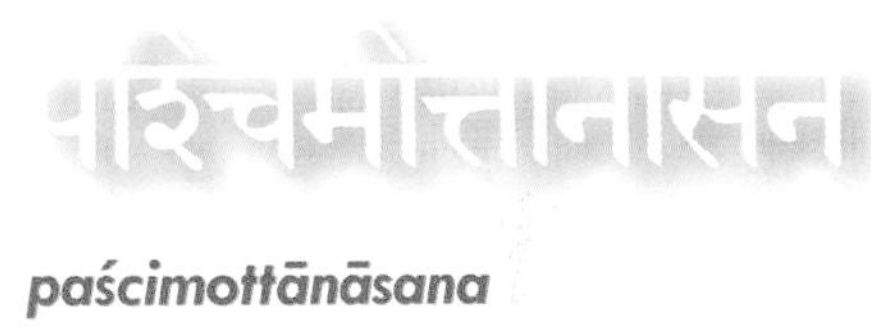

paścimottānāsana
Seated Forward Fold Pose

About the pose: Seated Forward Fold Pose is a good way to calm and nourish ourselves, appreciate our own beauty, and evoke humility. As we practice it, we are better able to refrain from comparing ourselves to others and instead notice our own beauty no matter what shape we are able to compose. This pose provides an opportunity to practice gratitude for a body that can do yoga poses, as well as a mind flexible enough to try yoga and a heart capable of expressing joy while doing it.

Instructions: Sit on the mat with your legs extended. Lean forward and gently pull the flesh of your buttocks back and out to find your sitting bones. If you feel a sagging in your low back or your low back is moving out behind you, sit on blankets, a sandbag, or a bolster (see figure 6.53). Start with bent knees and flexed feet on the carpet. Bend your knees

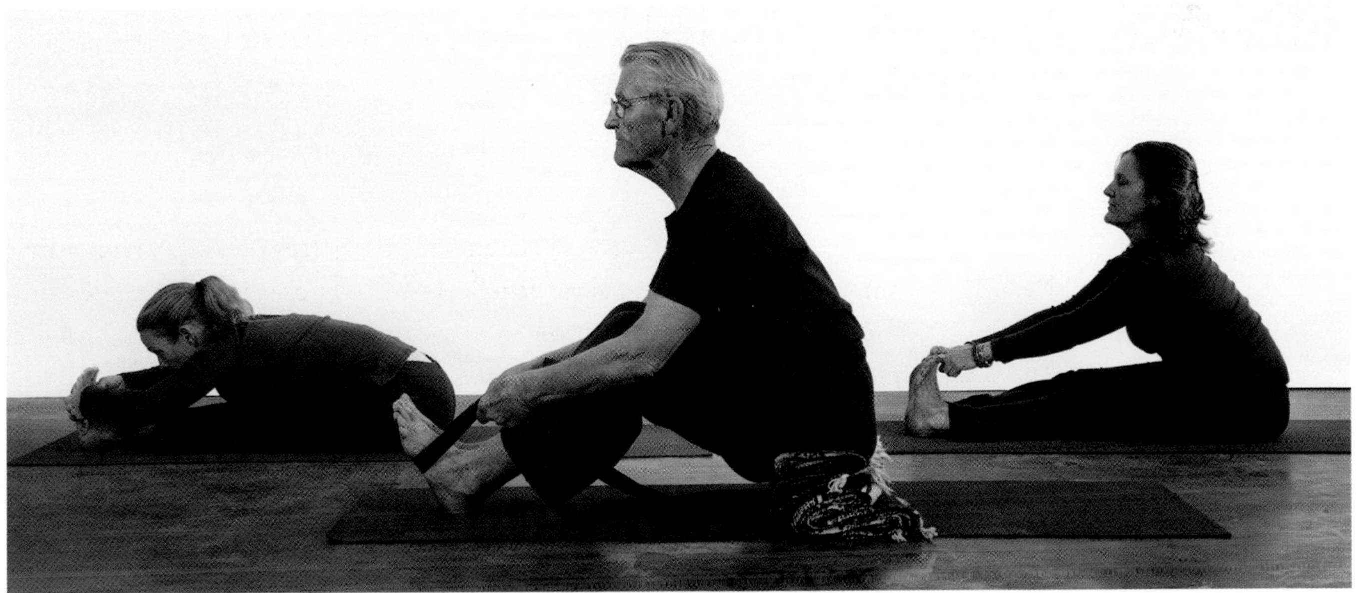

Figure 6.53. Seated Forward Fold Pose—Pascimottanasana

enough so you can feel that your torso or rib cage is touching your thighs. Put your thumbs at the base of your big toes or use a belt as you slowly begin to extend your legs, keeping your front rib cage and thighs touching, your heart and sternum lifted, and your back body long. Breathe slowly and deeply as you let your head rest on your legs, a bolster, or a block. When you are finished, sit up slowly and feel the sense of sitting upright on your sitting bones, engaging your core.

Knee to Head Pose—Janusirsasana

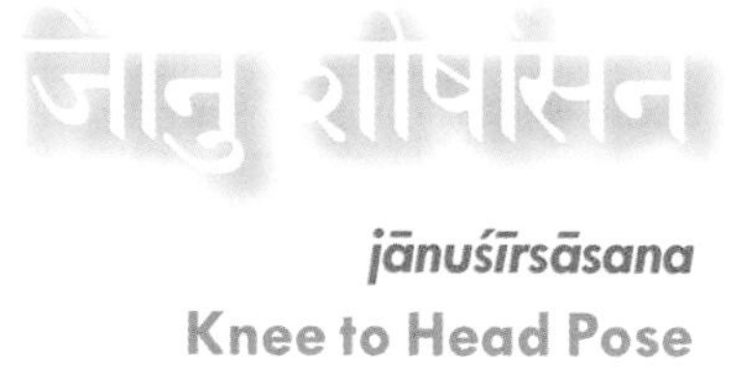

jānuśīrsāsana
Knee to Head Pose

About the pose: Knee to Head Pose can make you more aware of your inner self, that you are more than any external traits. The name of the pose indicates the direction in which to move rather than actually putting your knee to your head, especially not at the expense of your focus on lengthening your spine.

Instructions: Sit with your legs extended, pull the flesh of your buttocks back and out to find your sitting bones, and lean forward to come to the front rim of your sitting bones. Bend one knee and place the bottom of your foot to your inner thigh as close to the groin as possible with no knee sensation. If there is sensation in your knee, change your position. Inhale, lengthen your spine from your waist up, and exhale, turning toward the extended leg. Begin to fold toward the leg, letting your hands rest by the

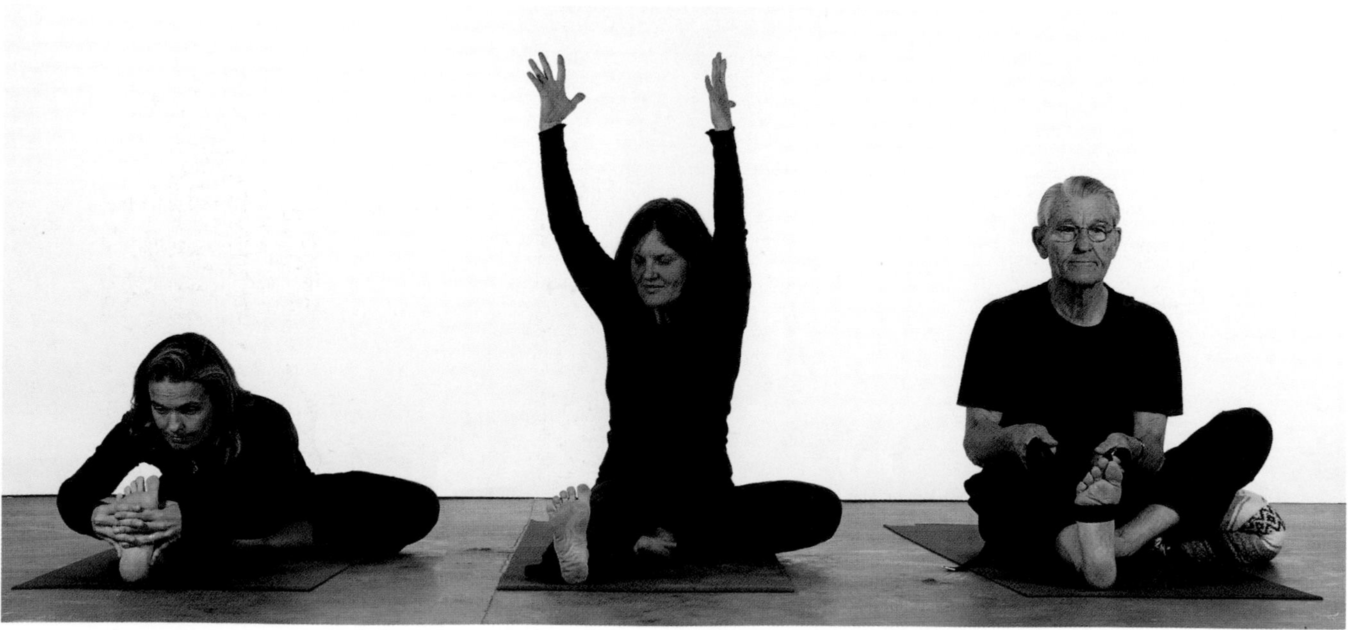

Figure 6.54. Knee to Head Pose—Janusirsasana

sides of your leg, and touch your foot or use a belt (see figure 6.54). Keep your shoulders on your back by bending your elbows slightly back and tilting your sternum forward. If you feel any pulling or sharp pain in your back, bend your extended knee and bring your rib cage next to your thigh, perhaps beginning to straighten your leg, breathing into the sensation and staying at the minimum edge for a number of breaths. Repeat on the second side.

Hero Pose—Virasana

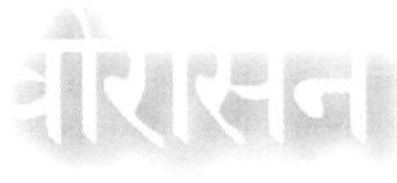

vīrāsana
Hero Pose

About the pose: This is an excellent pose in which to contemplate being a hero, according to your own definition. You could consider who your heroes have been in the past and are in the present, as well as what type of hero you would like to be. Hero Pose is the only pose that can be done with a full stomach as it aids digestion. You might even invite your family and friends to do the pose after a large celebratory meal. This pose lengthens the front thigh muscles (quadriceps), deepens the thigh in the hip socket, opens the ankles, and is a good pose to attempt to stay in for longer and longer periods of time as your body adjusts.

Instructions: Kneeling, bring your knees toward each other. First cross your ankles in back, noticing how your thighs roll out. Next bring your ankles directly behind your knees, and notice how your thighs are neutral. Then bring your ankles outside your hips and begin to sit down. If you

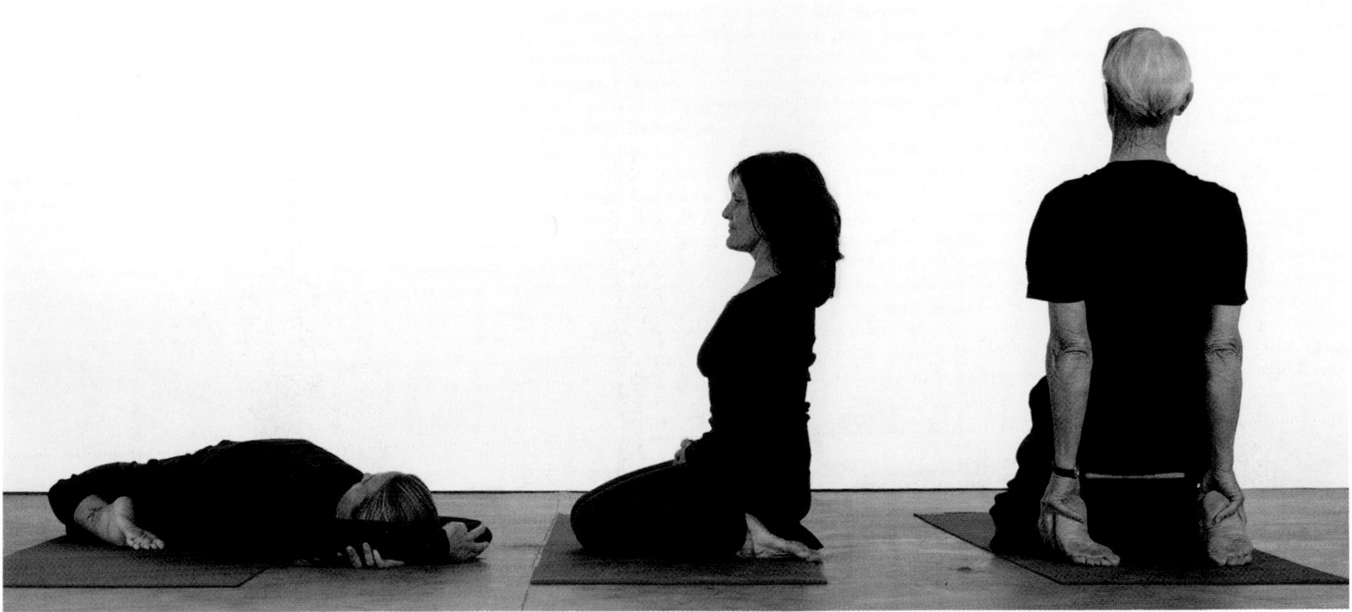

Figure 6.55. Hero Pose—Virasana (right); Lying Hero Pose (left)

can't bring your sitting bones (not just your buttocks) to the floor, use a prop, such as a block, blanket, or a sandbag, to sit comfortably (see figure 6.55). If your ankles are stressed, lift your hips higher with more props. Arm shape variations for the pose include lifting your arms, hooking your elbows, and putting your hands behind your back for reverse *anjali* mudra. Once your hips move closer to the floor you can change to **Lying Hero Pose—Sputa Virasana**, by lying on the floor without your legs lifting up, as demonstrated in figure 6.55.

Happy Pose—Sukkasana

sukkāsana
Happy Pose

About the pose: The name of this pose can also be translated as Easy Pose, and it should feel both easy and happy. Happy Pose can be used for practicing *pranayama*, meditating, or just feeling at ease, with props if necessary. The idea is to feel grounded from the hips down and light and open from the waist up, using the breath to find both feelings.

Instructions: Pull the flesh out from under your sitting bones and lean forward to find their front edge. Cross your ankles or try stacking them (see figure 6.56). If your low back is rounding or your knees are high, sit on props. You might lift yourself up and lean forward to find the front edge of your sitting bones and then release to the ground. Inhale and lengthen your

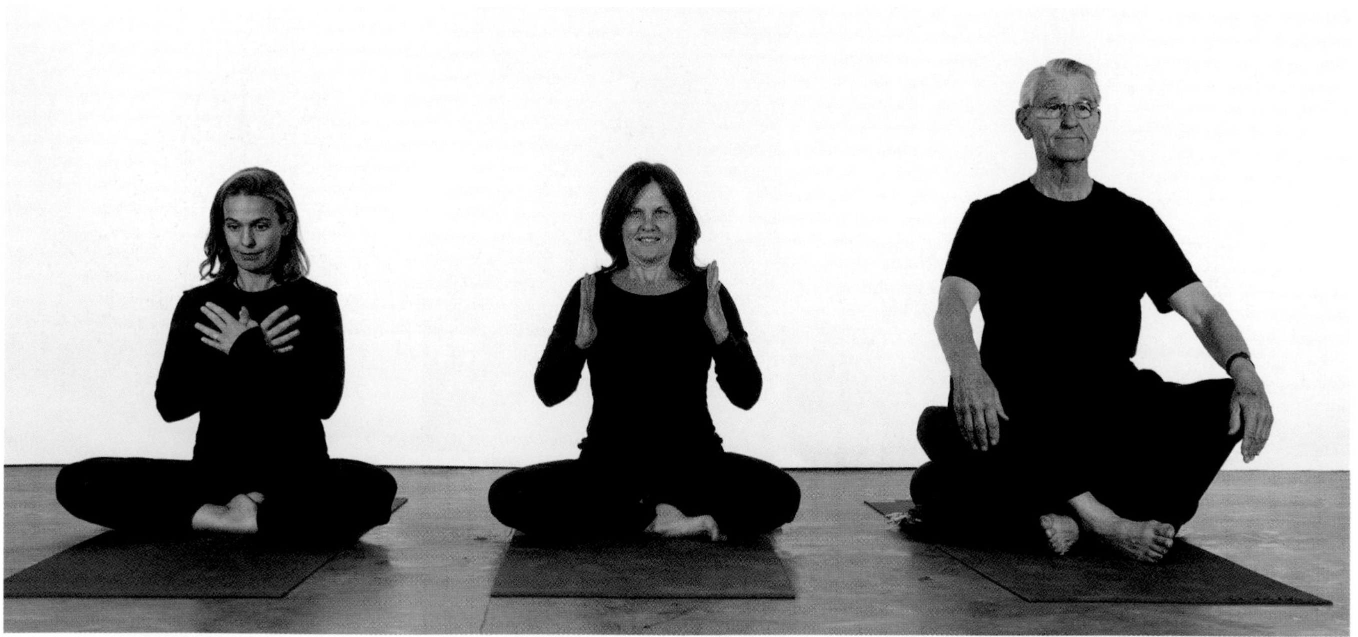

Figure 6.56. Happy Pose—Sukkasana

spine. Exhale and roll your shoulders back and slightly down, spreading your shoulder blades apart and feeling light in the torso. This is a terrific pose for practicing mudras, and you may start with *garuda* mudra (figure 4.17) at the heart to experience a sense of limitless possibility.

Seated Angle Pose—Upavista Konasana

About the pose: Seated Angle Pose may allow us to feel we are opening to a creative expression emerging from our inner core. To facilitate this connection, you may close your eyes, feel vibration in your body, and imagine what you would like to create.

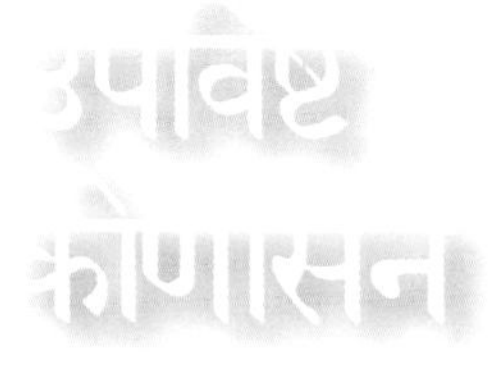

upaviṣṭa koṇāsana
Seated Angle Pose

Instructions: Spread your legs and bend your knees, lifting your flesh out from under your sitting bones and leaning forward. Keeping your knees bent, fold between your legs. Once you are at your lowest level, strongly engage your legs and begin to straighten them (see figure 6.57). Your knees should point upward and your legs stay active. You can use a belt for your legs or just fold forward in a gesture of surrender. Stay in this pose for minutes, breathing deeply, unless you experience discomfort.

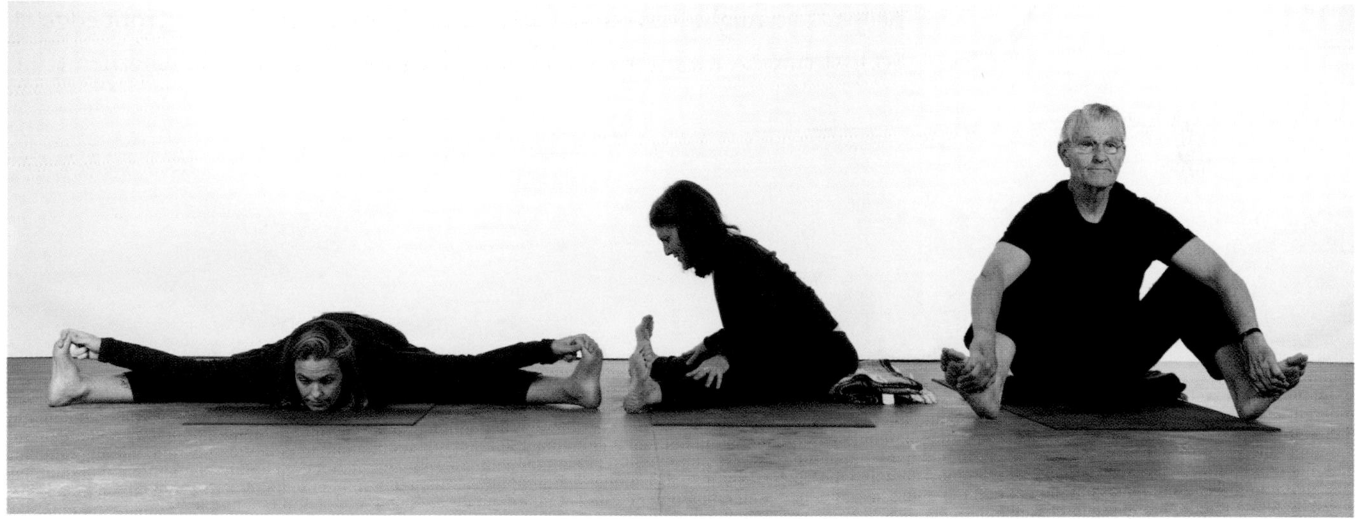

Figure 6.57. Seated Angle Pose—Upavista Konasana

Twisting Poses

Benefits: Twists help us develop more flexibility in the spine and massage the digestive organs. Doing them can make us feel like we are eliminating our anxieties and becoming freer. The more we twist, the better able we are to believe we can transform aspects of ourselves, initially at a physical level and increasingly at a spiritual one. When we are mentally and spiritually fatigued, twists give us the fresh energy to go on. As a result, they help us digest not only food but also the experiences of life.

Key Principles: Finding the wave of the breath as we move in twists helps us keep the rotation of the spine whole. When we breathe in a twist, lengthening and then moving, we experience the action along the entire spine, even if one part is relatively motionless. In twists, we lengthen the spine on the inhale, holding the length as we exhale, and twist beginning with the base of the spine then moving up with the exhale.

Key Anatomy: The side wraparound muscles are given some attention in these poses, so it is helpful to be able to visualize them as we practice twists. Figure 6.58[15] shows, from the rear, the muscles involved in Revolved Knee to Head Pose, Parivrtta Janusirsasana, as an example of how the *latissimus dorsi* and other muscles move in a twist.

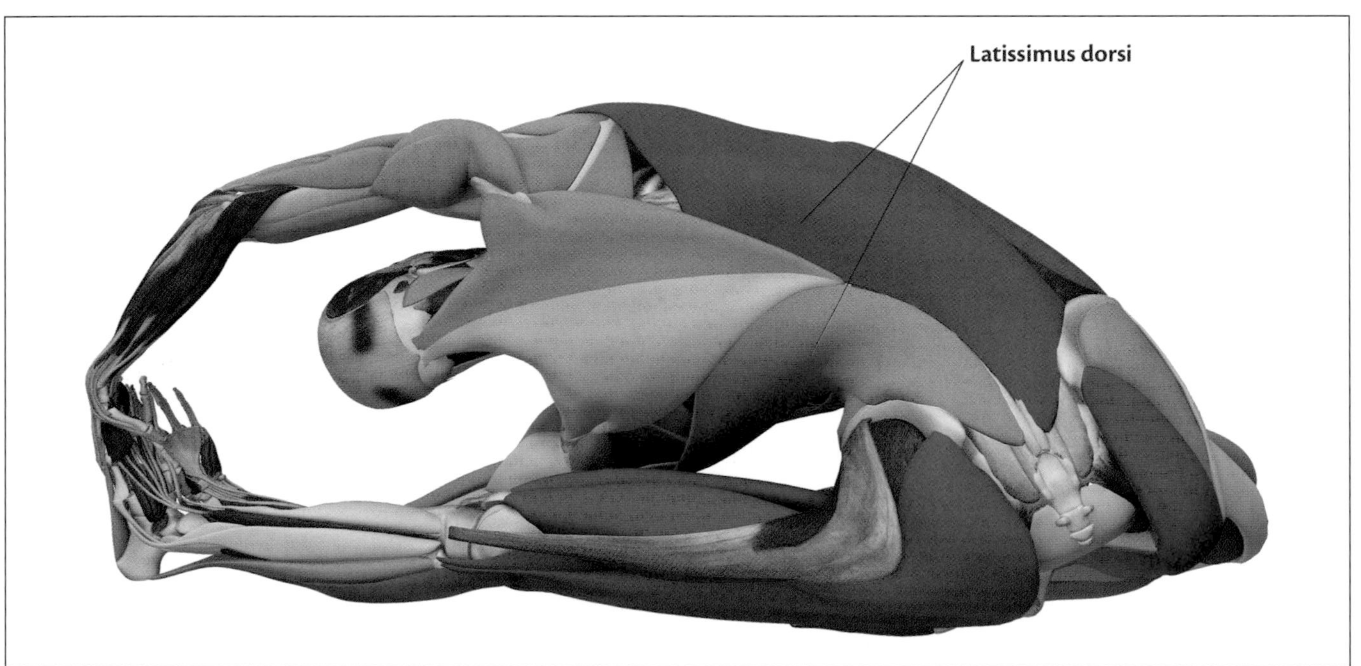

Figure 6.58. Seated twisting anatomy

Half Fish Twist Pose—Ardha Matshendrasana

About the pose: This pose is named after the great sage Matsyendra, who is regarded as a founder of hatha yoga. Use the breath to fill the belly and lengthen the spine on the inhale, and find strong core action on the exhale to twist. You can imagine that as you inhale, your spine is like a round toothpaste tube that hasn't been used, and as you exhale, your spine lengthens toward the sky like squeezing hard on the tube with the top off so the toothpaste shoots up.

Instructions: Cross one leg over the other and pull the flesh out from under your sitting bones so they are on the ground, using a blanket if necessary (see figure 6.59). Inhale and lift the arm opposite the crossed leg. Keep the length, exhale, and twisting toward the top knee, lightly rest the other hand behind you. Use your arms for leverage to facilitate the twisting action around the spine and the squeezing of the organs. Be sure not to jerk your shoulders as part of the twist. You can also bind your hand or extend your arm. Repeat on the second side.

अर्ध मत्स्येन्द्रासन

ardha matsyendrāsana

Half Fish Twist Pose

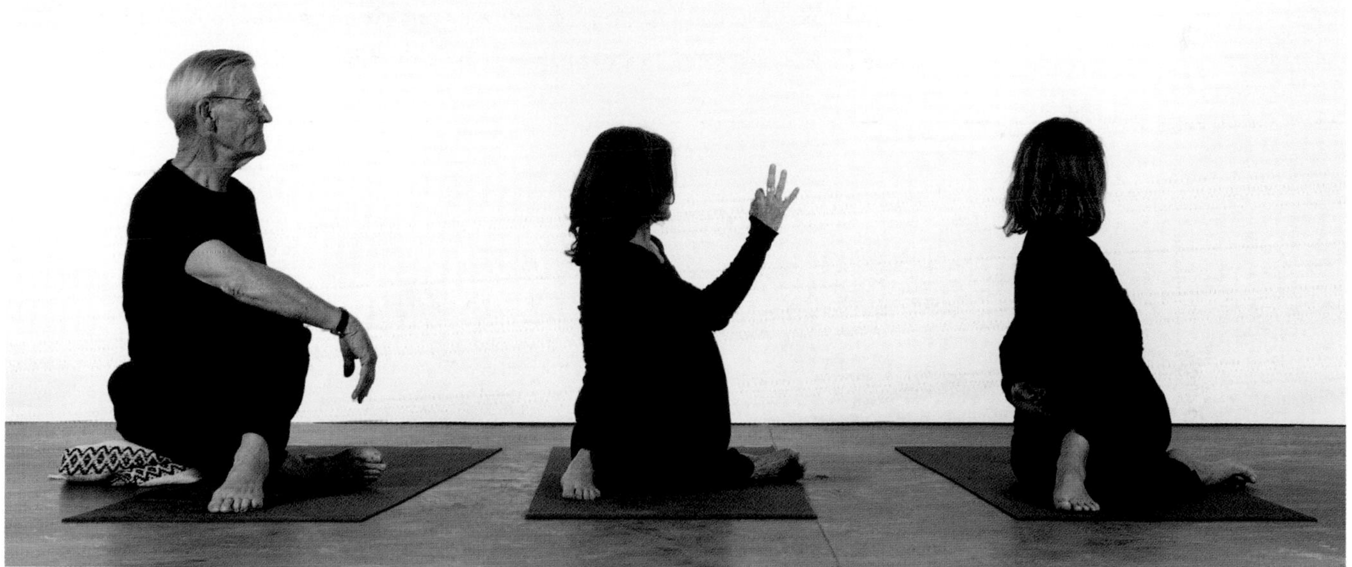

Figure 6.59. Half Fish Twist Pose—Ardha Matshendrasana

Revolved Knee to Head Pose—Parivrtta Janusirsasana

About the pose: This pose combines the grounded feeling of sitting poses and the more flighty feeling of twists. It is a good pose near the end of your practice as your body may feel simultaneously more awake and yet relaxed.

Instructions: Extend both legs wide, bend one knee, and bring the foot back to the opposite inner thigh. Dip your shoulder toward the same side knee as you slightly bend it (see figure 6.60). Inhale and press down with the bent leg. Exhale and deepen toward the floor with your shoulder as

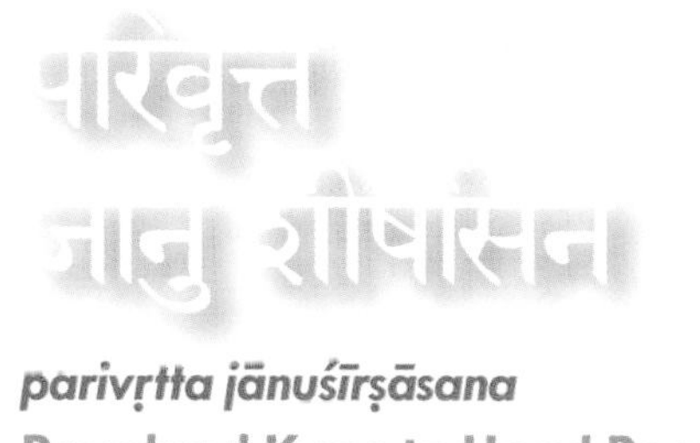

parivṛtta jānuśīrṣāsana

Revolved Knee to Head Pose

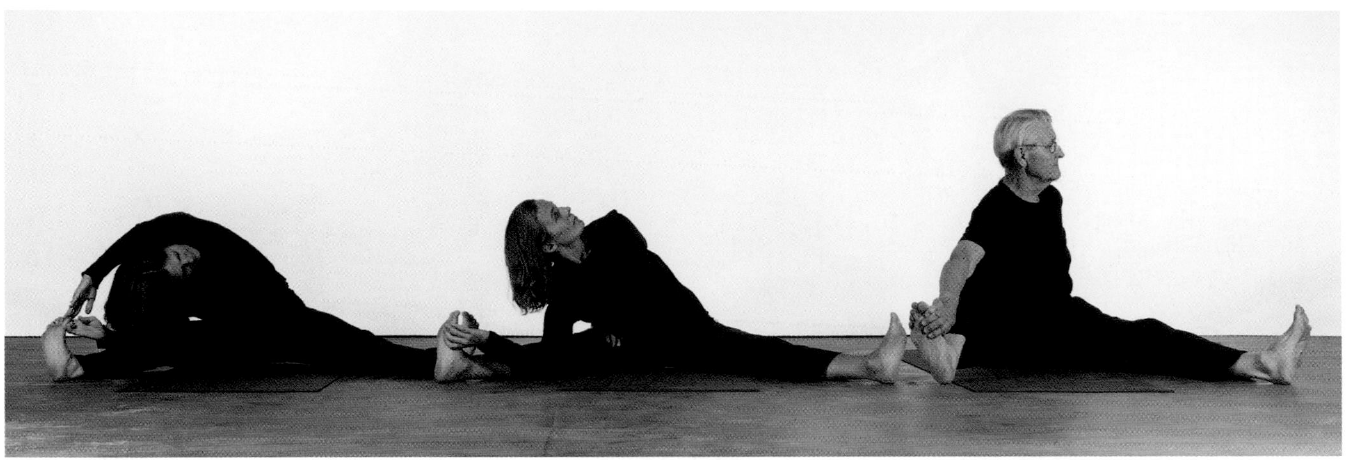

Figure 6.60. Revolved Knee to Head Pose—Parivrtta Janusirsasana

you turn your torso toward the sky. Use your knee as leverage to twist, and then slowly straighten your leg. Your top arm can be in various shapes, as long as you make sure that there is no shoulder or neck tension. Repeat on the second side.

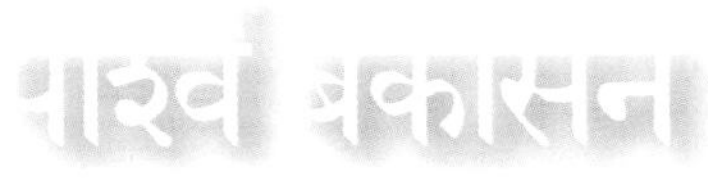

pārśva bakāsana
Side Crow Pose

Side Crow Pose—Parsva Bakasana

About the pose: Side Crow is achieved through trust. On the physical level, you find the necessary balance as you trust that you can move forward and support yourself, while on the spiritual level you build trust in being able to support yourself in whatever you are guided to do.

Instructions: Squat sideways on the mat with your heels lifted. Inhale and lift your torso. Exhale and twist toward the front of the mat, hooking your elbows initially at either end of your thighbone. (Later, you can hook the elbow closest to your knee.) Breathing deeply, lift your core as you move forward to balance on your arms (see figure 6.61). If you are concerned about falling forward, put a blanket where your head would land. You can also use the wall to practice the twist. Repeat on the second side.

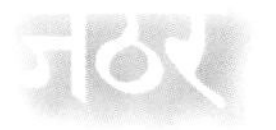

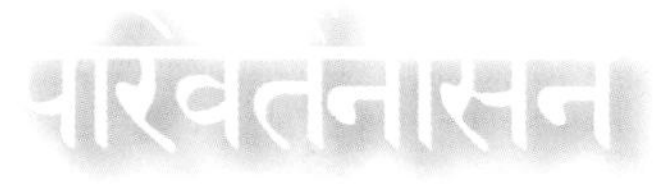

jaṭhara parivartanāsana
Lying Twist Pose

Finishing Poses

Lying Twist Pose—Jathara Parivartanasana

About the pose: Lying Twist makes us feel expansive and empowered to achieve our goals by allowing us to spread out on the ground and rotate around our central axis. For this reason, it is a good pose to do near the end of practice.

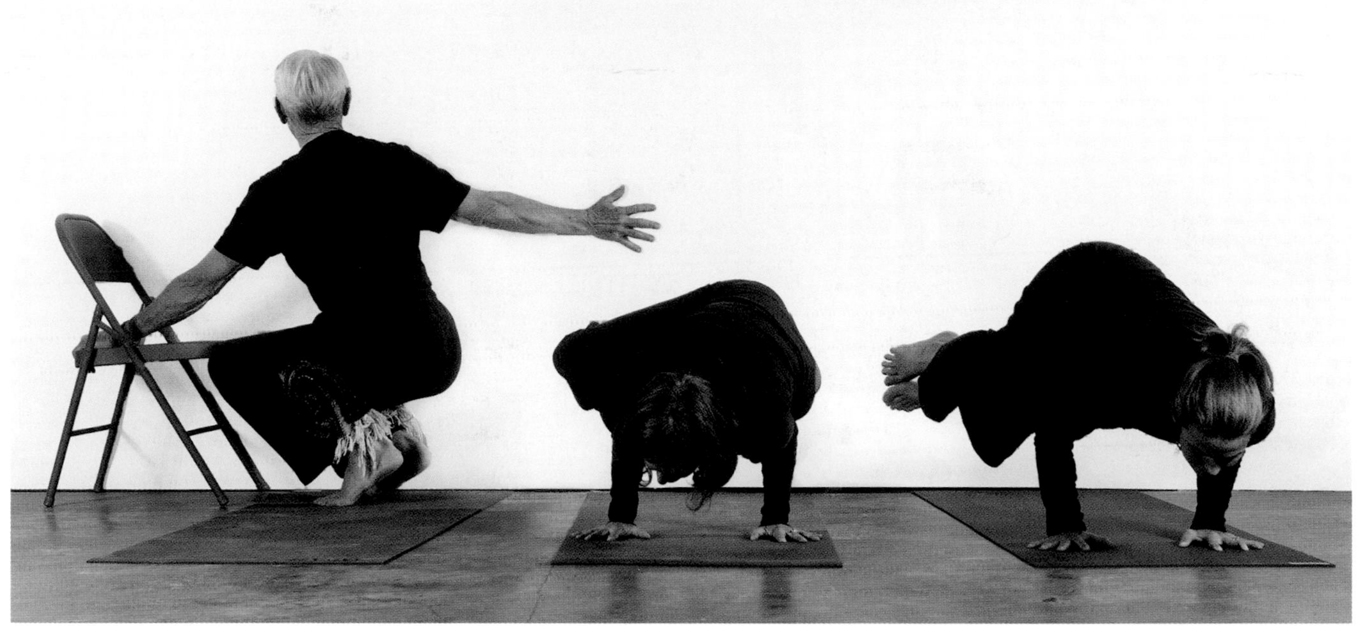

Figure 6.61. Side Crow Pose—*Parsva Bakasana*

Instructions: Lie on your back, inhale, and bring one knee to your chest. Exhale and cross that leg over your body, allowing your top hip to rotate over your lower hip (see figure 6.62). Variations include straightening your leg and reaching for both legs. Repeat on the second side.

Corpse Pose—Savasana

About the pose: Often called the most important and difficult of yoga poses, Corpse Pose is done at the end of class to integrate all the work of practice on physical and energetic planes, including poses, breath, and intention. As such, it is a good pose for practicing self-acceptance—the idea that you are perfect just as you are, that you have everything you need for enlightenment and bliss. The goal is to bring attention back to the present moment, the sensations of your body on the mat.

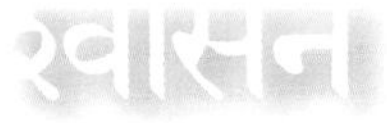

śavāsana
Corpse Pose

Instructions: Lie down on the mat, roll your legs out, close your eyes, let your shoulders drop, and relax so your whole body feels heavy. You may want a blanket under your head if your chin is lifting up, or under your knees if your lower back is sensitive (see figure 6.63). Breathe normally without control and watch as energy flows up and down the center channel of your body. Your mind may seem to be filled with thoughts that are like tetherballs going off in space on long cords, but they can be

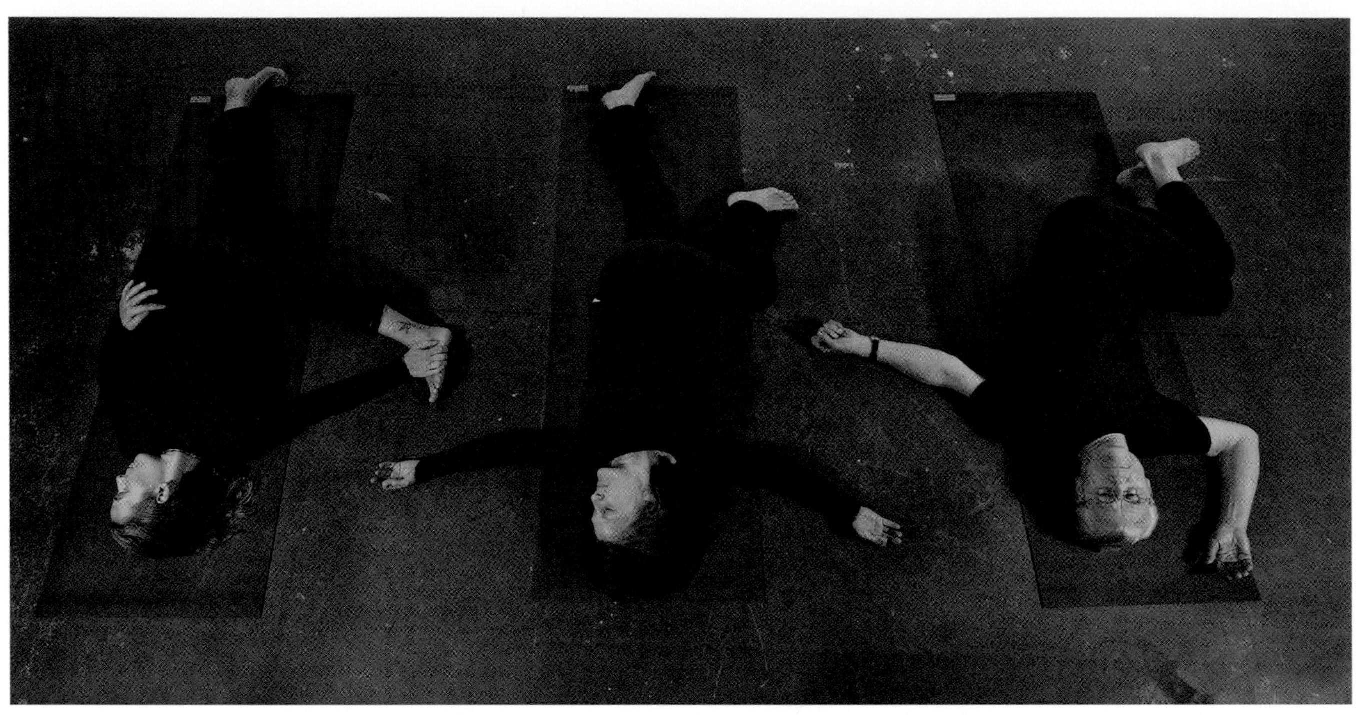

Figure 6.62. Lying Twist Pose—Jathara Parivartanasana

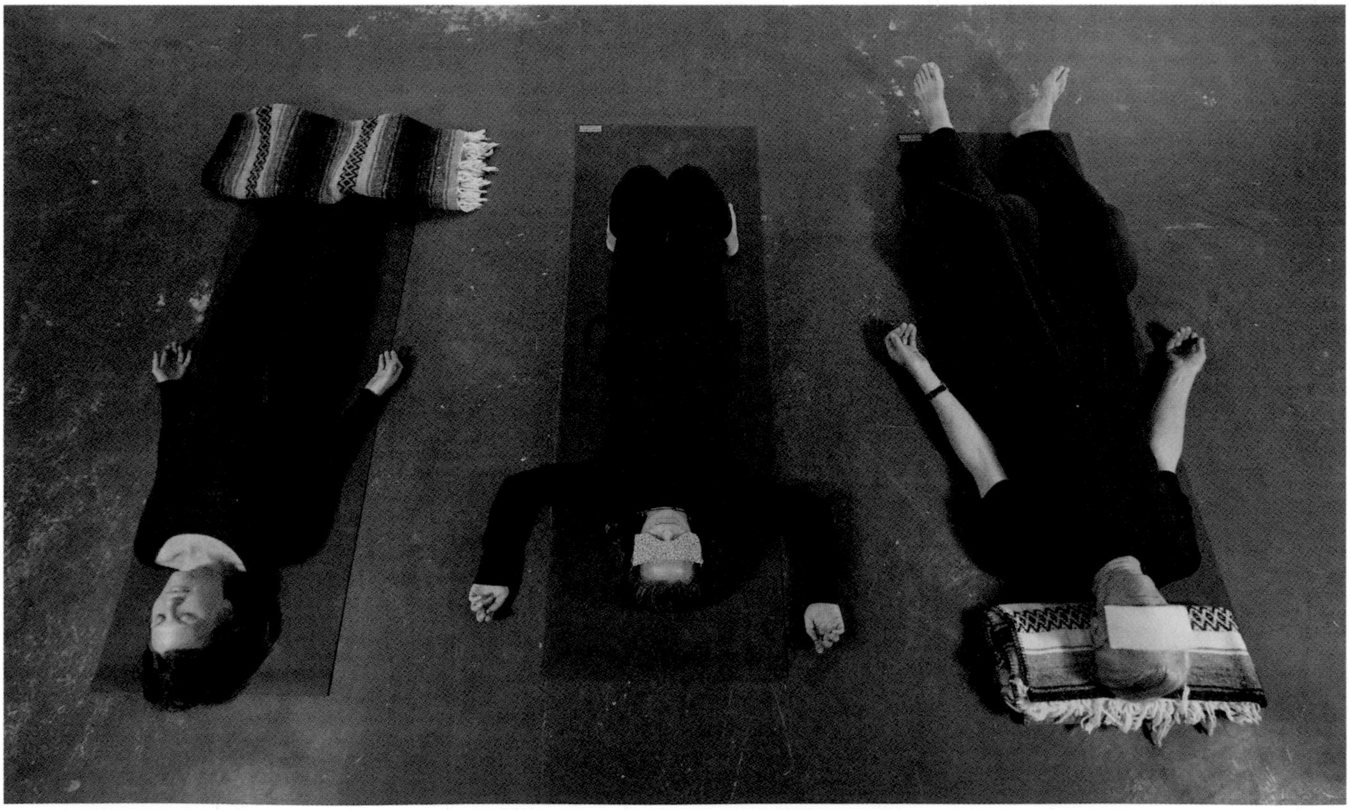

Figure 6.63. Corpse Pose—Savasana

brought back to the pole again through awareness of the "now." Practice Corpse Pose a minimum of ten minutes, although longer is preferable.

Flowing with the Poses and Breath

You can link poses together and move with the breath in the flowing style of yoga called *vinyasa*. There are limitless ways to connect poses and create a flow. Sun and Moon Salutations, popular forms of this style of yoga, represent different aspects of us: the sun relates to moving forward, building strength, achieving clarity and discernment, the male part of ourselves, and the left brain, while the moon is about transformation, flexibility, the female part of ourselves, and the right brain. The salutations can be done to honor those aspects of us, as well as to honor the natural world—the light and power of the sun and the luminosity and energy of the moon. Moon Salutations are often done on full moons or new moons, for example.

There are many versions of these salutations. An example of a Sun Salutation is seen in figure 6.64 and of a Moon Salutation in figure 6.65. Notice that with each movement there is a corresponding breath that matches the action, usually moving you away from gravity on the inhale and into gravity on the exhale.

Sanskrit Gem

***Vinyasa* means flowing sequence, arrangement.**

Figure 6.64. Traditional sequence of Sun Salutation

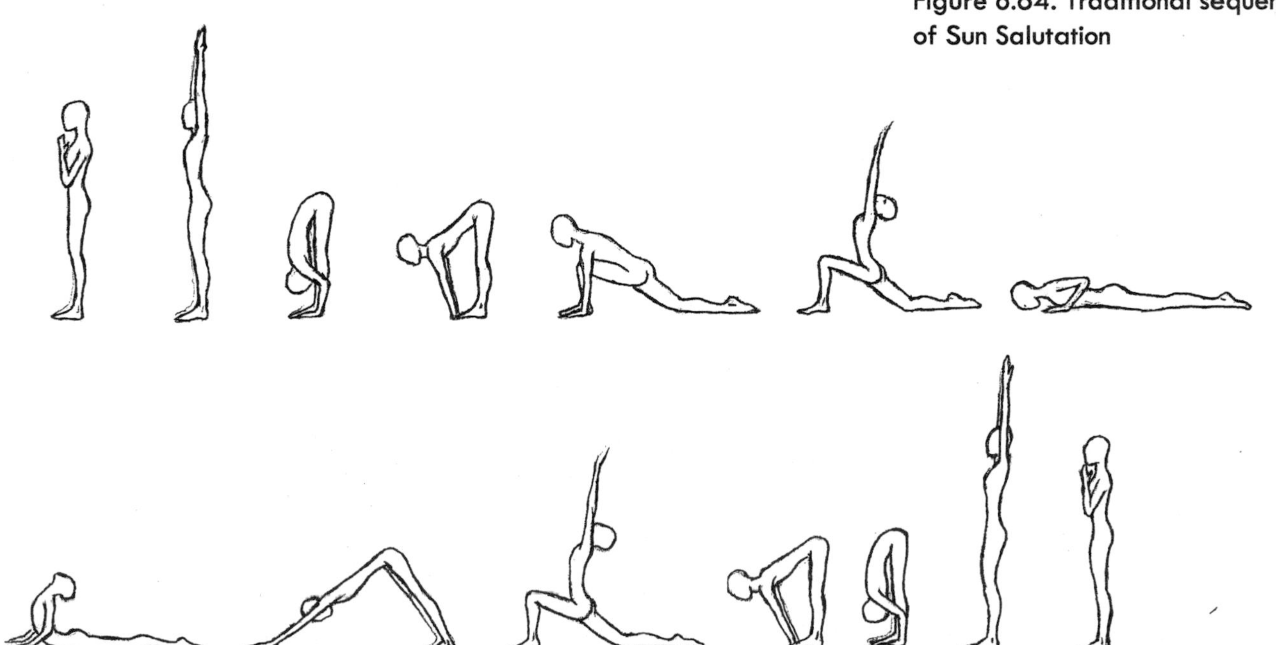

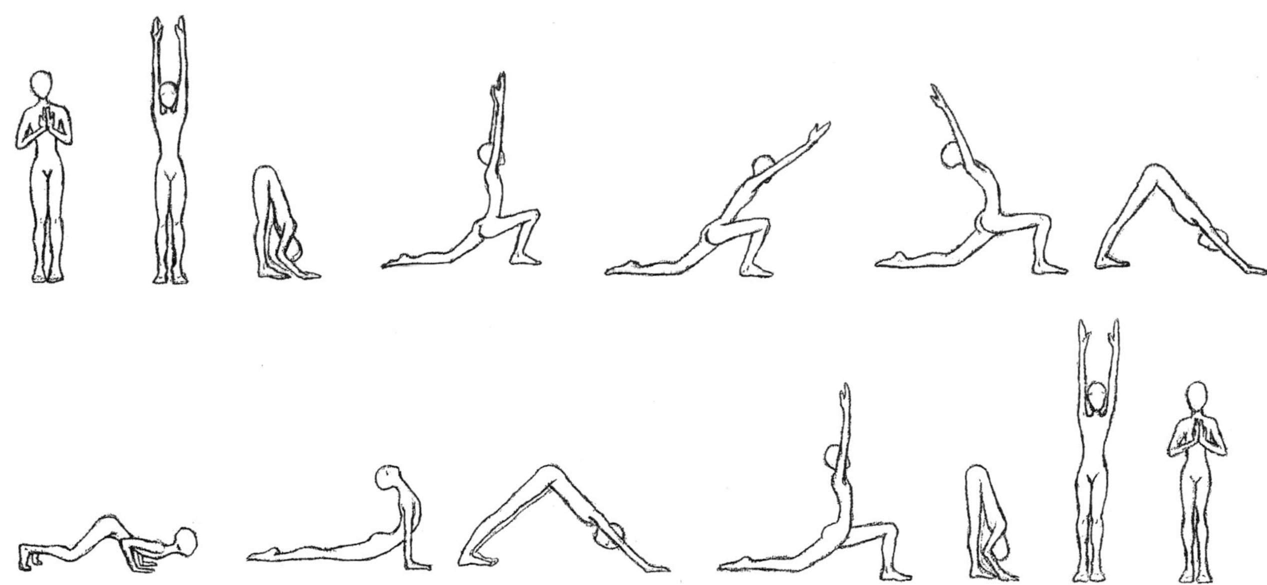

Figure 6.65. Traditional sequence of Moon Salutation

To begin vinyasa, find a series of poses that appeals to you either because of the movements or the teacher, or both. After gaining proficiency with that series and the Golden Rule of Practice—find your breath, follow your breath to the place of sensation, and listen intently to your experience—you can safely develop your own flow yoga.

Define your understanding of "abandoning unsuitable company." Reflect on your daily experiences to gain awareness of the types of people and situations that deplete or enhance your energy. Also, before meeting with an individual or a group, be aware of the energetic sensations and feelings in your body, heart, and mind, then reassess them after you leave the meeting. You might even assign a number from one to ten to your feelings, determining, for example, that before the meeting you felt very good, about a nine on the scale, while after the meeting you felt more like a four. Consider any person or group that lowers your number as "unsuitable company" and people with whom you have common interests and goals—such as a political agenda, community organizing, or working with youth—as "suitable company."

Set an intention and practice the first poses of each category; after mastering them, continue with the next poses. See how the poses feel in your body and how the intention feels after you've practiced.

Practice one neo-asana each week. Once you are comfortable with them all, work with the classical asanas in a way that adds no tension to any part of your body.

Practice one session not moving past the minimum edge for at least one minute, then slowly move deeper, noticing your sensations.

PART III

INTO THE WORLD

driving to a certain place to eat. But soon you begin to visualize the experience of dining there, and an inner voice tells you this is not really what you want to do. So maybe you pull over, listen, and hear your inner voice take you in a completely different direction, giving you a sense of control.

Or perhaps it's near the end of the day and you're very tired but have more work to do. You get a strong urge to smoke a cigarette and drink some wine. But then you listen to your inner voice telling you that if you do you'll probably never get your work done and that what you need is some rest and rejuvenation. Upon recognizing that underlying need, you may take a bath, call a close friend, or lie down for a few minutes. Soon you might notice that the urge to smoke and drink have completely disappeared and, feeling energized, you are able to finish your work so you can sleep more peacefully.

On a more interpersonal level, you may listen to your inner voice while conversing with your partner or while parenting your children. Doing so can alert you to options that make your family life more harmonious.

YOGA AS COMMUNITY

Yoga can be a constructive lead to supportive resources. One support resource that can help us use yogic principles in life is a *kalyana mitra,* or auspicious friend. A *kalyana mitra* is someone who also seeks *samadhi,* ecstasy, and wants to share experiences for mutual support, a relationship that can be beneficial to both seekers. In the words of one yogi: "I know whatever I'm working on, my *kalyana mitra* will support me and ask me penetrating questions, not as a critic but as a loving and careful holder of yogic principles. I definitely couldn't have gotten through my last year—including a breakup, a family crisis, and money problems—without her."

Sanskrit Gem

Kalyana **means auspicious, and** ***mitra*** **means friend.**

Another support resource is a yoga *kula,* an energetic community formed by yoga studio, class, or retreat participants. A yoga community can encourage you to use yogic principles in daily life and support you during difficult times. For example, yoga studios may offer special classes during traditional holidays, creating a sense of community and peaceful interaction in contrast to more stressful family gatherings. As one student remarked:

Sanskrit Gem

Kula **means community of the heart.**

> *Holidays always made me feel like I was left out and looking at everyone else doing something more fun than me. Now I come to yoga and I see there are other people who would rather start Christmas, New Year's Day, and the Fourth of July in a yoga class. It has shifted my*

experience of these occasions, and the rest of the day is always better, whether I do something traditional or not. I'm forever grateful to yoga, and it's not only because I can do a pose.

Sanskrit Gem

***Kama* means love, and *sutra* means treatise.**

YOGA FOR IMPROVING SEX

Yoga makes us more flexible, balanced, and stronger, as well as increasing the flow of *prana* in our bodies so we are more in touch with every part of our physical and emotional selves. Thus, not surprisingly, yoga can improve sex.

Yoga has long been associated with sex. The *Kama Sutra,* written between the first and sixth century CE, focuses on cultivating erotic pleasure and includes rituals to prepare yourself and your bedroom for erotic love; words that describe different kinds of kisses, embraces, and caresses; discussions on choosing a suitable partner; and advice on how a man can understand a woman when she's on top.[1] Images of sexual acts are on public buildings throughout India, as exemplified in figure 7.1. In addition, Tantra yoga encourages the use of sex as a powerful tool for spiritual enlightenment. An important distinction between the *Kama Sutra* and the views of Tantra yoga is that the former is concerned with cultivation of erotic pleasure, while the latter is about how to reach enlightenment through conscious sexual practices. You may want to consider advice from both sources, excellent translations of which are available.[2]

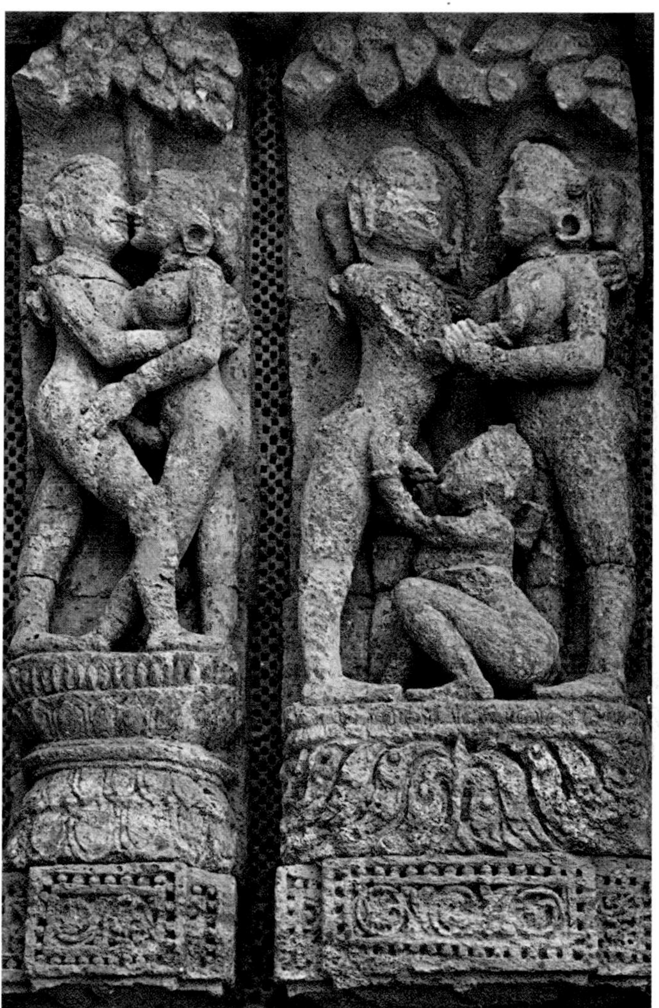

Figure 7.1. Detail of erotic carvings decorating the Surya Hindu Temple at Konark Orissa, India, built in the 13th century CE

Americans, coming from a different background, may be shocked by the use of explicit sexual language in such historical religious contexts. As Thomas Moore notes in his article "Sex (American Style)" and later book *The Soul of Sex,* Americans have issues around sex:

> *The body is our central embarrassment—merely having one, making love with one, or indulging in the human fascination for the sexual body. To all appearances, we'd like to be bodiless, and most of our recent inventions point toward that goal; they encourage us to sit in front of a*

screen and work, play, shop, and meet with old friends electronically. . . . We have yet to discover that sex is not physical love but the love of souls. You don't have to spiritualize sex to make it valuable, because by its very nature sex is a deep act of the interior life and always brings with it a wealth of emotional and spiritual meaning.[3]

Indeed, many yogis, experienced in witnessing their body off the mat as well as on it, note that as their practice of yoga has evolved, their experience of sex has become more satisfying, explorative, and fun.

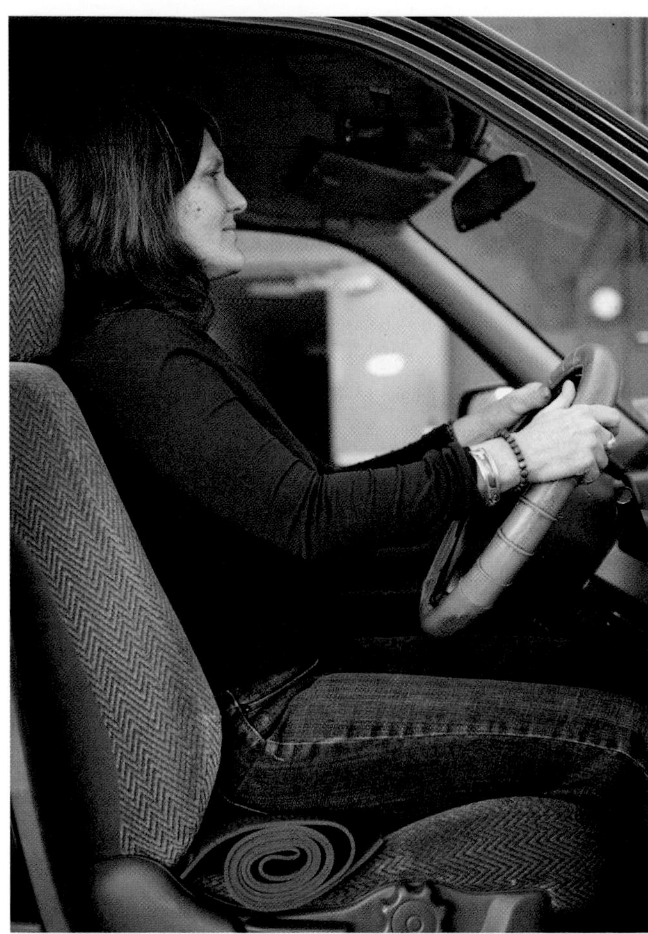

Figure 7.2. Seated against rolled yoga mat in car

YOGA IN A CAR

It is possible to do various types of yoga poses while either driving or parked, depending on the circumstances. When doing yoga in a car, make sure you are not rolling on your sacrum and are instead sitting up on your sitting bones. Since cars aren't designed for yoga practice, you might want to use props, such as a roll under your sitting bones as shown in figure 7.2. Also you can use the headrest to make sure your head isn't reaching forward, straining your neck and shoulders.

One way to practice yoga in a car is to do spinal twists while turning to look behind you before backing out of a parking lot. Just inhale, lengthen your spine, then exhale and twist, first in one direction from the bottom of the spine, pulling in your belly, and then in the opposite direction to be sure you are balanced.

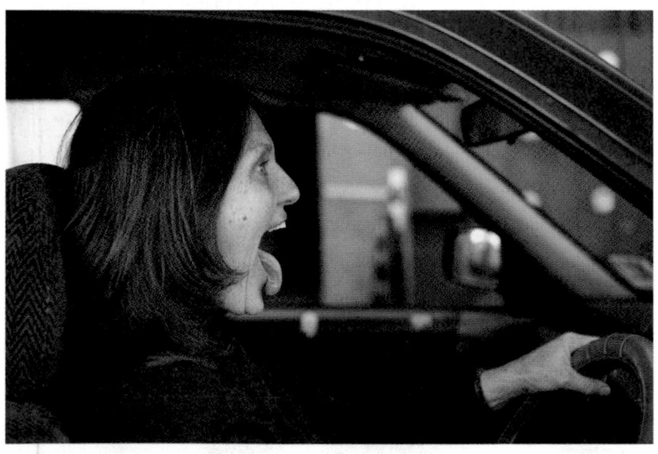

Figure 7.3. Lion Pose in car

Driving is also an ideal time to practice Lion Pose with sound, especially when your jaws have become tight with frustration. At a red light or while in stopped traffic, open your jaw wide, stick out your tongue as far as possible, and make a loud noise (see figure 7.3). When you are out of breath, pause and see how you feel. Then repeat if necessary.

An especially good yoga exercise to help deal with road rage is a game of projecting ideas onto objects to gain increased insight into the true nature of the mind. You can do this by imagining that every car you see is a manifestation of a thought. For example, when a car turns in front of you without signaling, you could tell yourself, *That's the thought I have of constantly changing my mind and not knowing exactly where to go.*

YOGA AT THE COMPUTER

Many variations on yoga poses can be practiced while using a desktop computer. First, consider standing up at the computer at least part of the time, to use your legs as support (see figure 7.4).

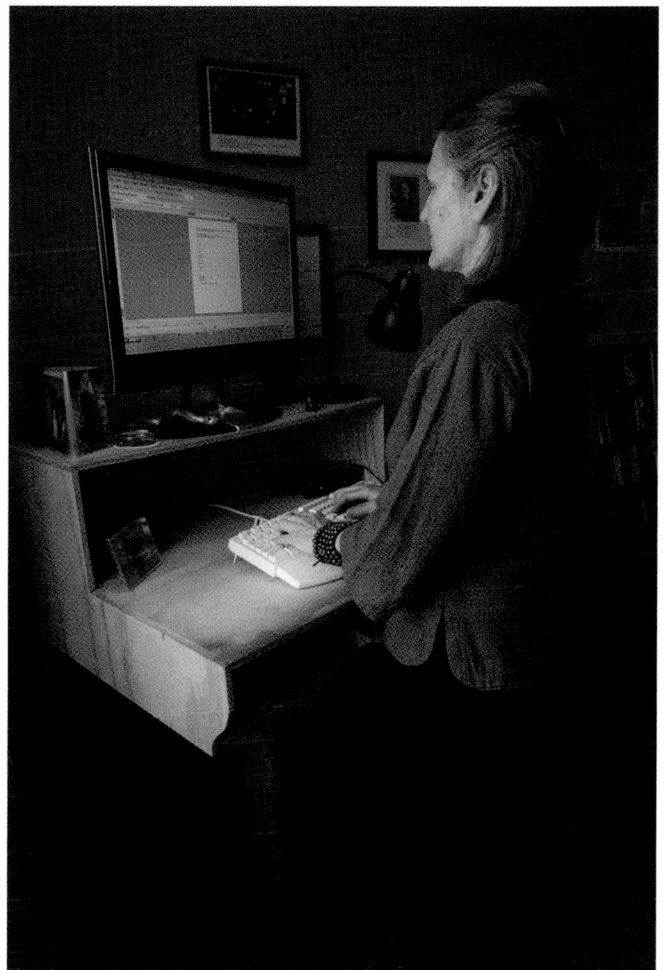

Figure 7.4. Standing at computer

While standing, you can also practice "Desk Dog," as shown in figure 7.5, to lengthen your spine and open your shoulders and hips. To do Desk Dog, put your hands on the desk and stand back from it. Bend your knees and lift your sitting bones up, with your inner thighs rolled toward the floor. Then slowly straighten your arms, letting your heart melt toward the floor. Move your hands wider if there is tension in your shoulders or neck. Take eight to ten long slow breaths. Slowly stand up, close your eyes, and see how you feel.

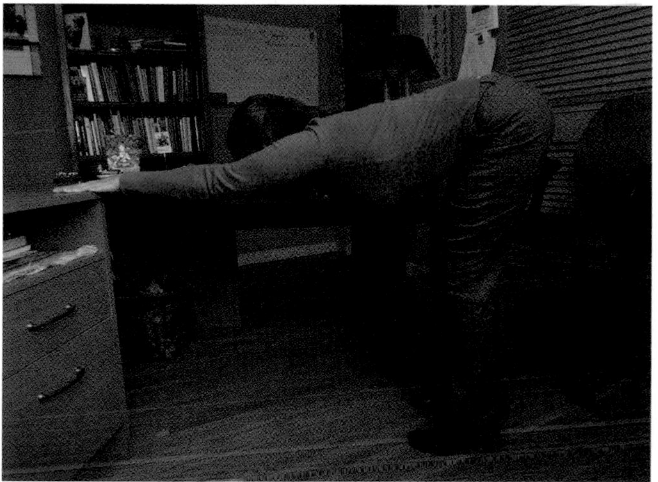

Figure 7.5. "Desk Dog"

While sitting at a computer, take breaks every forty-five minutes to walk around. If you begin to feel fragmented or overwhelmed but don't want to stand up or walk around, simply close your eyes and take several long slow breaths, lifting your root up and feeling your body physically and energetically. You may try practicing sense withdrawal, consciously shutting out the noise in the environment, perhaps even with earplugs, and just listening to your breath. After a few minutes, return to your work and smile.

Another practice you can do at your desk is to transform your view of e-mail. You know from meditating that an important practice is not being reactive to the mind, not taking every thought so seriously that you react. Treating e-mail as you would thoughts, instead of immediately replying or reacting to messages as soon as you receive them, become an observer, distancing yourself from their implications. You could also limit the number of times you check your e-mail each day—or simply refrain from checking it until you've done your meditation practice, then consider how you might respond differently.

YOGA WHILE STANDING

While standing and doing routine tasks, such as waiting in line at the grocery store, the bank, or the post office, washing dishes, talking on the phone, or chatting with a coworker, it is possible to do yoga without anyone noticing. You can do Mountain Pose (figure 6.20, page 142) even if your arms are in soapy water or holding vegetables. Plant your feet firmly on the ground, with your legs engaged and stable, then strongly engage *mula bandha* and let that lift your belly. Keep breathing, and smile as you build strength and connection to your body.

Or suppose you are standing in a slow checkout line at the grocery store and the woman in front of you looks like she'll be a problem. It would be easy in this situation to just grin and bear it, but you have another choice besides reading the celebrity magazines displayed nearby—you can practice Mountain Pose. Breathe and say to yourself: *Everything is exactly as it should be; I have the perfect amount of time and the perfect moment to experience it.* Then, as you breathe and relax, amazingly the world may change as you do. The woman in front of you may smile and initiate a pleasant exchange. Suddenly what was a barrier to your day has enhanced it.

While standing, you can also practice Tree Pose (see figure 7.6). First find Mountain Pose, then keep your eyes on a single point of focus. You might withdraw one of your senses, or your peripheral vision, then lift one leg and put it in a comfortable position, perhaps just below your other knee. Next lift your abdominal core and breathe, counting breaths. Or perhaps look around you and see how to balance as you shift the direction of your gaze. Repeat on the second side.

YOGA WHILE SHOPPING

To ease tension during a shopping spree, yoga can be done in a fitting room or restroom. I discovered the benefits of this while buying dresses for my daughters, Shona, then thirteen years old, and Bella, ten. Usually such an experience caused frustration, as my two independent girls have their own ideas about style, and it isn't unusual for them to spend hours trying on clothes at every appropriate shop in the mall, only to come away empty-handed. On this occasion, there was no wiggle room as Shona's Bat Mitzvah was in two weeks and the girls each needed two dresses with just the right amount of formality, hipness, and comfort.

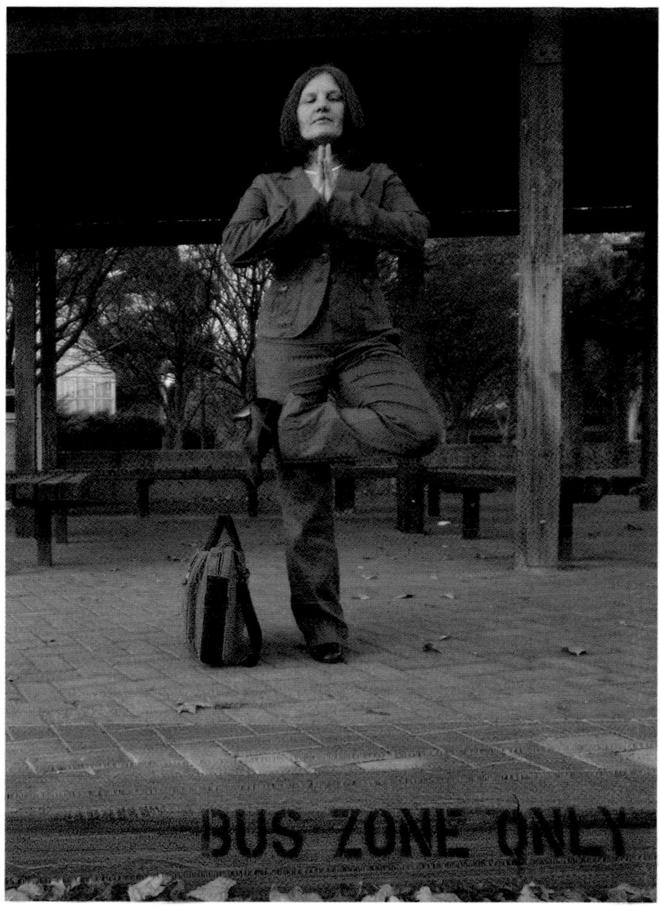

Figure 7.6. Tree Pose at bus stop

So we went to a department store with the largest selection of girls' clothes, and I started picking up dresses and saying, "Look at this. This is great!" The girls would scrunch their faces with repulsion and reply, "Oh yeah, right, Mom, you wear that," or just look at each other and roll their eyes. I could see I was useless as a fashion consultant to my daughters and needed to relax. I lay down on the carpeted floor of the fitting room, put my hips against the wall, brought my legs straight up the wall with flexed feet, rested my arms a few inches from my body with palms up, closed my eyes, and breathed deeply from my belly, even reaching to *mula bandha*. As I replenished my body, mind, and spirit, the world became a beautiful, peaceful place again.

The girls came and went, trying on clothes, asking my opinion only when they already knew what they wanted. They were a bit embarrassed to see their mother doing yoga in that semi-public area, but since no one could actually see me they did not protest much. Bella only sighed and said, "We know, Mom, everything revolves around yoga."

Yes, for me, everything does revolve around yoga. I'm always looking for opportunities to do yoga in my everyday life because no matter how much I do on the mat, it's really the yoga I do off it that impresses me with the transformative value of yoga.

THE UPSIDE OF SQUATTING

Although it's uncommon in the United States, people in many other cultures around the world squat as a comfortable way to relax. Because it opens the hips and lengthens the lower spine, this position feels good physically, as well as making you feel more grounded and connected to the earth—as do many yoga poses.

It can be especially helpful to practice squatting while doing something else. You can squat against a wall for more ease, for example, while taking a telephone call (see figure 7.7) or while watching the news, peeling potatoes, or brushing your teeth. Be sure to look for the oppositional energy so that as your hips descend you lift the root and low belly. If you feel sensation in the knees, move up high enough to eliminate it.

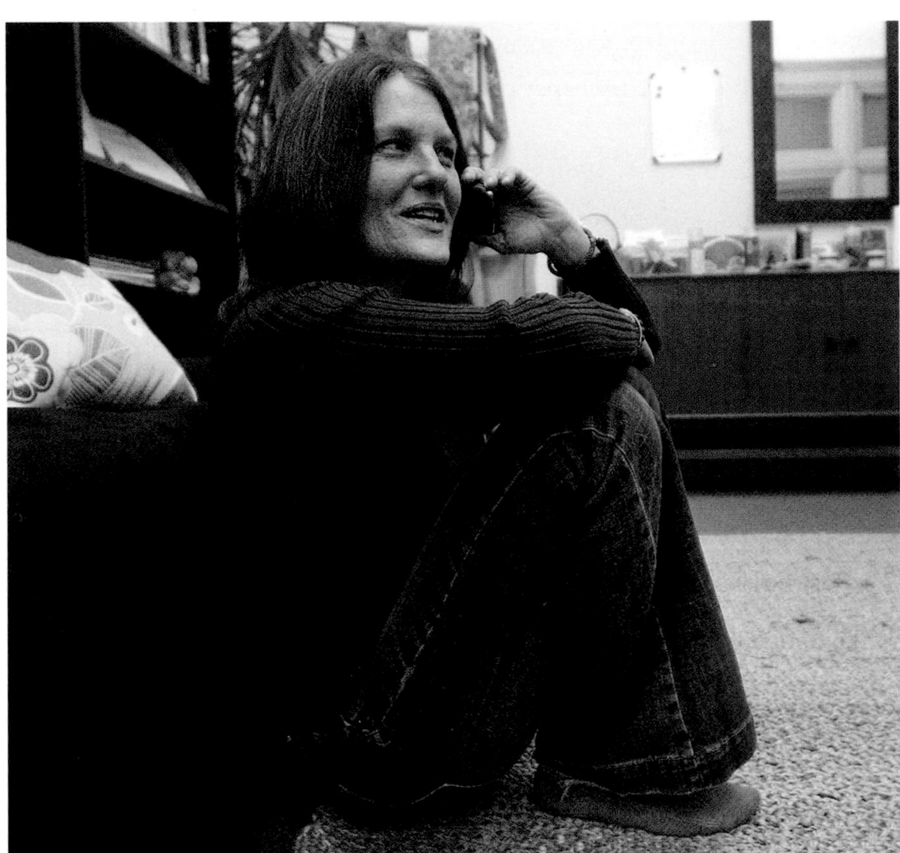

Figure 7.7. Squatting while on the phone

STEALTH YOGA

When you are in a place where any visible yoga posture would feel obtrusive yet you must wait while uncomfortable or bored, you can always practice "stealth yoga," which is an invisible but powerful form of yoga that can be done in daily life. One type of stealth yoga is to work with the soft palate. Just move your tongue behind your upper teeth and slide it along the roof of your mouth to the soft palate. Next, release your tongue down and visualize your soft palate opening like a parachute, becoming softer and more expansive. Then imagine your face relaxing, your jaw slackening, your head becoming lighter on your neck. One yoga student described such a scene in the following way:

> *I was sitting in the waiting room of my surgeon's office. I knew I was going to be called in at some point and the doctor would perform some really painful and invasive postoperative procedures on me. At first I was feeling anxious. Then I remembered the soft palate practice. I felt the soft palate with my tongue and immediately imagined my entire face softening, feeling loose and heavy. Soon my whole body was relaxed, and by the time they called me in I had lost the tension in my body and mind.*

Breathwork is another type of stealth yoga that can be done to avoid reacting negatively and instead gain a positive outlook. For example, a yoga teacher realized her purse had been stolen just before students arrived for class. This was unnerving, especially as she had been saving for a trip and there was a sizable amount of cash in it. Nonetheless, she wanted to be present with her students and not ruin their experience of yoga. So she practiced stealth yoga: she breathed up and down her spine slowly, felt her soft palate expand, and then honestly hoped that whoever got the money used it to generate happiness in their life. Finally, she calmly shared the incident with the students and even managed to find humor in the situation, telling them she hated the way she looked in her driver's license picture and could now get a new one.

After class, a number of the students told her how impressed they were that she could remain so composed after the theft. Some of them subsequently gave her money to replace what had been stolen, as they wanted her to go ahead with her plans. In the end, she felt so supported by them that she decided the theft's purpose had been to impress upon her the value of yoga and community.

THE NONVIOLENT COMMUNICATION MODEL

A tool helpful for implementing the important yogic principle of nonviolence in daily life is a model for creating peace and harmony developed by Marshall Rosenberg called Nonviolent Communication (NVC),[4] or compassionate communication. Its purpose is to enhance our ability to

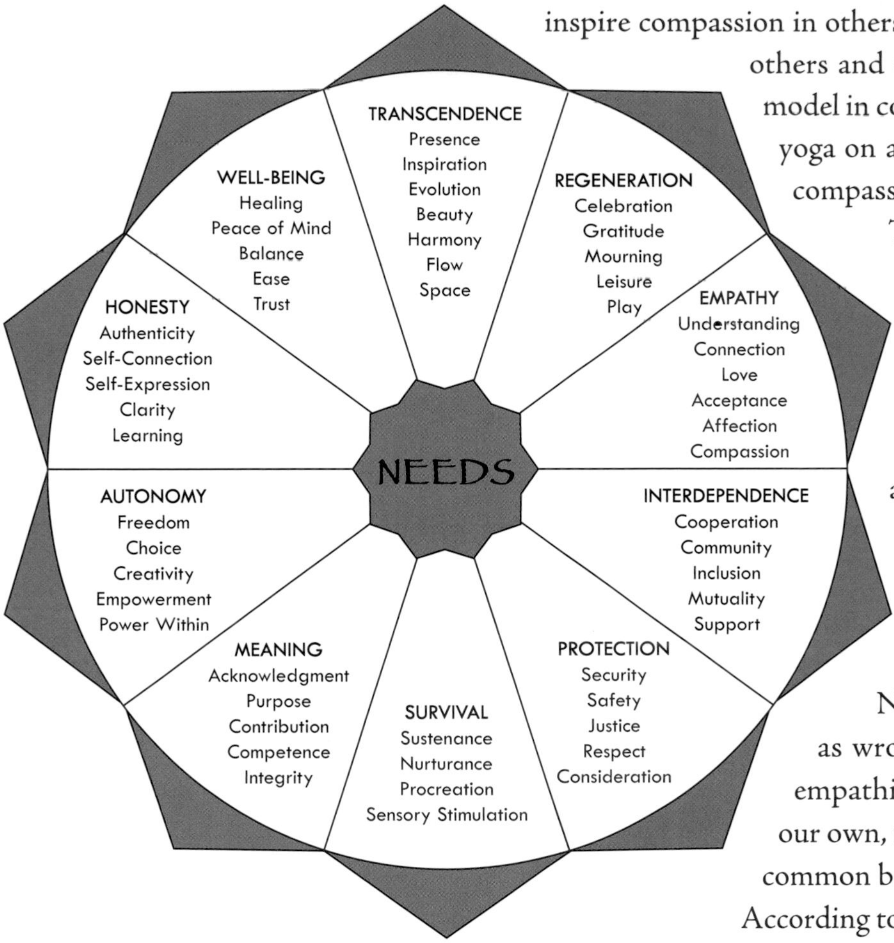

Figure 7.8. Basic human needs in Nonviolent Communication model

inspire compassion in others and to respond compassionately to others and to ourselves. We can use the NVC model in conjunction with the first two limbs of yoga on a daily basis to practice truthfulness, compassion, and peaceful communication.

The NVC model helps by reframing how we express ourselves and hear others by focusing on what we are observing, feeling, needing, and requesting so we can make conscious choices about how we will respond and behave. This approach to communication regards the motivation for action as compassion rather than fear, guilt, shame, blame, coercion, or punishment. In the NVC model, rather than seeing others as wrong, guilty, or blameworthy we look empathically for their underlying needs and our own, then connect with them based on our common bond of trying to satisfy basic needs.

According to the NVC model, we all have universal basic needs, as illustrated in figure 7.8. Feelings arise when our needs are either satisfied, making us feel fulfilled, or not met, making us feel unfulfilled. We often cover up our feelings (based in the body) with thinking (based in the mind), however, which keeps us unaware of them. Yoga helps us realize this as we practice observing our mind and feelings.

Sometimes our difficulty in identifying what we feel can interfere with our ability to understand our needs and those of others. Consequently, the NVC model provides lists (see tables 7.1 and 7.2) that can help us pinpoint our feelings and corresponding needs so we can communicate with others more nonviolently and compassionately.

This model can help us embody the foundations of yoga in our personal and professional relationships. For me, it was very useful in dealing with a teacher who was giving classes at my yoga studio. The teacher, who had just moved to town, had expressed enthusiasm for teaching a class and workshop at my studio. She signed a contract, and her class and workshop were put on the schedule and the Web site. After a month, however,

Affectionate
compassionate
friendly
loving
openhearted
sympathetic
tender
warm

Confident
empowered
open
proud
safe
secure

Engaged
absorbed
alert
curious
enchanted
engrossed
entranced
fascinated
interested
intrigued
involved
spellbound
stimulated

Excited
animated
ardent
aroused
astonished
dazzled
eager
energetic
enthusiastic
giddy
invigorated
lively
passionate
surprised
vibrant

Exhilarated
blissful
ecstatic
elated
enthralled
exuberant
radiant
rapturous
thrilled

Grateful
appreciative
moved
thankful
touched

Hopeful
encouraged
expectant
optimistic

Inspired
amazed
awed
enchanted

Joyful
amused
delighted
glad
happy
jubilant
pleased
tickled

Peaceful
calm
centered
clearheaded
comfortable
content
equanimous
fulfilled
mellow
quiet
relaxed
relieved
satisfied
serene
still
tranquil
trusting

Refreshed
enlivened
rejuvenated
renewed
rested
restored
revived

TABLE 7.1. A list of feelings people have when their needs are satisfied.

she realized the drive from her home was too far, given the increased gas prices, and class attendance wasn't as high as she'd hoped, although we had discussed the time it might take for the community to get to know her and enroll in greater numbers. She also saw that her real desire was to open a private office and see clients individually.

At first I was disappointed since she'd signed a contract, but I could see her heart wasn't in it. So I considered what my needs and hers were,

Afraid

- apprehensive
- dreading
- foreboding
- frightened
- mistrustful
- panicked
- petrified
- scared
- suspicious
- terrified
- wary
- worried

Angry

- enraged
- furious
- incensed
- indignant
- irate
- livid
- outraged
- resentful

Annoyed

- aggravated
- dismayed
- disgruntled
- displeased
- exasperated
- frustrated
- impatient
- irked
- irritated

Averse

- appalled
- contemptuous
- disgusted
- disapproving
- hateful
- horrified
- hostile
- repulsed

Confused

- ambivalent
- baffled
- bewildered
- dazed
- hesitant
- lost
- mystified
- perplexed
- puzzled
- torn

Disconnected

- alienated
- aloof
- apathetic
- bored
- cold
- detached
- distant
- distracted
- indifferent
- numb
- removed
- uninterested
- withdrawn

Disquieted

- agitated
- alarmed
- discombobulated
- disconcerted
- disturbed
- perturbed
- rattled
- restless
- shocked
- startled
- surprised
- troubled
- turbulent
- uncomfortable
- uneasy
- unnerved
- unsettled
- upset

Embarrassed

- ashamed
- chagrined
- flustered
- guilty
- mortified
- self-conscious

Fatigued

- beat
- burned out
- depleted
- exhausted
- lethargic
- listless
- sleepy
- tired
- weary
- worn out

Pained

- agonized
- anguished
- bereaved
- devastated
- grieving
- heartbroken
- hurt
- lonely
- miserable
- regretful
- remorseful

Sad

- dejected
- depressed
- despairing
- despondent
- disappointed
- discouraged
- disheartened
- forlorn
- gloomy
- heavyhearted
- hopeless
- melancholic
- unhappy
- wretched

Tense

- anxious
- cranky
- distraught
- distressed
- edgy
- fidgety
- frazzled
- irritable
- jittery
- nervous
- overwhelmed
- restless
- stressed out

Vulnerable

- fragile
- guarded
- helpless
- insecure
- leery
- reserved
- sensitive
- shaky

Yearning

- envious
- jealous
- longing
- nostalgic
- pining
- wistful

TABLE 7.2. A list of feelings people have when their needs are not satisfied.

then arranged for a discussion, in which I explained: "I want you to know that my underlying desire is to create an environment of mutual respect and dignity and to treat teachers and students with respect and dignity. That relationship is most important to me, more so than money. I look for mutual cooperation and fun in my relations at the studio. I know how talented you are, what a gift your teaching is, and how much you also share love of community and yoga."

The teacher immediately agreed and complimented the studio and students. The resulting sense of connection and goodwill we shared eased the communication that followed, when I said: "I know you have discovered that it doesn't work for you to drive to the studio, and I understand you were new in town when you made the commitment. So even though you signed a contract I'm willing to let that go. I realize you've opened your own office to work privately with clients, and I know you'll help many people. How about we just cancel the classes and workshop at the studio. If someone calls looking for what you have to offer, I will send them your way. Would you be willing to give me a percentage of fees from any clients I send to you?"

The teacher was happy to do that and to continue our relationship in a positive way. She even stopped by the studio and brought me a lovely note and small gift as a token of her goodwill.

In most circumstances in life, when we understand what our needs are and truly consider those of others before interacting with them, we can figure out how to satisfy both parties. The NVC model can help us learn such skills. Groups teaching and practicing NVC can be found in many towns.

YOGIC FOOD

Yoga encourages us to eat with awareness and conscience. What, when, and how much we eat are very important concerns for yogis. We believe that the food we eat plays a large role in determining our degree of health and happiness. For an example of how the ancient Upanishads address ways in which food produces earthly creatures, see "Sages Say."

Individuals must decide for themselves what role yogic philosophy might play in their diet. Our decisions about how we eat can be well informed by the first principle of yoga, nonviolence. This could mean various things, from choosing not to kill animals for food to making sure

refine as you teach. And when problems arise, you can refer back to your statement to maintain stability and clarity. Following is an example of a statement of purpose for teaching yoga:

> *I teach yoga to help students discover their own unique beauty and gift to the world, honoring individuals as part of the diverse whole of humanity. I aim to create an environment that is welcoming and safe for all students. I am committed to a lifetime of learning and skill development through continual personal exploration. I am dedicated to the belief that healing and transformation are possible for us all. Yoga is the ultimate playground, a place to explore our bodies, hearts, and minds, to push and move our edges; and especially, to have fun.*
>
> *I look for success, not just in terms of financial viability but also in the quality of my teaching, the way I show respect for students and teachers and the human spirit, and my overall commitment to the greater community.*

Once you have clarity of intention, the next step is to find the right training. Today there are many teacher training programs around the country. Some are residential programs where you live for a period, programs where you can go to exotic places to study, intensive two- and three-week programs, and programs offered in local towns that you can attend on weekends.[3] You may want to choose the training that is most affordable and easiest to attend; on the other hand, you may want to take time away from your regular life and immerse yourself in yoga. The effort you put into the training will always affect the results you receive, but be sure to investigate the main teachers and their styles to see if they suit your preferences.

After you have trained and fulfilled the requirements for teaching yoga, you can apply for Registered Teacher Status with the Yoga Alliance, a national organization that sets minimum educational standards and requirements for teachers and schools offering training.[4] You can teach without the Registered Teacher Status, but it is becoming required in more and more yoga class locations.

You also need to prepare an ethical code of conduct document that reflects the underlying philosophy of yoga and your teaching approach. The Yoga Alliance requires the following pledge of its teachers:

As a Registrant of Yoga Alliance and as a Registered Yoga Teacher (RYT) or representative of a Registered Yoga School (RYS), I agree to uphold the ethical goals set forth in the following Code of Conduct:

1. Uphold the integrity of my vocation by conducting myself in a professional and conscientious manner.
2. Acknowledge the limitations of my skills and scope of practice and, where appropriate, refer students to seek alternative instruction, advice, treatment, or direction.
3. Create and maintain a safe, clean, and comfortable environment for the practice of yoga.
4. Encourage diversity actively by respecting all students regardless of age, physical limitations, race, creed, gender, ethnicity, religion affiliation, or sexual orientation.
5. Respect the rights, dignity, and privacy of all students.
6. Avoid words and actions that constitute sexual harassment.
7. Adhere to the traditional yogic principles as written in the Yamas and Niyamas.
8. Follow all local government and national laws that pertain to my yoga teaching and business.[5]

The Yoga Alliance states: Our mission is to lead the yoga community, set standards, foster integrity, provide resources, and uphold the teachings of yoga. We do not claim to represent yoga in the United States, but do represent our registrants and support all yoga teachers, whether or not registered with our organization.

When a school has met the standards of the Yoga Alliance, it is awarded the Registered Yoga School (RYS) status. Students can earn two levels of training: 200-hour Registered Teacher Status and 500-hour Registered Teacher Status.

You can begin by taking the 200-hour RYT training and teach at that level. If you want to continue your study, you can add the 500-hour level by taking a 300-hour level, offered at many schools. It may be most useful to take the 200-hour training and then teach for a while before doing additional training, as you will have new insights and questions based on your experience.

Both 200 and 500 RYT training include time in each of these categories. "Techniques Training/Practice" includes asanas, *pranayamas*, *kriyas*, chanting, mantra, meditation, and other traditional yoga techniques. "Teaching Methodology" includes principles of demonstration, observation, assisting/correcting, instruction, teaching styles, qualities of a teacher, the student's process of learning, and business aspects of teaching yoga. "Anatomy & Physiology, Yoga Philosophy/Lifestyle, and Ethics for Yoga Teachers Practicum" includes practice teaching, observing others teaching, and giving and receiving feedback.

Sages Say

"Many of my students have wrist problems, such as weakness and carpal tunnel syndrome. Do you have any ideas for strengthening wrists?"

—*Betty*

Dear Betty,

Clearing wrist problems is not only a matter of strengthening the wrists; a high percentage of wrist problems have their origin in shoulder misalignments, too. The first thing to do is to open and balance the shoulders through a variety of poses performed with good alignment.

The next key therapeutic step for the wrists is to strengthen the flexor muscles of the forearms (the muscles on the underside of the forearm). Do this through isometric actions in basic positions, while bearing light weight on your hands. It is essential to place your hands on a firm surface, with the four corners of each palm anchored on the firm surface, shoulder-width apart; also make sure the creases of your wrists form a straight line, and your fingers and thumbs are evenly spread.

To build isometric strength in the flexor muscles, claw your hand on the firm surface so that the tips of your fingers and the four corners of your palms press down, and draw back toward your shoulders. Keeping your finger pads down, bend your fingers slightly and lift the center of your palms up without lifting the four corners of the palms. The flexor muscles should firm as you attempt to move the head of your arm bone backward in relationship to your torso.

It is important to note that wrist problems will be aggravated if:

- Your weight falls to the outside of your hands.
- Your index finger knuckle lifts away from the foundation.
- Your weight collapses to the heel of your palm.

Basic positions include an L-pose with hands on a tabletop; Child's Pose with the arms extended forward; bearing your weight on all fours with hands in front of your shoulders; and Adho Mukha Svanasana (Downward Facing Dog).

Start with poses that bear less weight, then increase the weight on your wrists as you are able to maintain good alignment and proper muscular action. With regular therapeutic asana practice, carpal tunnel syndrome and other common wrist issues can usually be eliminated.[6]

—*John Friend*

Once you are teaching yoga, you may still need a mentor to address concerns that may come up in your classes. As preparation for this, when you are searching for a teacher training school, ask if teachers will continue to be available for mentoring after you graduate. Also, online communities serve as forums for answering questions and providing instruction. For an example of an online exchange via the *Yoga Journal* Web site, see "Sages Say."

When teaching, it is important not to overwhelm students with instructions but to give enough so they can experience a pose from inside the body, using words to communicate sensation and awareness. Because there are many possible instructions for each pose, it is advisable to identify three points you would like to teach and perhaps add an additional focus appropriate to the skill level of a class. For example, you may want to emphasize the shoulder placement because a number of students mentioned tense shoulders when you checked in with them at the beginning of class. Instructions should have a reference point for action, such as pressing the feet toward the floor as you lift the thighs up toward the waist.

Ashtanga Limbs	Teaching Application
Yama	
Ahimsa—nonviolence, love	Teaching students not to push into pain but to respect their edges and love themselves
Satya—truth	Teaching students to be truthful with themselves in their poses; instructing students honestly, neither inflating nor deflating them with kindness
Asteya—nonstealing, generosity, honesty	Never stealing a student's effort by diminishing them in any way
Brahmacharya—boundaries, protection of creative life forces	Respecting the student-teacher relationship and never taking advantage of a student's love of yoga and you as a teacher to indulge in a romantic relationship
Aparigraha—nongrasping; awareness of abundance, fulfillment	Releasing expectations of what students or your teaching plan should do, teaching in the moment what each student requires
Niyama	
Sauca—simplicity, cleanliness, purity	Presenting yourself in a clean and professional manner; teaching students to treat the environment with respect and care, including putting props away with mindfulness

TABLE 8.1

While teaching yoga, you can apply experiences you have gleaned from work, family, or relationships. For example, my teaching is informed by my previous experiences in corporate and university teaching. I developed and directed a program at Arthur Andersen & Co. to prepare entry-level staff for their new management responsibilities. I also taught large undergraduate classes with diverse students from farms in Indiana and the plains of China. In all situations, I learned how to teach using multiple methods, words, pictures, and hands-on practice. These skills help me teach yoga because yoga students also vary in age, experience, body awareness, and openness to practicing this discipline.

Santosha—contentment	Teaching students to be content and pleased with poses as they are able to currently do them
Tapas—self-discipline, fire	Encouraging students to stay in poses as a means of building discipline rather than reacting to the mind's messages to stop; exhibiting passion for practice, to inspire students
Svadhyaya—self-study, study	Bringing in sacred yogic texts to teach the wisdom of the day's practice, and encouraging students to study
Isvara-pranidhana—devotion and surrender	Reminding students that they can practice yoga and find support, that they can surrender to a higher power rather than trying to control all aspects of their lives
Asana	Teaching other limbs of yoga through poses, understanding alignment principles, basic anatomy, and oppositional energies
Pranayama	Introducing breathing techniques at the beginning or end of an asana class, or suggesting their use during poses, such as recommending *kapala bhati* during a backbend
Pratyahara	Teaching withdrawal of the senses by asking students not to look at others, having them use earplugs for part of the class, during a special sequence of poses, such as Sun Salutation
Dharana **Dhyana** **Samadhi**	Having students direct their attention to a specific point on the wall or ceiling during a pose, concentrate intently, then perhaps slide spontaneously to ecstasy

TABLE 8.1 CONTINUED

TEACHING SPECIFIC POSES

Learning the best ways to make specific adjustments in classes, whether with more instructions or a demonstration, takes forethought and practice. Some schools of yoga advise making adjustments that cause the body to feel it is being manipulated by a strong force. Other schools don't suggest any hands-on adjustments, while still others propose lightly touching students

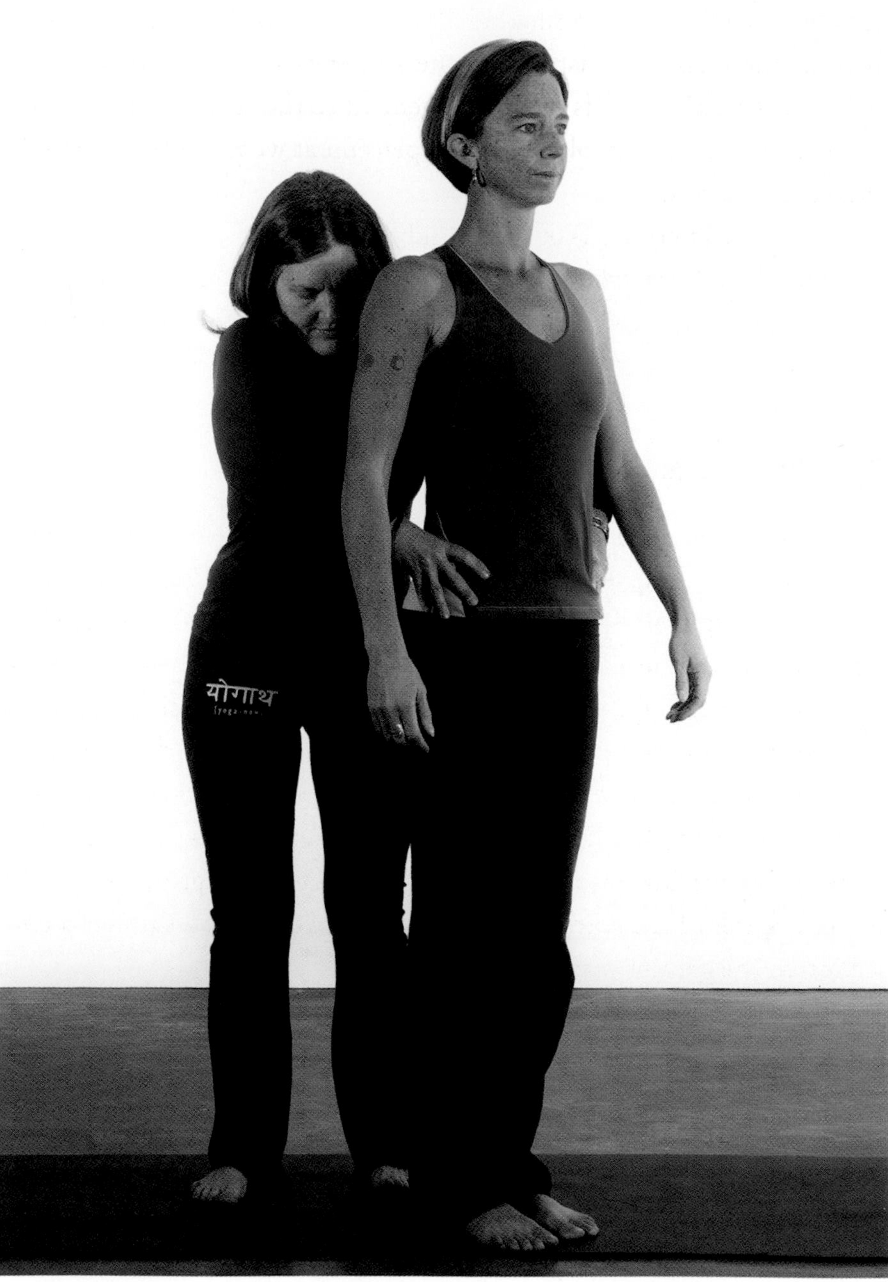

Figure 8.2. Encouraging downward pressure on hips for Mountain Pose

to encourage a flow of energy. Over time I have found that for me the most effective adjustments—those that my students consider helpful—entail asking them to perceive a potential transformation in the part of the body under consideration, perhaps adding a physical adjustment. Students who observe an improvement are much more likely to remember it.

Whatever methods you decide to use in making adjustments, be sure to arrive at them with respect for the students. Always prepare by envisioning your students as beautiful, complex human beings, and not an aggregate of bones and muscles. Many times, the best way to inspire an adjustment isn't by instructing the student to change a pose but by smiling or speaking words of encouragement so the student gains greater confidence. In focusing solely on body placement we risk overlooking the person for the pose.

Below are descriptions of specific adjustments and common issues for each pose described in chapter 6. Consider them a starting point for teaching, while remembering that students have their own inner gurus and that learning from the students' experience is as important as instructing them.

Standing Poses

Show students where the hips are pointing to help them understand instructions for each pose. Have the students find their hip points, noting that in Mountain and Warrior I poses they are facing toward the short end of the mat, while in Triangle Pose they are facing toward the long side of the mat. Encourage students to feel the power of standing poses and imagine their own strength manifesting in whatever way they currently need. Often having students focus on the feet helps establish grounding. Asking students to feel the four continents of connection of the feet (ball mount of big toe, little toe, inner heel, outer heel) and to grow roots down into the center of the earth metaphysically moves students to feel a connection to the greater whole.

Mountain Pose

Students practicing this pose (figure 8.2) often have their knees hyperextended. For an adjustment, have them put even pressure on the hips and feel their body weight moving from the waist down toward the floor as they lift their core and spine up toward the heavens.

Warrior I Pose

When students in this pose (figure 8.3) have their leg extending back rather than facing forward, consider advising them to lift their back heel or make their leg stance wider and shorter. An adjustment for students who are not keeping their front knee moving toward the middle of the foot, just over the ankle, might be to provide hand pressure to encourage their knee to assume the correct alignment or to encourage their shoulders to relax

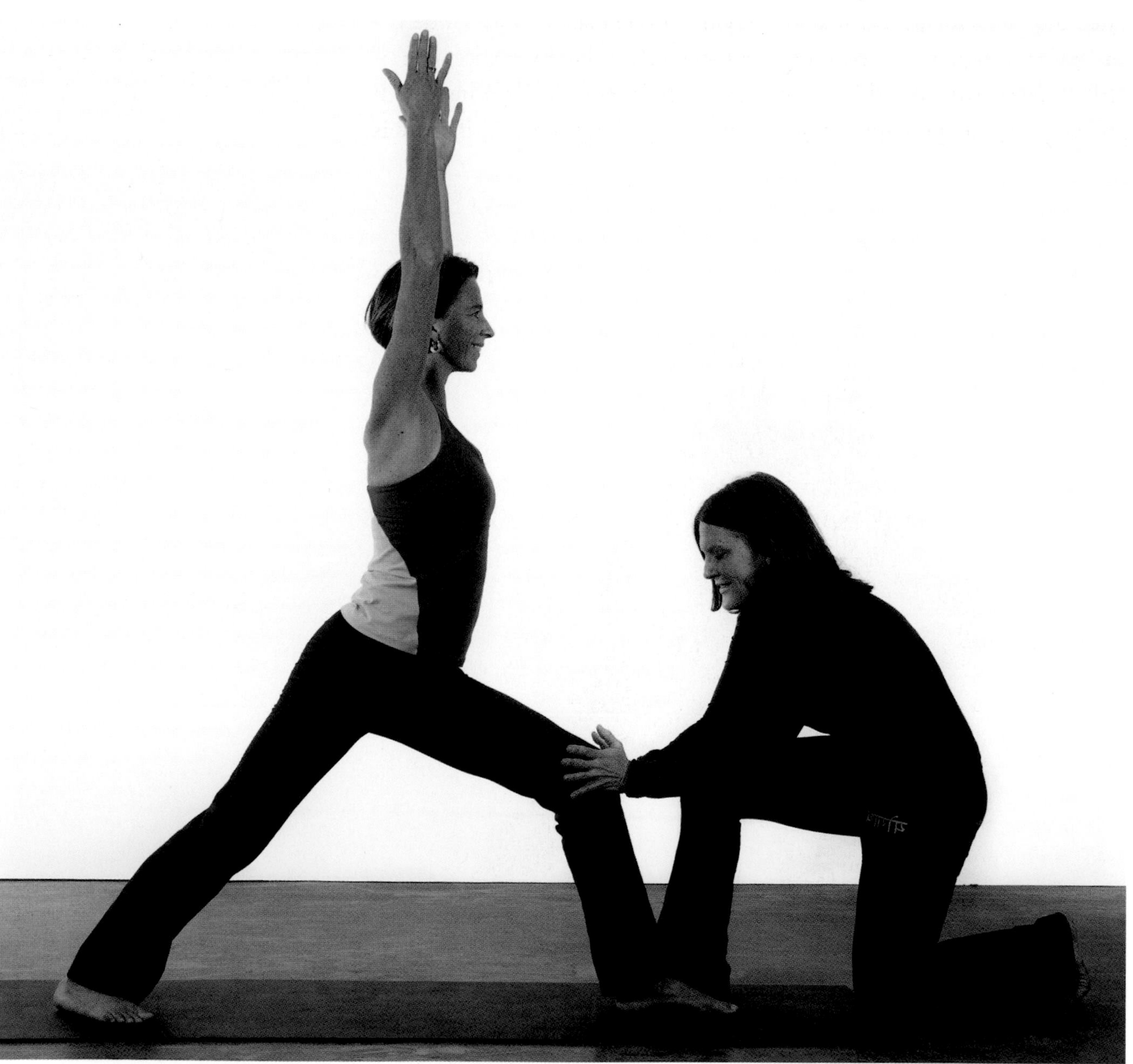

Figure 8.3. Aligning front knee toward outer edge of foot for Warrior Pose

with a featherlike or firm touch, depending on the student. To all students in this pose you might talk about Arjuna, the warrior in the Bhagavad Gita, reminding them that we are warriors for our true purpose on earth.

Triangle Pose

Students often reach down so low in Triangle Pose (figure 8.4) that the body folds forward instead of staying in one plane. This can be adjusted by bringing the hand up on a block or on the body while externally rotating the front thigh. Suggest that students move their head with the entire spine, perhaps looking down and tucking the chin if there is

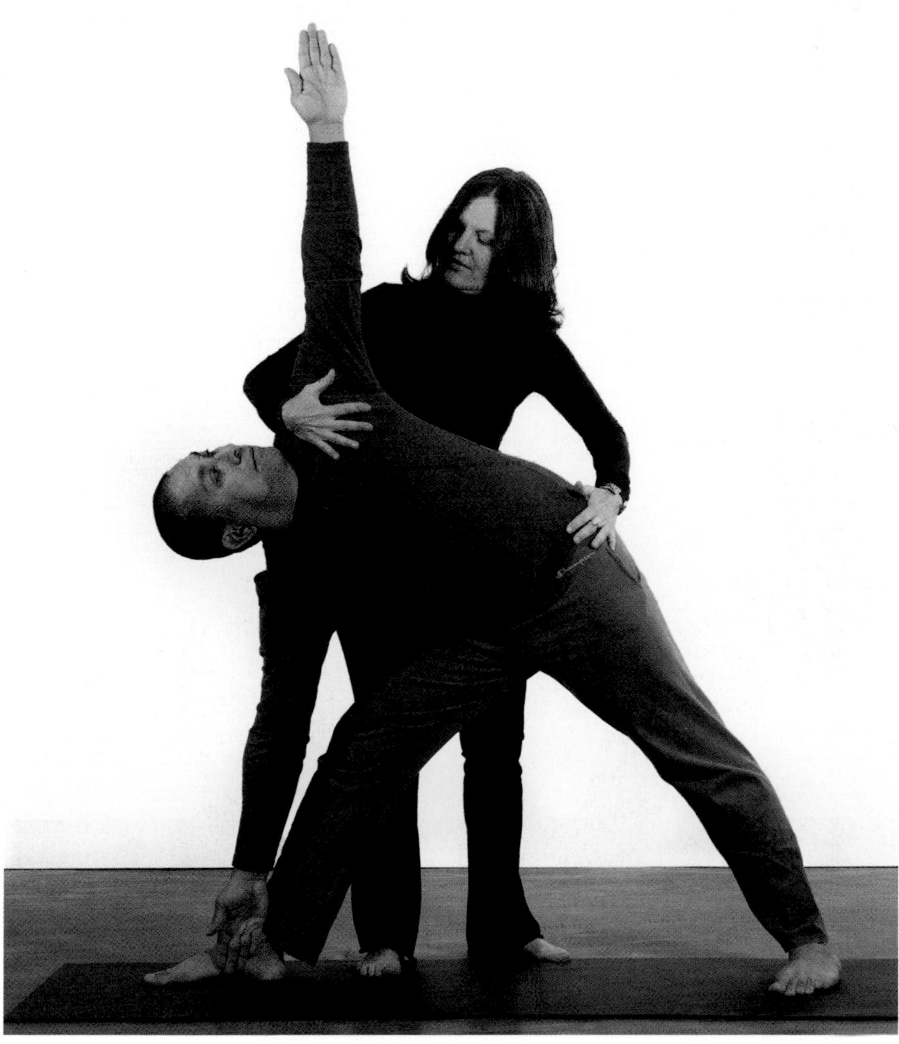

Figure 8.4. Adjusting Triangle Pose from behind

sensation in the neck. Another adjustment is to stand behind the student and, on the exhale, gently help the rib cage rotate toward the sky.

Downward Facing Dog Pose

Beginning students working on this pose (figure 8.5) often struggle with getting their weight back on their legs and off the wrists. A helpful adjustment is bending the knees and shifting the sitting bones up, as well as energetically lifting the wrists. Another good adjustment is to press the hips back either from the front or the back, or use a strap from the back and lean away from the student.

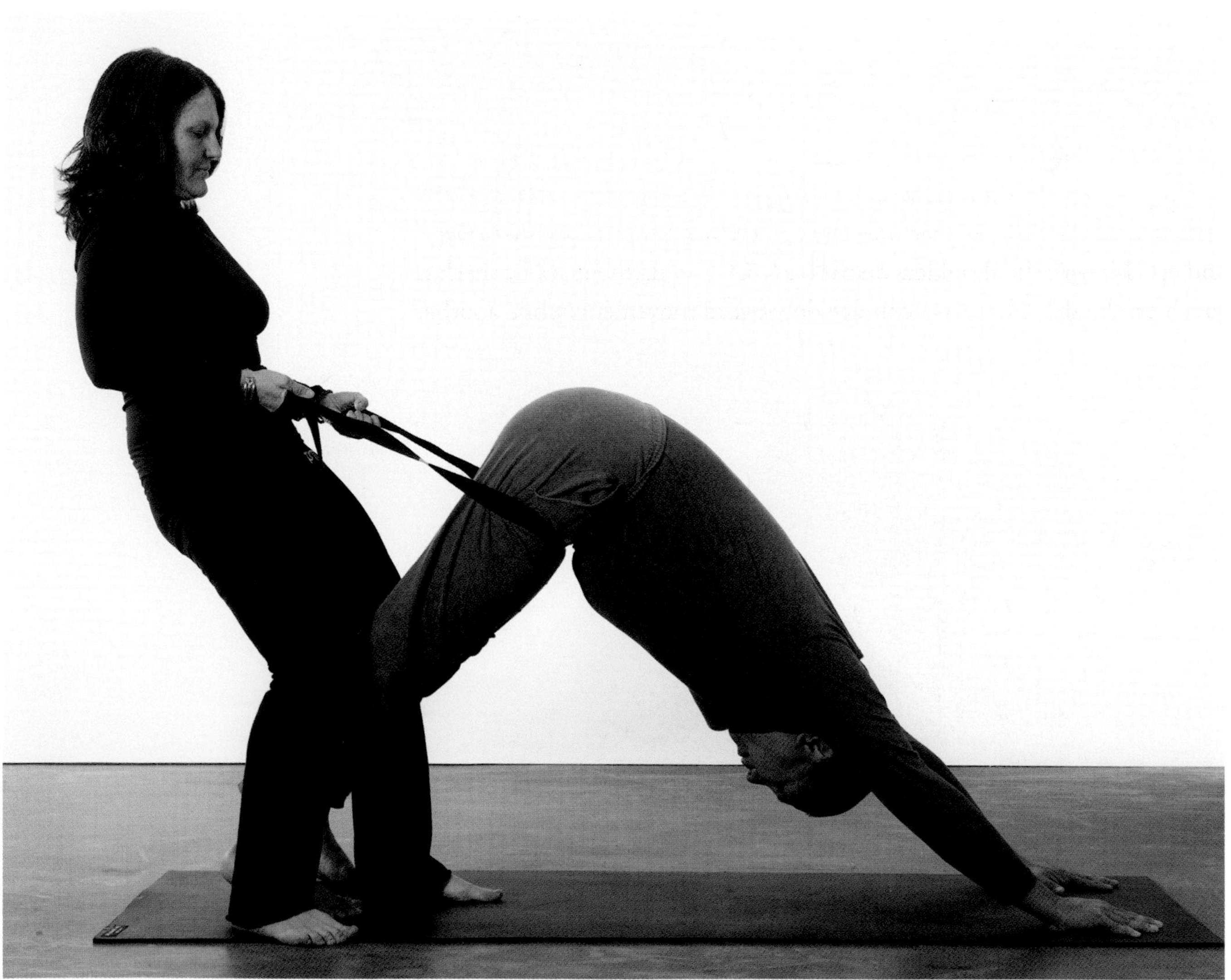

Figure 8.5. Shifting energy and weight back with strap for Downward Facing Dog Pose

Backbends

It can be helpful to have students palpate their sternum, or breastbone, before practicing backbends so they have a tactile sense of what you are asking them to move when you instruct them to curl the sternum forward, thereby opening the spine. Have students find their lower front rib cage and touch the middle spot, called the ziphoid process, then feel the sternum all the way up to the top (see figure 8.6), making them aware that in the back body, the mid-spine, or thoracic spine, curves as well, but it is harder to feel. Additionally, since backbends are often scary and difficult for students, to inspire practice of them point out how they can fix all that has collapsed forward during the day and refresh the spirit.

Cobra Pose

Students often mistake this horizontal backbend (figure 8.7) for a big pivotal lift from the low back instead of a forward curling of the sternum, with shoulders lifted. Suggest that students come down lower and slide forward and up a bit with the shoulders on the back. One adjustment is a featherlike touch on the shoulders to encourage downward movement, while another

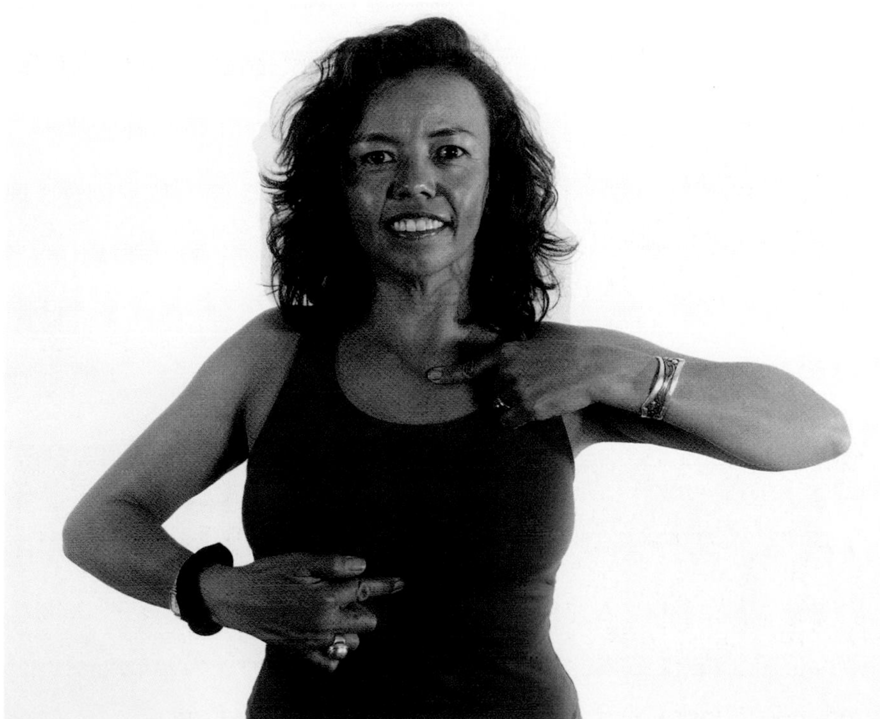

Figure 8.6. Palpating top and bottom of sternum for backbends

is a firmer touch to put weight on the sacrum and move it toward the feet as students lift and curl the sternum forward and up. Also, you might point out how graceful a snake is as it slithers across the ground and see if students can feel that same gracefulness as they curl their sternums up.

Camel Pose

Students may experience low back pain or other negative sensation in this pose (figure 8.8) if their hips move back and there is too much pressure on the low back. As a precaution, suggest that they lift themselves up (with their hands on blocks or the back of the waist) and move the hips forward. A very helpful adjustment is to have students face a wall, pressing the hips toward the wall as the sternum peels away from the wall. To offer further support, press down on the sacrum as students lift the sternum up. Additionally, you can ask students to contemplate the camel's ability to survive a long time by storing water and how they could "store," or maintain, what they need to thrive.

Figure 8.7.
Supporting shoulders in Cobra Pose

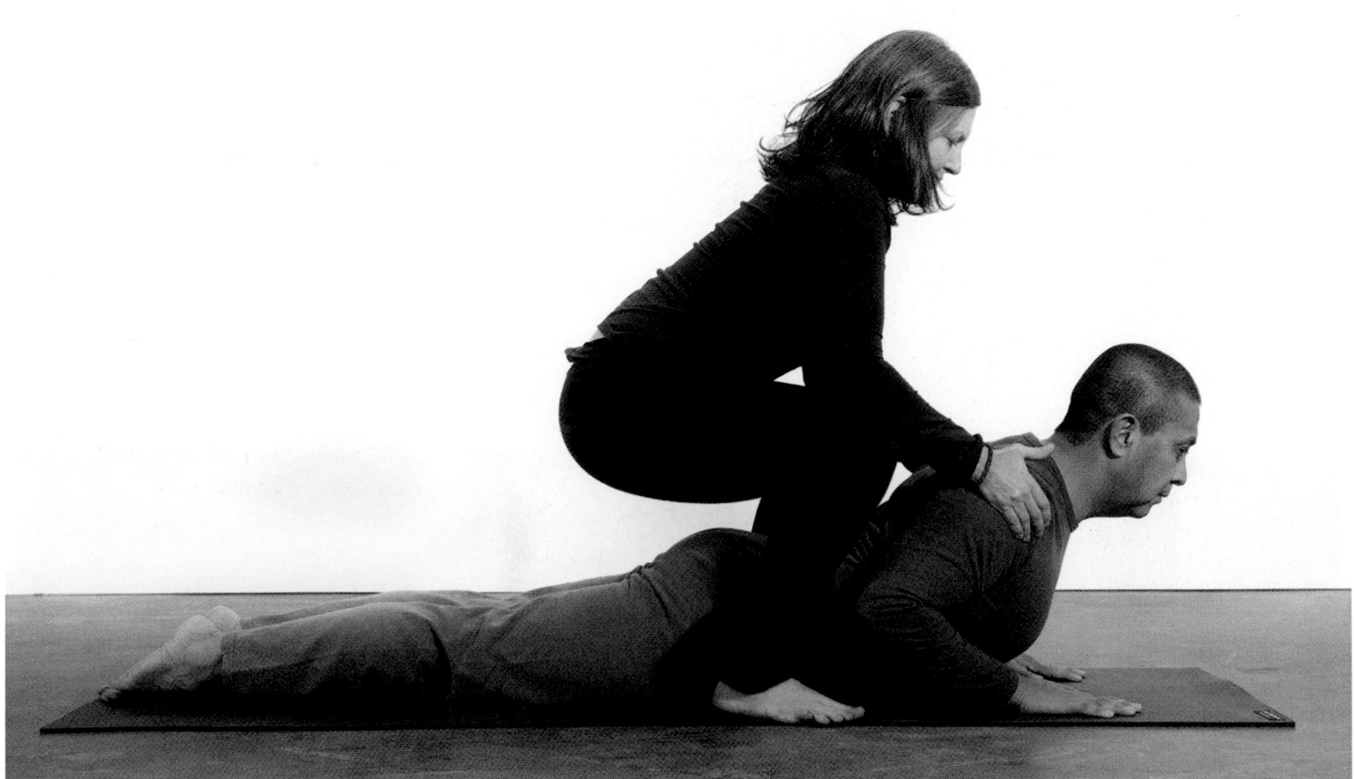

Upward Bow Pose

When doing this pose (figure 8.9), students commonly let their elbows roll out to the side as they prepare to lift their body off the floor. To prevent this, suggest that there is a string between the elbows, keeping them moving toward each other as their hands are set on the floor. Adjustments include placing blocks by the wall for the hands, to reduce pressure on the wrists; making a featherlike motion to encourage the inner

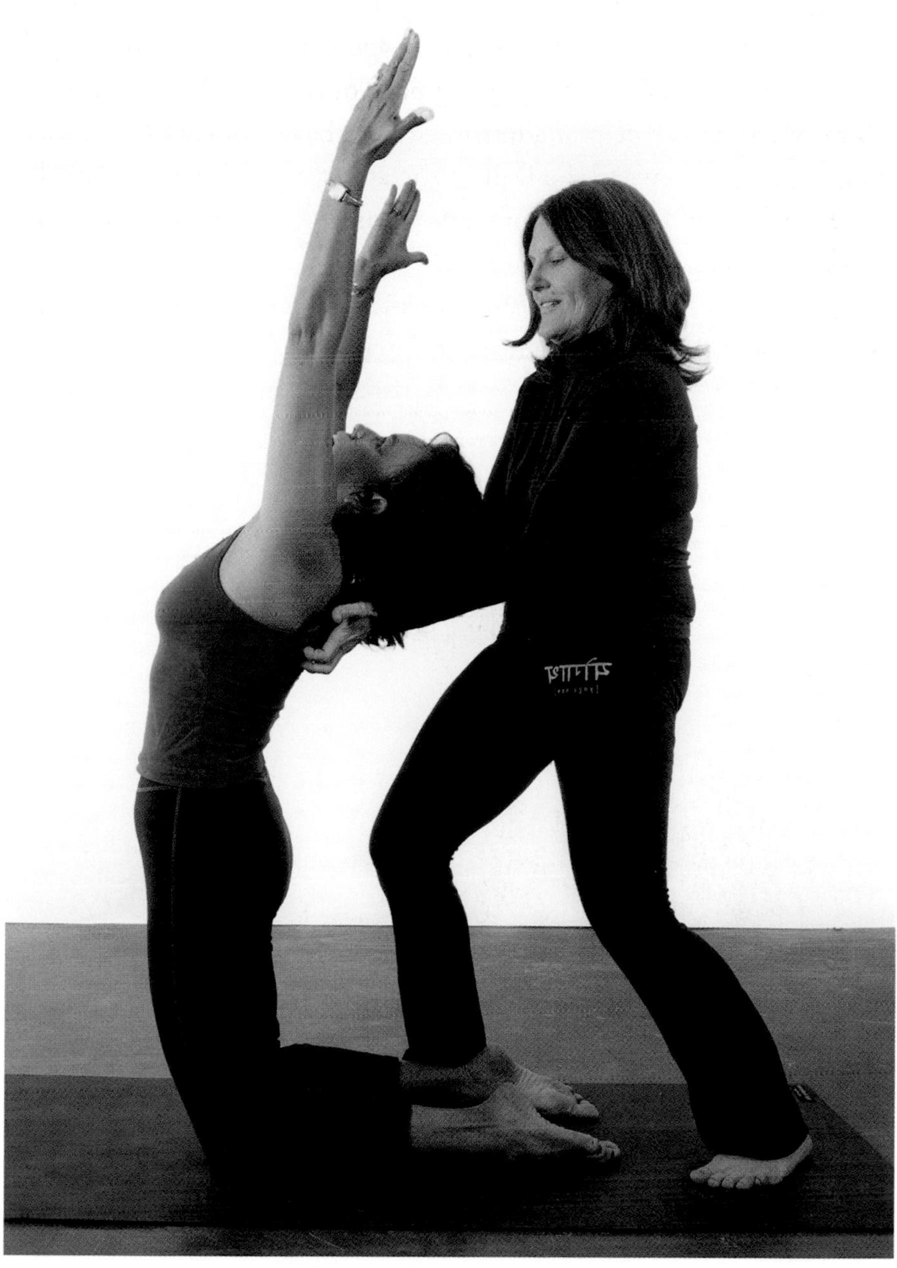

Figure 8.8. Supporting lifted shoulders in Camel Pose

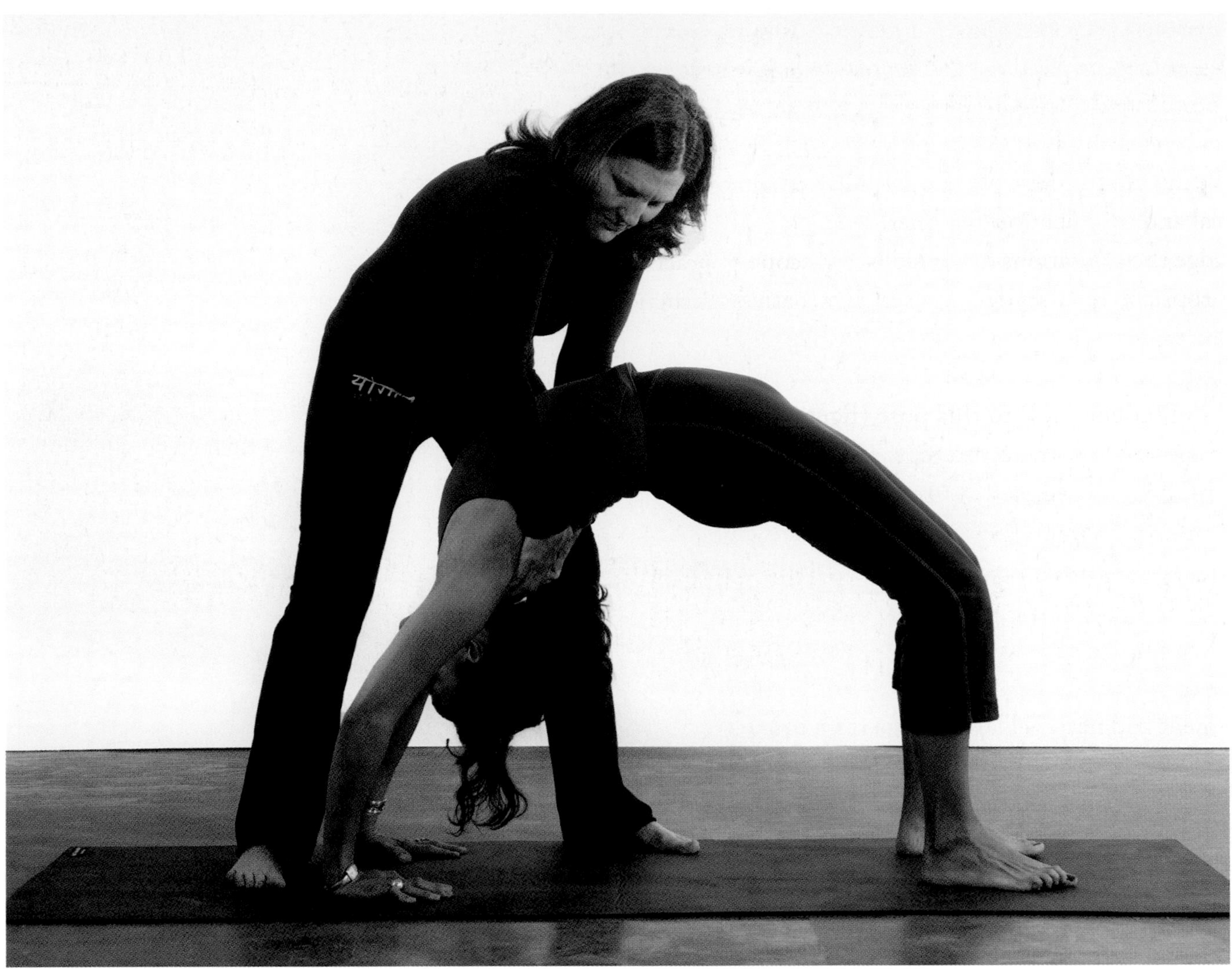

Figure 8.9. Supporting shoulders and spine in Upward Bow Pose

thighs to roll down; and providing firm support for the shoulders as students work to straighten the arms. Upward Bow Pose can remind us to eliminate habitual body actions and thinking by focusing on the unusual movements. While students are doing this pose, you can ask them to consider how much of what they do is habit and which physical and mental habits they would like to change.

Inversions

When teaching inversions, always encourage students to do as little or as much as they are guided to do and offer specific substitutes. Students may not want to practice inversions in a given class for various reasons such as having their period, suffering from a headache, or feeling light-headed. A good alternative pose is a supported **Supine Bound Angle Pose** as shown in figure 8.10. To encourage seeing the world in these new ways, ask students what would look better upside down or what they would like to see shaken up.

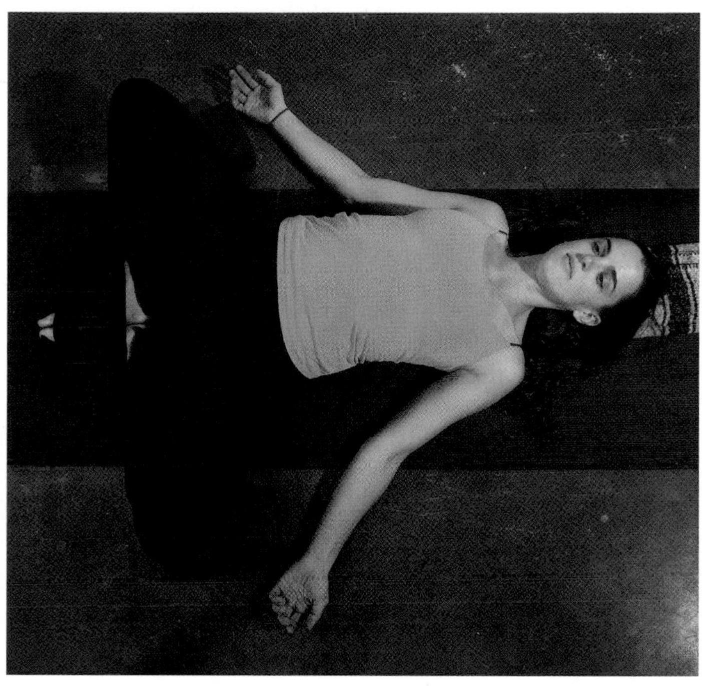

Figure 8.10. Using props to adjust Supine Bound Angle Pose

Legs up the Wall Pose

Students new to this pose (figure 8.11) often cannot figure out how to get their hips right next to the wall, even after a demonstration. If you notice students far from the wall, sit on the floor next to them and show them how to start sideways and roll the legs up the wall. Adjustments include putting a sandbag on students' feet and softly touching their shoulders to encourage dropping them to the floor.

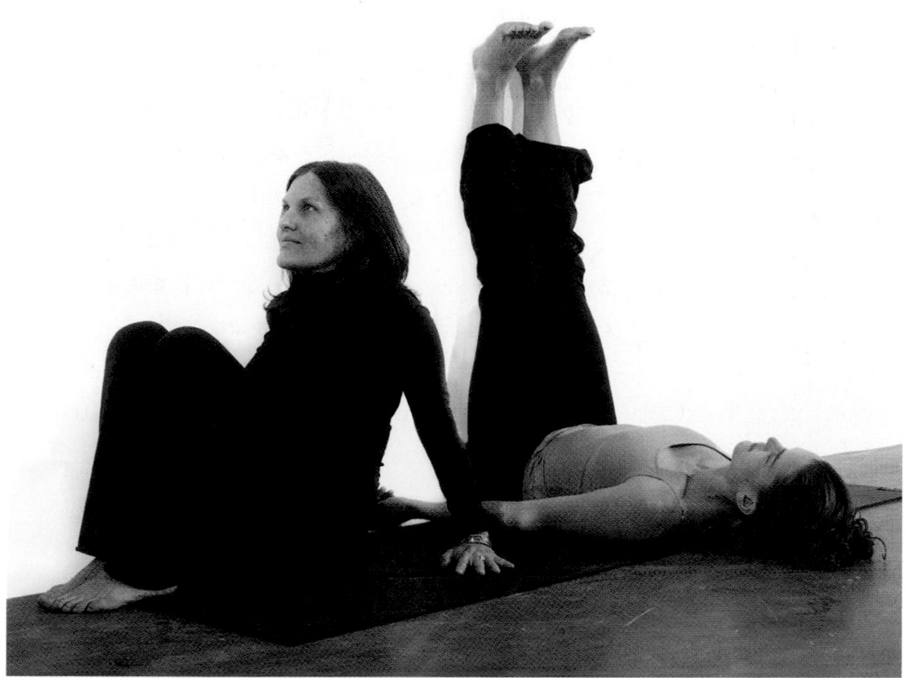

Figure 8.11. Sitting sideways next to the wall (left), and swinging the legs up (right) in Legs up the Wall Pose

Headstand Pose

In this pose (figure 8.12), a common misalignment is that the elbows are placed wider than the shoulders, interfering with sufficient shoulder stability. To adjust, have students come down and reset their elbows closer together, then return to Headstand, pressing down on their elbows, forearms, and hands, and feeling the lightness in their head. Generally, if students cannot lift their head off the floor they don't have the necessary strength to hold the pose for longer than a couple breaths. Staying in Headstand can only be safely done when students have enough core, shoulder, and arm strength to support their body.

Figure 8.12. Supporting lifted leg to help the body rise in Headstand Pose

Always have students count breaths, which reminds them to breathe and not hold the pose longer than five to ten breaths in the beginning, gradually

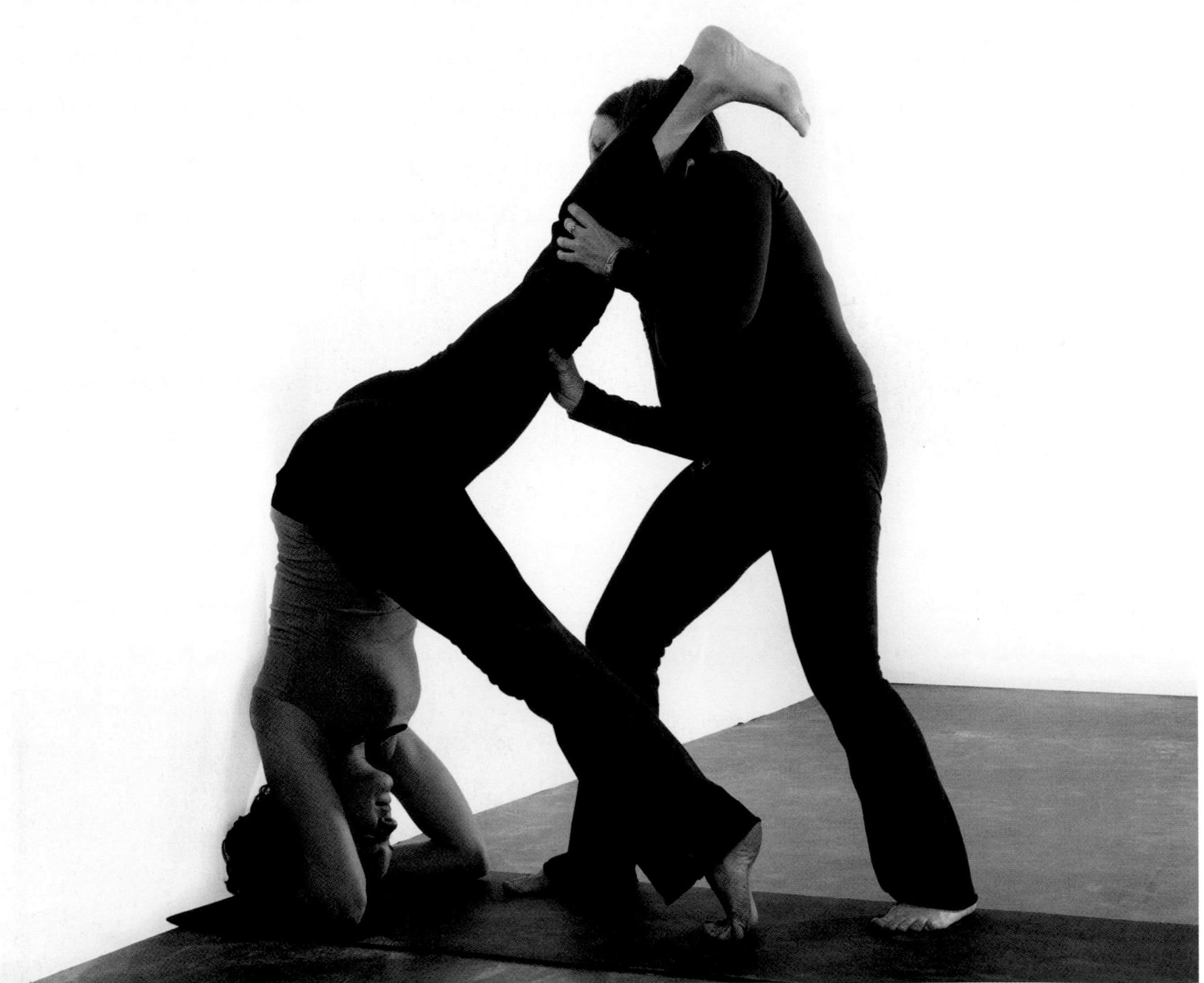

building endurance. An adjustment for the pose is to have each student lunge and lift the extended leg; then take the lifted leg and tell the student to press down on it as you guide it up toward the wall. Additionally, keeping in mind that Headstand prepares us for risk taking and connects us to the earth with our head and to the sky with our feet, you can have the students consider what they might do if they were fearless and how connection with the larger realms of earth and sky changes their perspective of themselves.

Table and Handstand Pose

When doing Table Pose (figure 8.13), students often round their back away from the wall. Suggest bending the knees, moving the heart

Figure 8.13. Lifting hips and moving mid-spine to wall in Table Pose

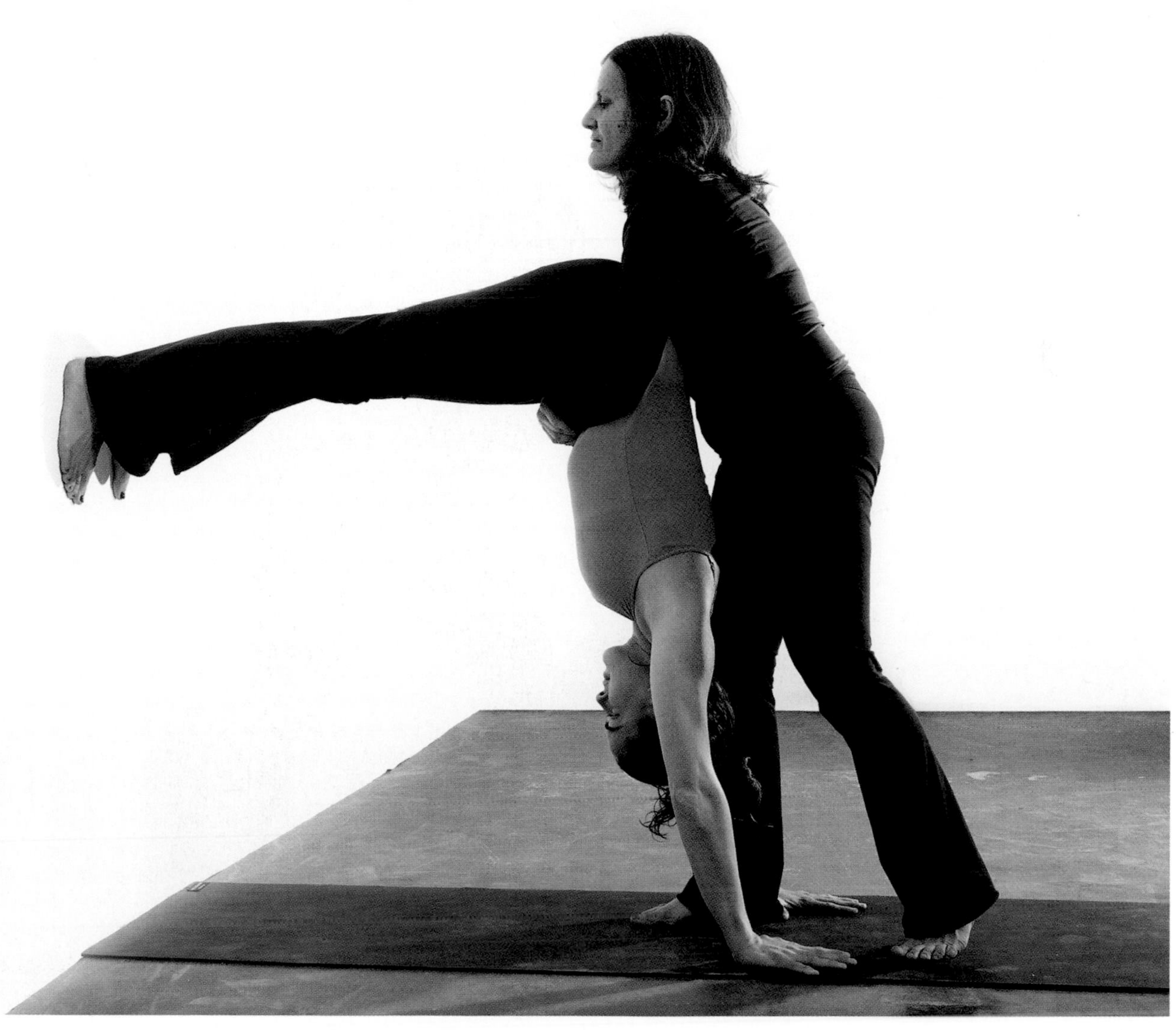

toward the wall, and then engaging the core. When doing Handstand, students can have a banana-shaped back, which puts too much pressure on the low back and doesn't elongate the front and back planes of the body. An adjustment for Table Pose is to tell students to push down on the hands as they lift the hip girdle up. An adjustment for Handstand is to demonstrate how lifting the head can result in a banana-shaped back and how looking toward the belly can help eliminate it.

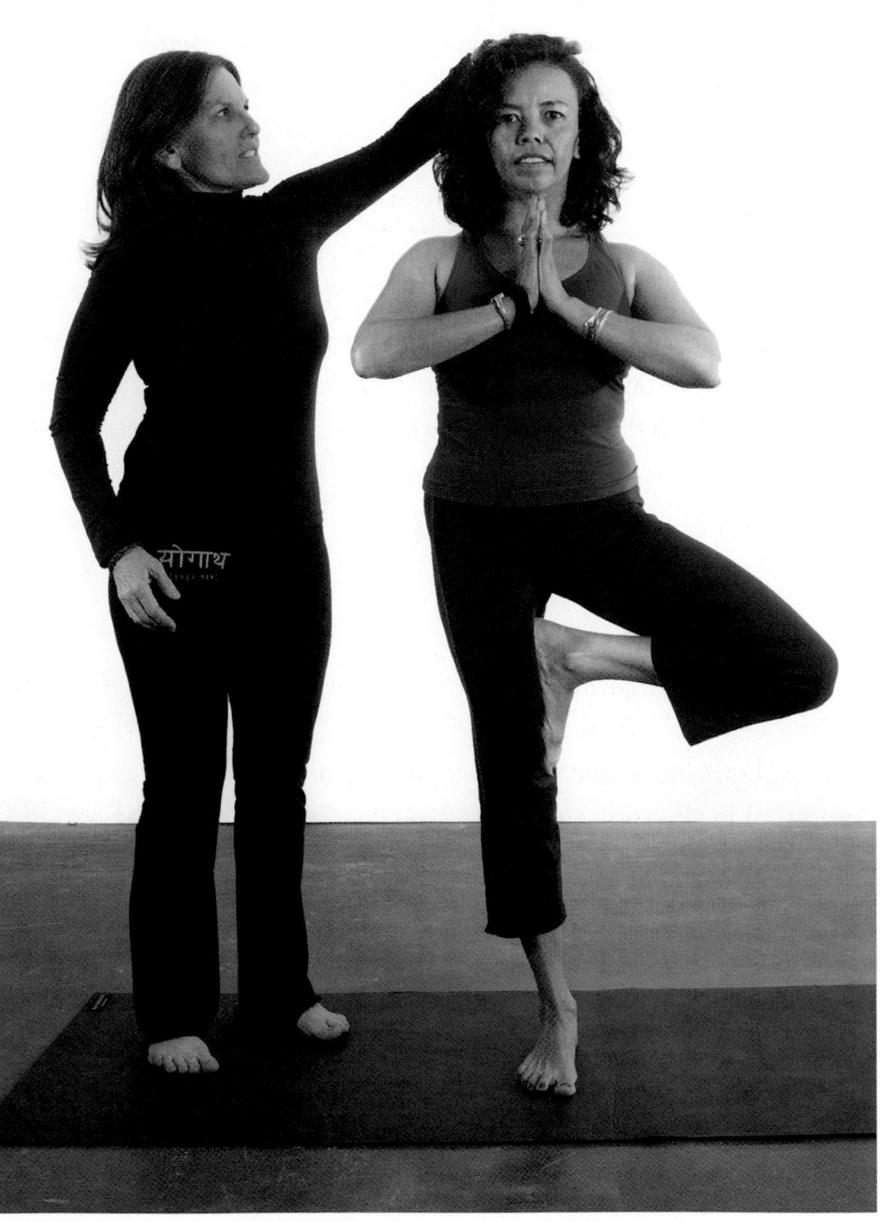

Figure 8.14. Lifting head to encourage feeling length in Tree Pose

Balance Poses

Remind students that balance isn't something you have or don't have but something that everyone can attain with practice. Techniques you can use to improve balance include: keeping the eyes very focused; lifting the core to cultivate power; remembering that balance is dynamic, that there is always movement as the body finds balance; and looking for the opposing aspects to find the point of stillness. As students practice, you may ask them to consider what it is in life that throws them off balance and whether any part of the balance poses can help them maintain emotional and spiritual balance in daily life, such as keeping the eyes steady when they feel off balance at home, as in Tree Pose.

Tree Pose

When doing Tree Pose (figure 8.14), students sometimes have difficulty keeping their foot to the inside of their leg, which depends on finding oppositional energy and is unrelated to the fabric of clothes or sweatiness of the body. Suggest that students press the foot firmly to the leg and resist with the leg pressed back, to find stability between these two forces. Also advise students that they can get support by using a wall or pressing the hands together.

Half Moon Pose

In this pose (figure 8.15), students have more difficulty finding balance when the hand on the floor is too close to the standing leg. Suggest that students move that hand forward from the foot about eight inches and outside the foot about eight inches (where the hand would fall under the shoulder) and use a block. Also tell students they could get extra support by using a wall, or stand behind them, making it easier for them to gain stability and open their heart to the sky.

Crow Pose

In this pose (figure 8.16), students often bend the elbows out instead of back and are nervous about falling forward. You can demonstrate the correct way to bend the elbows. As support, you can have students use the wall for

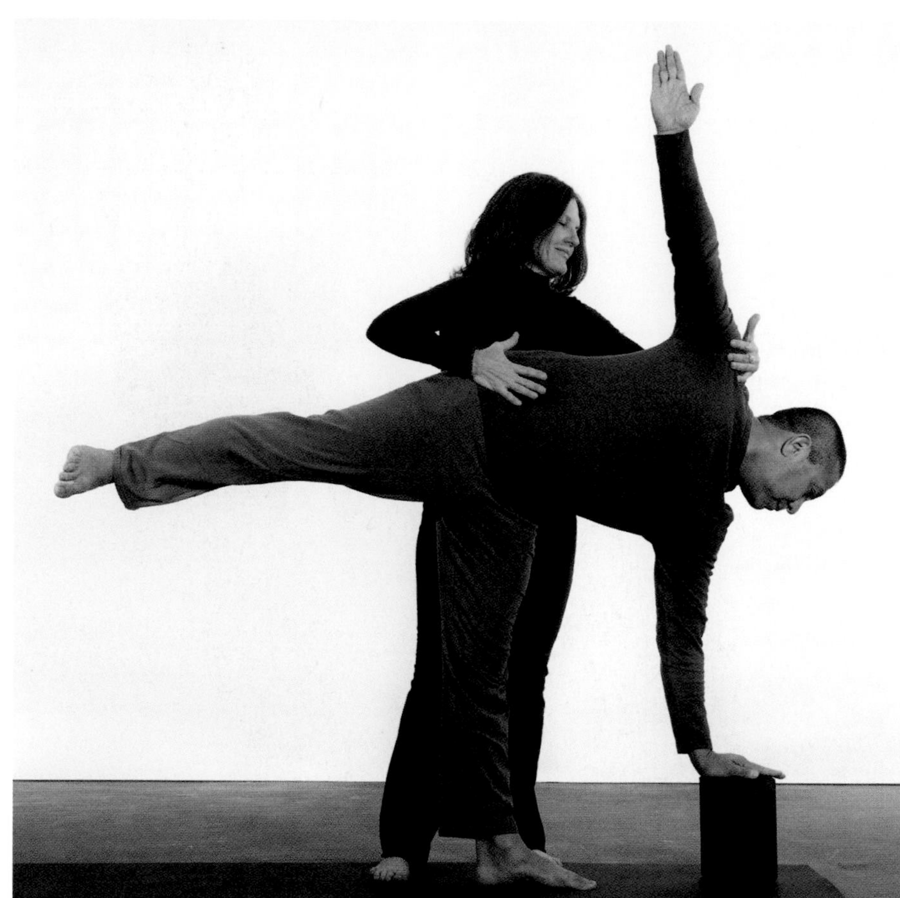

Figure 8.15. Supporting top shoulder and hip from behind in Half Moon Pose

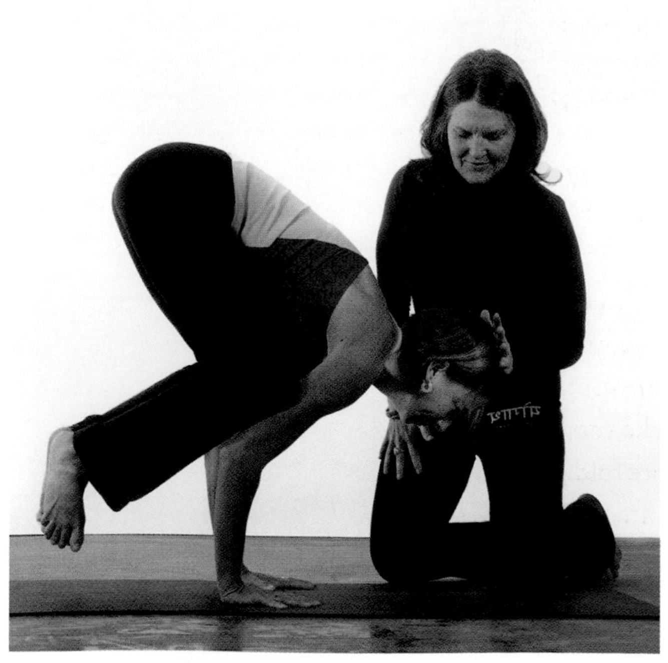

Figure 8.16. Supporting head to adjust balance in Crow Pose

their feet, experimenting with proximity by lifting one foot and adjusting the distance. You can also have them set a blanket on the floor to provide a soft surface in case they roll forward. Since the crow, which is often on the ground but also flies, can teach us how to be grounded yet aspire to heights, you could also have students consider how they might manifest these characteristics in life.

Seated Poses

With seated poses, the basic challenge for students is to keep the spine lengthened as they fold and not round over as they attempt to touch the toes. It is helpful to demonstrate using props and show how bending the knees at first helps.

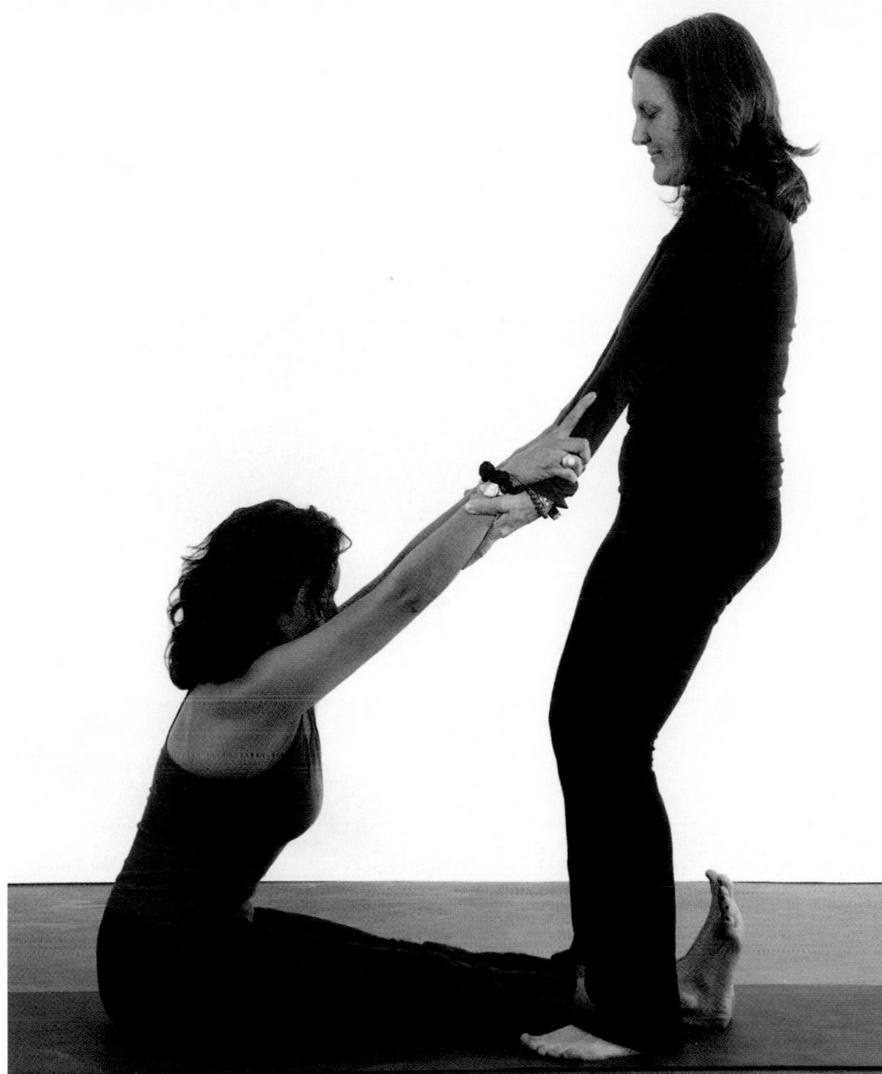

Figure 8.17. Lifting arms up and away in Seated Forward Fold Pose

Seated Forward Fold Pose

In doing this pose (figure 8.17), students commonly remain rounded and experience no rotation of the hip girdle. Encourage them to either use a belt or put their hands on the floor beside their legs with knees bent, then feel the rib cage next to their thighs and slowly move forward. Support for the pose can be to put downward pressure on the hips and legs as they spiral inward. Another means of support is to take the student's arms and help lengthen the torso away from the hips before folding. Since Seated Forward Fold is about being at peace with who we are, when we are stressed by external responsibilities and bombarded by relentless media images of perfection, the pose can help us remember that our real home is inside and we are perfect just as we are.

Knee to Head Pose

When doing this pose (figure 8.18), students often remain rounded and experience no rotation of the hip girdle, as with Seated Forward Fold, and also do not properly twist toward the extended leg. You may have students lift the torso completely and do only moderate forward folding, as well as bend the knees. Support for the pose can be to take the student's arms and on the inhale gently lift them up and out, then on the exhale lower their torso by moving their arms down.

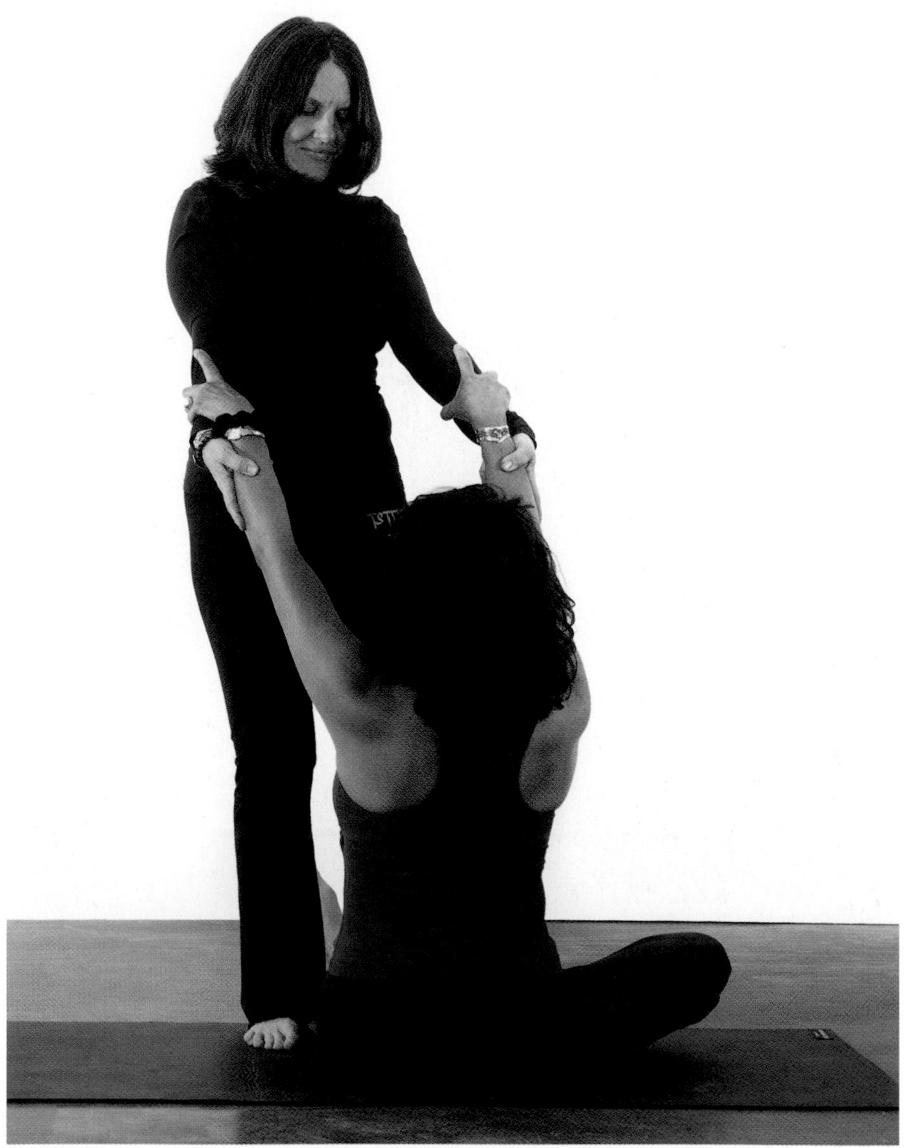

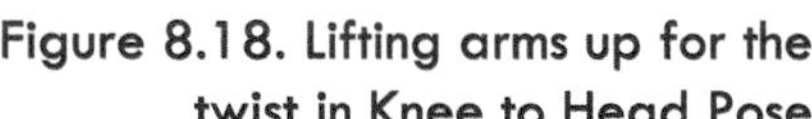

Figure 8.18. Lifting arms up for the twist in Knee to Head Pose

Hero Pose

Knee and ankle discomfort are common complaints in this pose (figure 8.19), so encouraging students to use more than one block is helpful. If the students have a rounded low back, you could suggest they use a thin block to support the spine in creating the natural lumbar curve. Additional support can be provided by the weight of sandbags on the thighs or your hands on the thighs while you do a modified Downward Facing Dog, if it is not invasive to the student. Because the name of this pose can inspire students to cultivate a positive self-image, you can ask them to recall moments of success in the past when they felt proud of their accomplishments, their heroism.

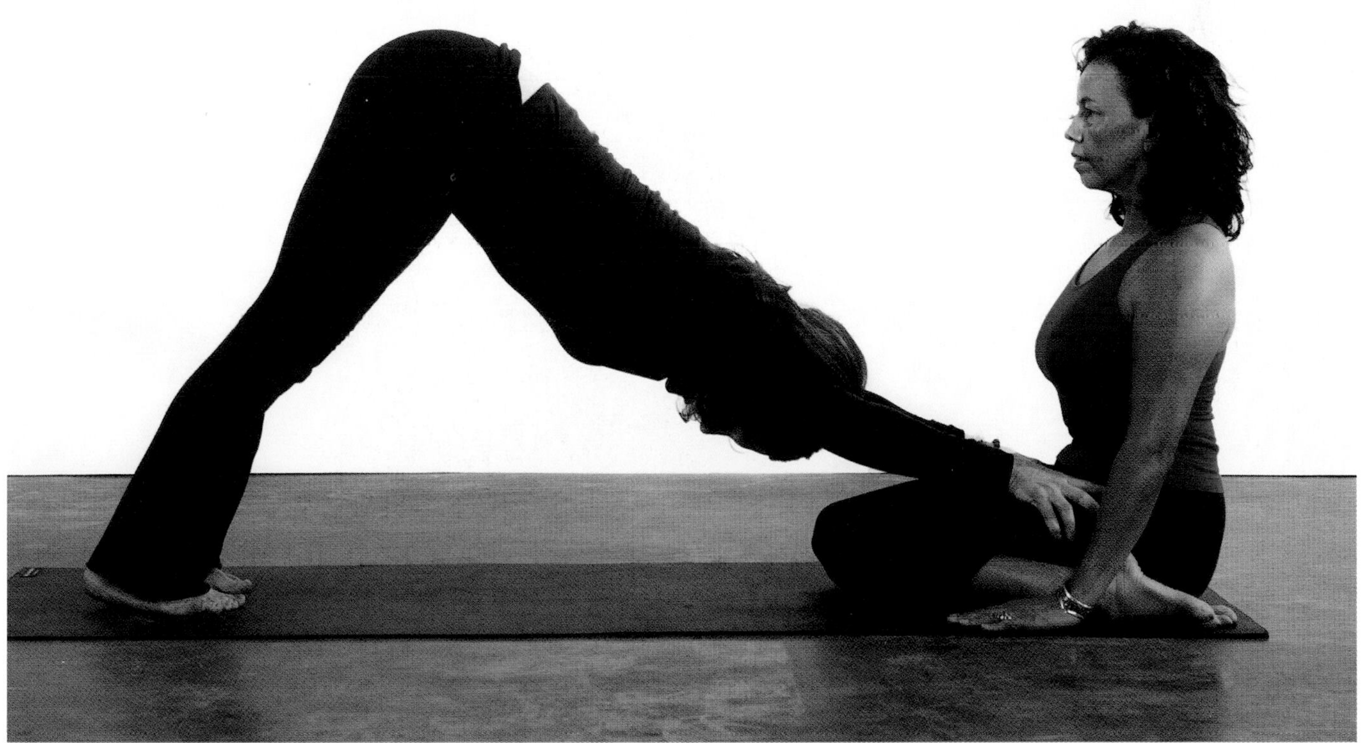

Figure 8.19. Applying pressure on thighs to support grounding in Hero Pose

Twists

In doing twists, it is important for students to elongate the spine before moving it. Emphasize that the twisting action originates in the lower spine and is done by finding the abdominal core strength to pull in and lift up. You could also point out that although getting all twisted up has a negative connotation, twisting allows us to see from multiple angles and to experience full movement, both physically and in our lives. This can help students use twisting poses to forget the past and generate new ideas.

Revolved Side Angle Pose

When doing this pose (figure 8.20), students commonly experience problems with rounding the back and leaning over the hooked leg. Both problems can easily be adjusted by having students come up a bit higher and lean back. As a further adjustment, you can have students inhale and

Figure 8.20. Encouraging twist from behind in Revolved Side Angle Pose

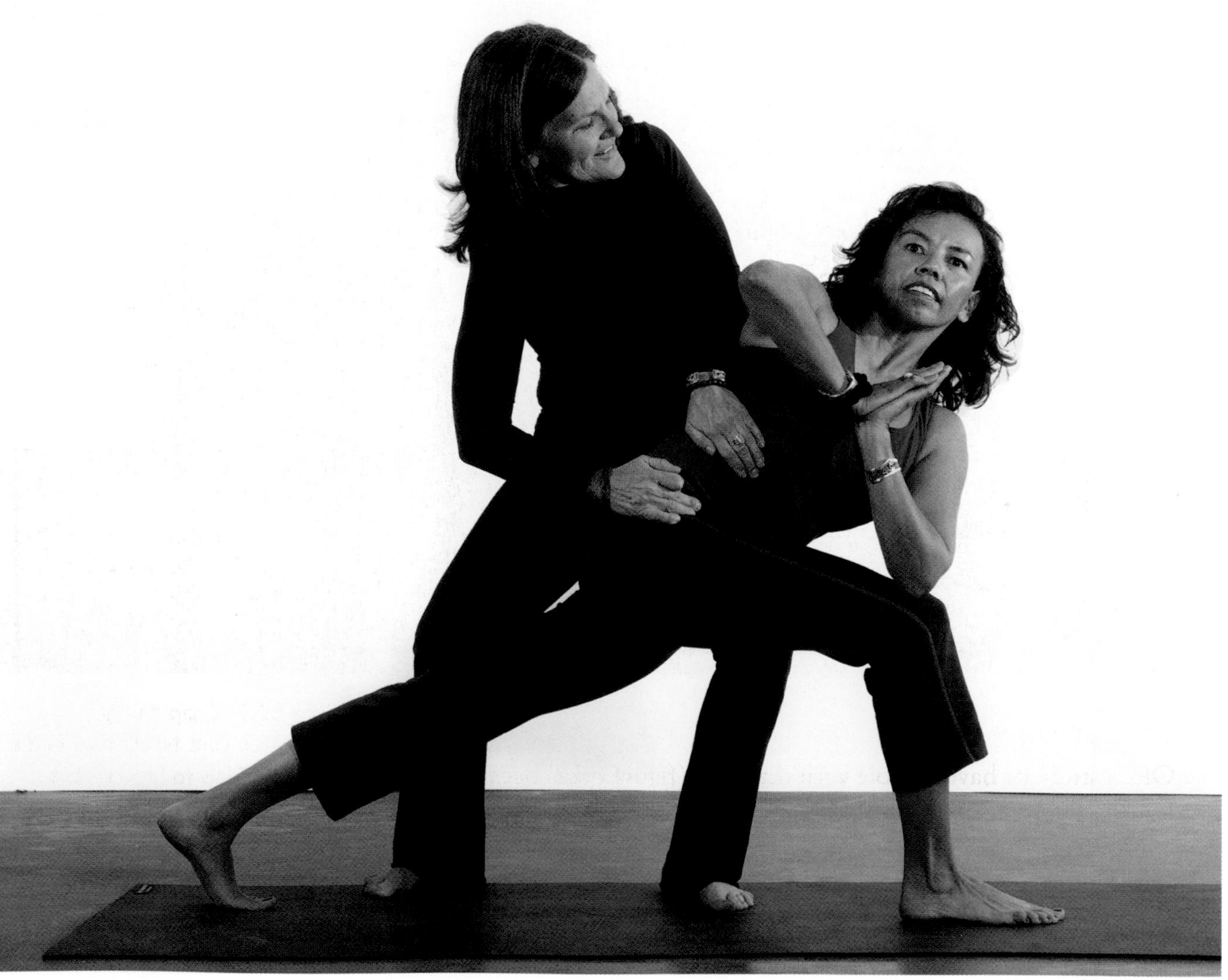

lengthen the spine then exhale as you support rotation of the rib cage. Another adjustment is helping to lift the students' sacrum up and into the body to lengthen the spine.

Revolved Knee to Head Pose

In this pose (figure 8.21), students can reach for the foot and fold forward instead of rolling upward. Also, if the hand is holding the foot the back can round. In both cases, advise students to lift their torso up more and then twist. You could help lengthen the spine by holding their arms. Or you could put a leg behind their back, then on the inhale have them lift and elongate, while on the exhale assist their revolution.

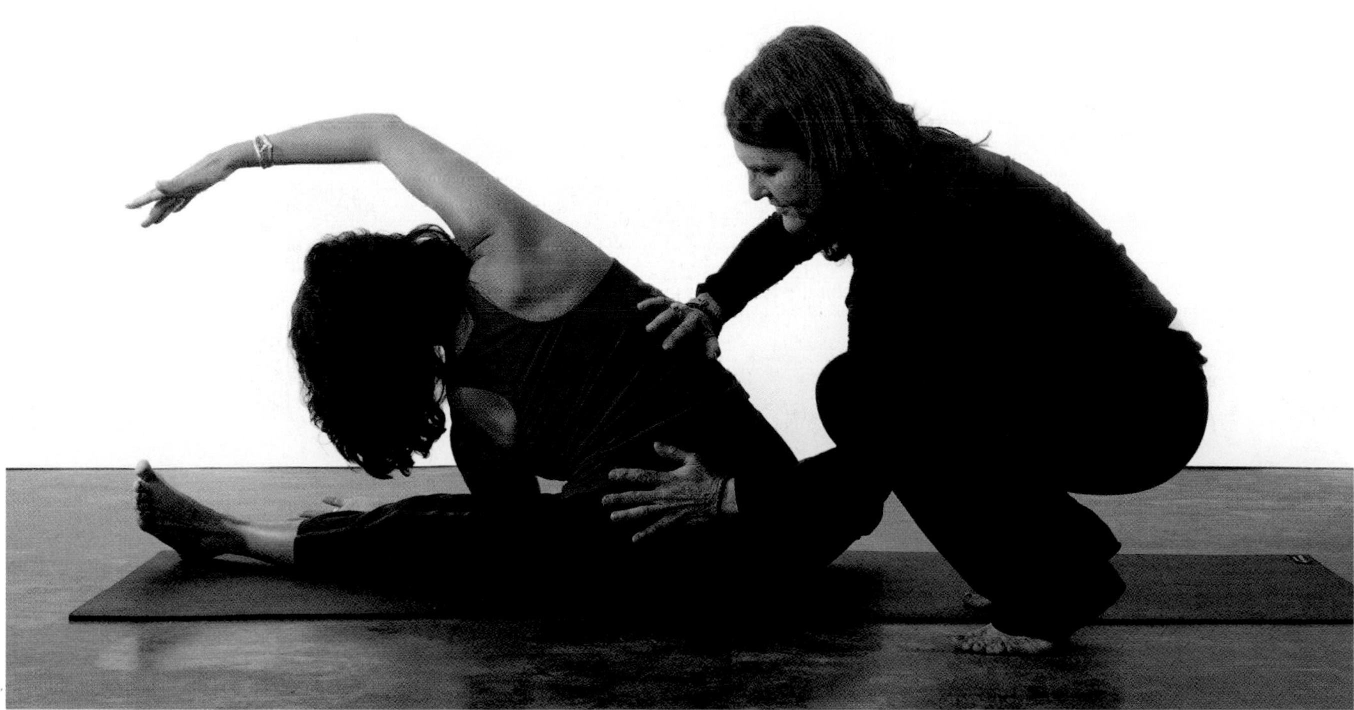

Figure 8.21. Supporting lengthening and twisting of spine in Revolved Knee to Head Pose

Side Crow Pose

Often students have trouble with this pose (figure 8.22) because they don't lean far enough forward. Demonstrating the amount of forward movement will assist students in seeing the balance point. Suggesting they put a blanket under their head may help provide a softer landing platform. For further support, advise students to use both elbows or arms rather than only one.

Figure 8.22. Use of a blanket under the head for arm balance in Side Crow Pose

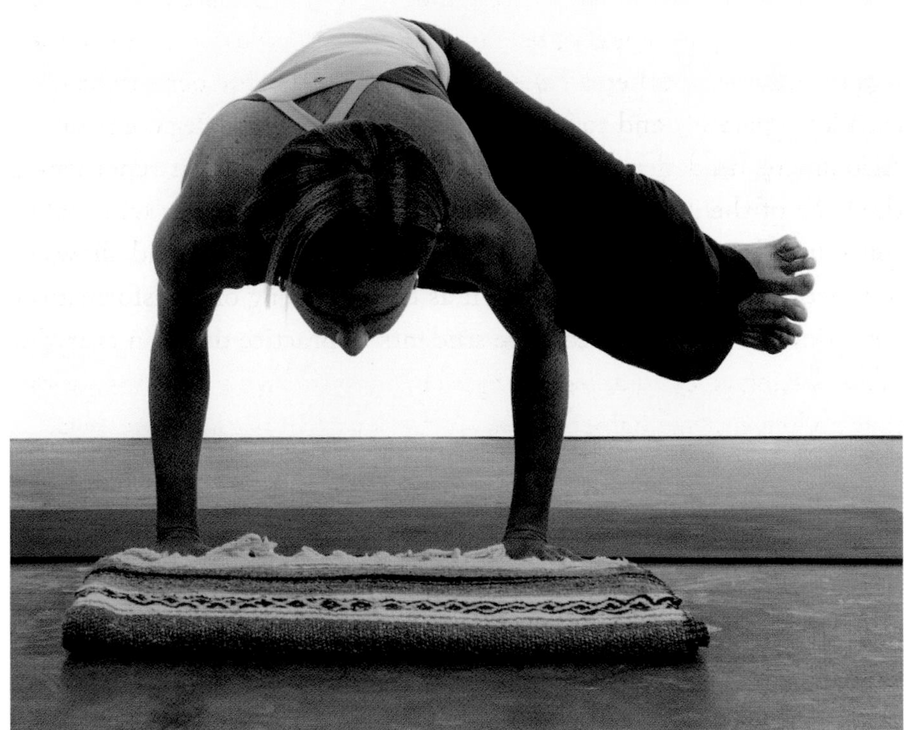

Figure 8.23. Gently pressing the shoulders to support relaxation in Corpse Pose

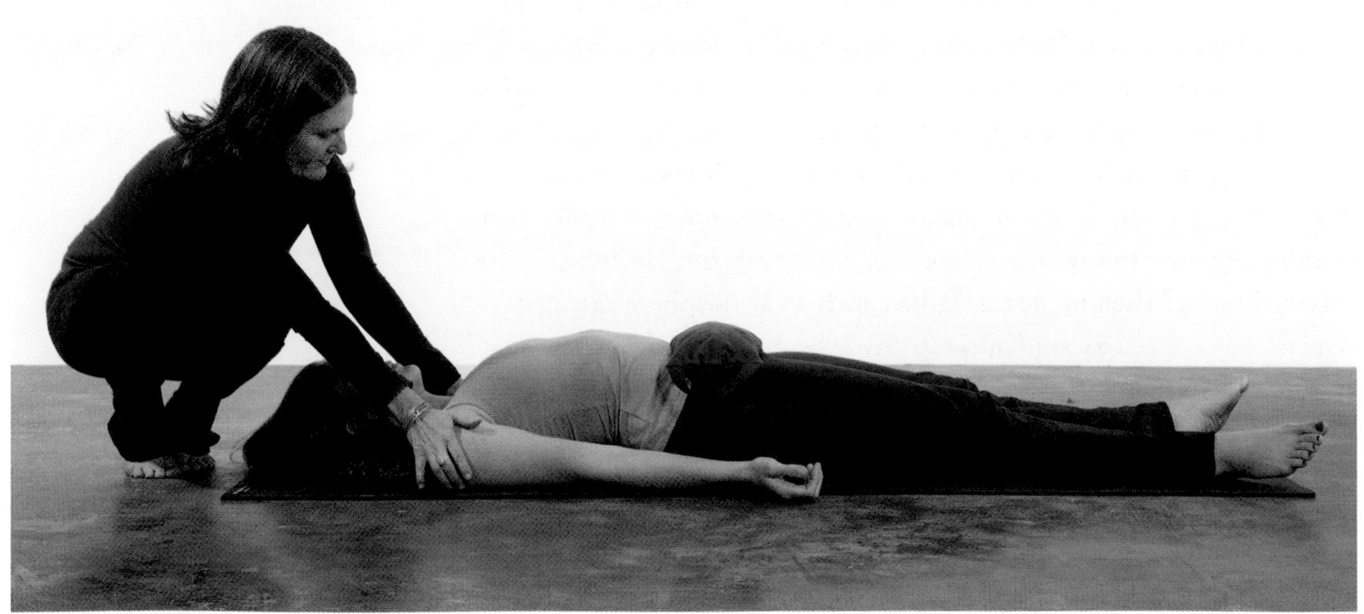

Corpse Pose

Even in this relaxing surrender pose (figure 8.23), some students feel unable to release. You can use props to aid them: prop their knees or legs with a chair or put a blanket under their head (if their chin is lifted and the back of their neck is shortened). You can also have students roll their legs in and out and then let the thighs roll out. For further support, lift each leg separately and roll it in circles and then let the leg come down. Also lift the head; gently rock it side to side; bring it down, lengthening the back of the neck; and press the shoulders to the floor with palms rolled up. Corpse Pose reminds us of our inevitable death and allows us to practice death and learn to see it as the beginning of transformation, by letting go. You can encourage students to practice death in everyday life by letting go of what is no longer useful to them, such as possessions they no longer need, habits that don't support their growth, or a negative self-image that has kept them in a job they hate or an abusive relationship.

DESIGNING A CLASS

One important aspect to consider while designing a class is the setting. Selecting the teaching setting requires careful consideration as it affects the general atmosphere and effectiveness of the class. Whether it is your living room, the lunchroom at your job, a gym, or a yoga studio, be aware that the space should be made sacred and peaceful in support of focus and meditation, and a place where differences are honored and students feel safe and sheltered from the concerns of the external world. Additionally, the atmosphere should create a sense of community, which is one goal of yoga. Such a sense of community doesn't happen necessarily because students talk among themselves, although friendships are often established in yoga classes; it occurs because students and teachers are working together toward the auspicious goal of creating inner peace first in ourselves and then in others. When such an atmosphere exists, it can be readily perceived by students and gives them a sense of belonging and of doing sacred work. Joining together to do sacred work in a peaceful place supports students as they move beyond the mat into the world to create positive change for our planet.

When designing a class it is also crucial to keep in mind that yoga is more than asanas, so stress underlying themes of what you are teaching, whether it is a limb of yoga, a pose, or a meditation. To help students bring more than their bodies to the practice, first offer a group intention, perhaps inspired by an ancient yogic text or modern yoga book. Then give students time to set a personal intention, or *sankalpa,* before you begin teaching poses.

Realize, too, that the order of poses you introduce helps determine the students' success with them and basic feeling of accomplishment. In general, the order in which poses are presented in this book—standing poses, backbends, inversions, balance poses, seated poses, and twists—is beneficial. Above all, be sure to follow a sequence that opens the body for the most challenging pose, or pinnacle pose, if there is one. For example, if you want to teach Headstand as a pinnacle pose, first introduce poses that elongate the spine, open the shoulders, and allow students to access core strength. If you teach practices that follow a preset order of poses, such as Ashtanga and Bikram, the design of the class should focus on what you will teach in addition to the poses, including principles you want to emphasize. An example of the primary series taught in Ashtanga is shown in figure 5.10. For help in designing classes, refer to the many books that include already designed classes with sequences of poses listed in the bibliography.

As you gain confidence in teaching, designing classes will become more creative and enjoyable. You will also learn to adjust your class designs in the moment based on watching the energy and expertise of students during their practice.

TYPES OF CLASSES: GENTLE, LEVEL 1, MIXED LEVEL, AND FLOW

There are many ways to define different class levels, and each studio generally posts descriptions in their literature or on their Web site. Usually these is some variation of Gentle, Level 1, Mixed Level, Levels 2 and 3, and Flow. Students may have to attend a few classes to find their correct level. They may also choose different classes depending on how they feel at the time—whether they have lots of energy or are exhausted, for example. If students are tired or confused, they might benefit from the deep movement of a Gentle class. On the other hand, if they have excess energy and are feeling overwhelmed a Flow class might work best that day. If they are new to yoga and have never done anything physical before, they might start with Level 1. If they are new to yoga and have participated in many physical activities, however, they might go to a Mixed Level.

In general, **Gentle** classes are not only for beginners but also for students who want to move slower yet with precision and power, and with attention to therapeutics (for information on therapeutics, see chapter 9). One such student described this level in the following way:

> *Gentle yoga made yoga accessible to me. It moved slowly enough that I could do everything to some extent, and I have made unbelievable progress. I came in with a cane and lots of problems. Now I don't use a cane, and although I may still have some of the same problems they don't bother me as much.*

An example of a Gentle class is one I taught last summer. Many of the students arrived in class that day with complaints of low back pain, and this class was designed to both lengthen and strengthen the spine and develop abdominal core strength. The spiritual intention was inspired by the Bhagavad Gita, and the following quote was read at the beginning of class as students were finding their breath while in Lying Release Pose: "The whole world becomes a slave to its own activity, Arjuna: if you want to be truly free, perform all actions as worship." After the reading, the class was invited to share the group intention as they practiced and then to set their personal intention to enhance their lives before proceeding with the following sequence of poses:

- Lying Twist Pose
- Lying Release with Leg Lift Variations
- Easy Wide Leg Bent Knee Twist Pose
- Cat/Cow Pose
- Low Lunge Pose with arms lifted (or not, depending on ability)
- Step forward to Mountain Pose
- Upward Facing Hands Pose
- Standing Forward Fold Pose with blocks or chairs for height
- Modified Warrior Poses I and II
- Modified Triangle Pose
- Modified Pyramid Pose
- Tree Pose at the wall for stability, if needed
- Camel Pose at the wall, hands on hips
- Table Pose or Legs up the Wall Pose
- Modified Seated Forward Fold Pose

Level 1 classes are for students just beginning yoga and should start with fundamentals. Ideally such students would sign up for a series of classes, each building on the previous one, so at the end they would have a body of knowledge. This does not generally happen, however, as Americans tend to come to yoga classes only when possible. An example of a Level I class, as well as a Mixed Level class and Flow class, appears in Appendix 3.

Mixed Level classes, or All Levels classes, are for beginning, intermediate, and advanced students. In these classes, students learn from one another and work with a variety of modifications, according to their abilities. Although it is important that beginning students not push beyond their limits, they often benefit from seeing more variations on a pose than they can currently do.

Flow, or vinyasa, classes are extremely popular, as they move with the breath and can feel almost like dancing. As a teacher, you want to emphasize that taking breaks, in Child's Pose or in Corpse Pose, is always an option as injury can occur if students move too forcefully. In Flow classes, usually each movement is choreographed to an inhale or an exhale, and poses are commonly not held for longer than twenty breaths.

In addition to the usual types of yoga classes, it is possible to teach specialty yoga classes aimed at specific groups, such as prenatal yoga, yoga for teens, yoga for prisoners, yoga for the military, yoga for golfers, yoga for tennis players, and yoga for runners. Such classes are often taught by instructors who have a special interest in these areas. If you want to teach specialty classes, research related organizations to find out what classes already exist and how your offerings might fit in. You might try volunteering at first to see if you enjoy teaching this specific group. In the case of prenatal yoga, to prepare to teach in safe, skilled manner first enroll in one of the many specialty trainings available. Regardless of how you begin teaching yoga, it is a worthwhile and joyful experience.

> **Design** a Gentle class with a theme of your choice and teach it on a volunteer basis to family, friends, or coworkers. Offer a group intention from one of the eight limbs of yoga, perhaps on *ahimsa*, nonviolence toward the self.

Design a Mixed Level class and teach it on a volunteer basis to family, friends, or coworkers. Offer a group intention from one of the eight limbs of yoga, perhaps on *pratyahara*, withdrawal of the senses, encouraging students to not look at others in the class. See appendix 3 for a sample Mixed Level class.

Practice every pose described in chapter 6, giving yourself instructions either out loud or silently. Be aware of your experiences as you experiment with moves that work.

CHAPTER NINE

Yoga Therapy Training and Yoga As a Profession

YOGA THERAPY

For thousands of years, yoga has been used therapeutically to heal illness in the body, mind, or spirit, which according to ancient texts occurs because of ignorance of the nature of the true self. Despite this long tradition, only recently has yoga therapy emerged as a separate field of study. Today, in addition to yoga teacher training programs that include therapeutics, some of which offer yoga therapy at the more advanced 500-hour level, there are separate yoga therapy programs that offer specific training in using yoga to heal.[1] Because these programs have existed for only about thirty years and the graduates are only now beginning to establish yoga therapy centers in a variety of global locations, including hospitals, schools, and community centers, it is too soon to assess how yoga therapy will develop or be integrated with other healing professions in the future. Certainly, medical professionals are increasingly acknowledging the healing power of yoga and recommending it to clients.

Although the question of how yoga therapy differs from ordinary yoga is still discussed in many circles without general agreement, the working definition of the International Association of Yoga Therapists is: "Yoga therapy is the process of empowering individuals to improve health and well-being through the application of the philosophy and practice of yoga."[2] From the perspective of yoga, pain occurs because *prana* has been constricted, and so yoga postures and breath help open the energetic channels, the *nadis*. Usually yoga therapy is done one-on-one between teacher and student with focus on a particular injury or challenge the student is facing. This is in contrast to a private yoga session, where a student doesn't have a particular injury or problem but prefers individual attention instead of, or as a supplement to, classes.

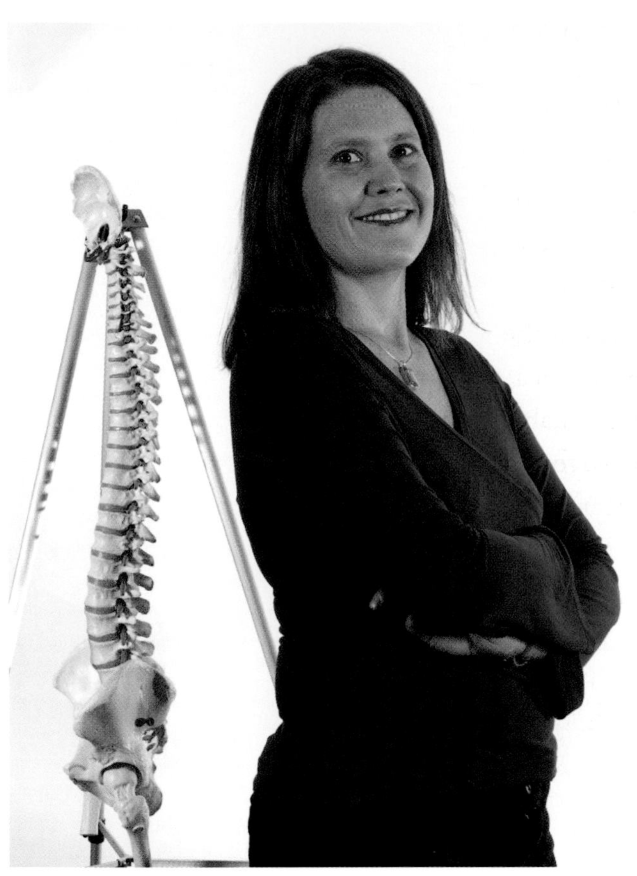

Figure 9.1. Kelly Coogan, chiropractor and yogi

Because the arena of yoga therapy is not well defined, it is important to create clear boundaries between the roles of student and yoga therapist, as well as distinctions between a yoga teacher-therapist and other health-care professions. Yoga helps people feel so much better that sometimes students project extraordinary power onto their yoga therapist, so it is necessary to remain honest about the limitations of yoga therapy. Students might like to find a healer who will give them poses instead of pills to eliminate their pains and problems, but a yoga teacher-therapist is not a doctor, physical therapist, massage therapist, chiropractor, psychologist, or social worker.

Compared to other health-care professions, yoga therapy has the advantage of connecting people to their inner world, experienced through breath and awareness of sensation. To achieve healing, yoga therapy employs not only poses, but also self-study, *svadhyaya*, all the *yamas* and *niyamas*, sense withdrawal, meditation, mudras, and chanting according to student needs and abilities. These potent tools provide an amazing resource for assisting students in recovery from a multitude of problems.

Further, yoga can be used therapeutically in conjunction with a wide variety of other practices. Medical doctors often recommend Gentle yoga after surgery and for the 30 million Americans suffering from back pain. Therapists recommend yoga for clients who suffer from depression and post-traumatic stress disorder (PTSD), especially returning war veterans. Also, chiropractors use yoga in conjunction with their work (see figure 9.1). The goal of chiropractic work, like yoga, is to create ease and increased function in any given part of the body, especially the spine. For an example of a chiropractor's use of yoga, see "Sages Say."

Even though yoga is used with a wide variety of other practices, it is crucial to keep in mind that it is not a substitute for medical treatments, and your role as yoga therapist does not include Western medicine or pharmacology. Always take into account the fact that students may be working with other medical professionals. Require that students' doctors

Sages Say

The chiropractic and yoga approaches have a few things in common. They both recognize that a healthy, aligned, and flexible spine is conducive to better health. Both disciplines also acknowledge that when the energies in the spine are freed, the tissues of the entire body are better controlled by the higher centers of the brain. In my own chiropractic practice, I teach yoga postures as an adjunctive therapy that the patient can do at home to enable their body to hold the adjustment I have given them. I have found that this approach not only allows the patient to feel better faster and longer, but it gives them a tool they can use when they have any feeling of dis-ease in areas with chronic problems. Yoga asanas work to help strengthen as well as elongate the tight tissues around old injuries or postural imbalances that people may have had for years. Yoga practice also includes breathing techniques that calm the mind, as well as allow the body to receive much-needed oxygen in all tissues for healing.

—Kelly Coogan

have released them to practice yoga or to take yoga therapy, and never prescribe medications for a student.

GENERAL PRINCIPLES OF YOGA THERAPY

The beginning step in practicing yoga therapy is to watch and listen to students. Often the best tool yoga therapists have to help students is to show them how to connect to the wave of their breath and elongate their spine. Generally, begin with Lying Release Pose, giving detailed instruction to initially find the three-part yogic breath and work with spinal elongation and movement (see techniques for Lying Release Pose and three-part yogic breath in chapter 4). In working with students who have been injured, be sure to have them practice first with the minimum edge, looking for ways the breath and inner attention can shift the minimum edge nearer to the maximum edge but never to the point of experiencing pain.

Joint Pain

The first principle of working with joints is to stabilize them before moving them, including shoulder, hip, and elbow joints. When pain occurs in a specific joint, look to the joint above it for the contraction of *prana*. For example, if a wrist is painful, stabilize and strengthen the elbow and shoulder. If a knee is in pain, look at the hip placement and thigh rotation. The second principle is that since joints are meant to move the bones—not to bear body weight, which is the job of the muscles—strengthening and lengthening muscles around joints helps put less stress on them and may help eliminate pain.

Low Back Pain

One of the most common complaints today is low back pain, which yoga can help reduce. As a yoga therapist, you want to help students find the underlying cause of low back pain, so ask them to consider the way they use their body during the day and see if this sheds light on the reason for their pain. Often the major muscles that connect the legs to the torso, the psoas muscles (see figure 9.2), cause low back pain because we spend so much time sitting, when in a car, at a desk, and while eating. And

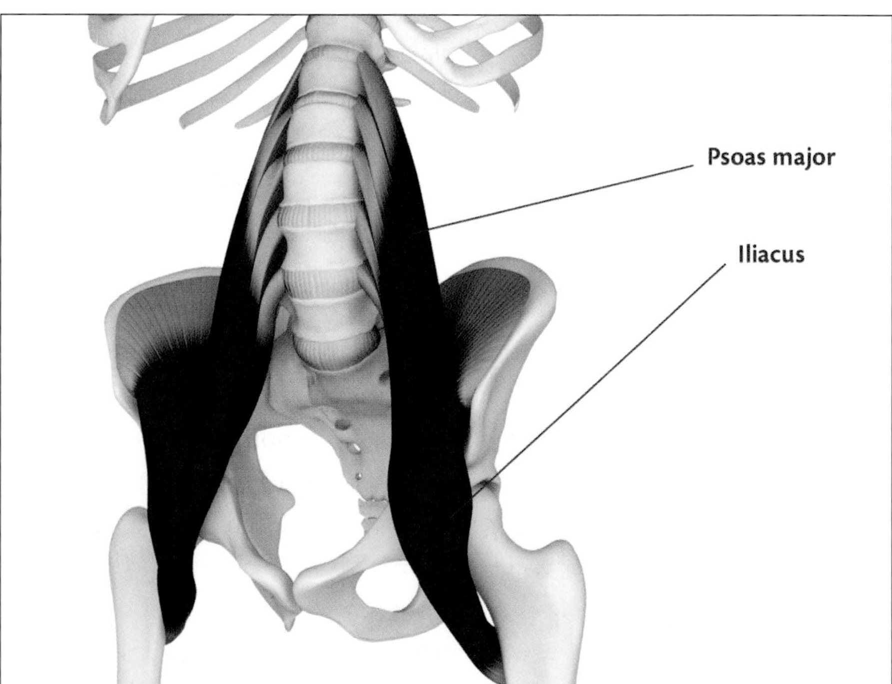

Figure 9.2. Psoas muscle group

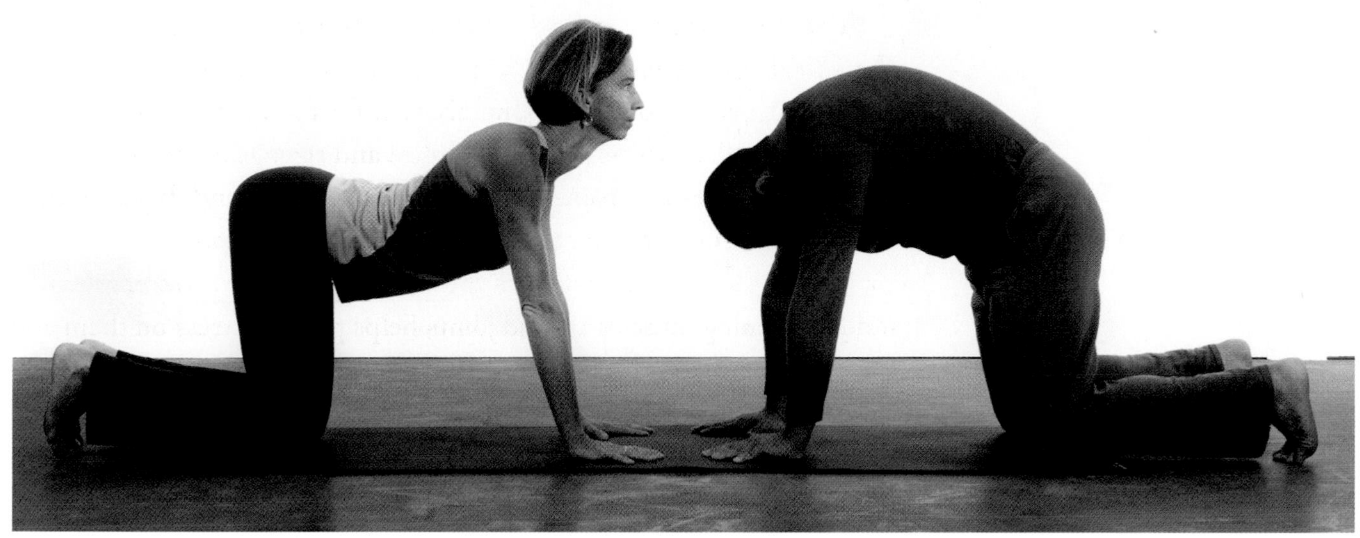

Figure 9.3. Cow (left) and Cat (right) for Cat/Cow Pose

frequently, instead of sitting on the sitting bones (*ishial tuberosities*) people sit rounded over and more on the sacrum, which was not designed to hold the body's weight. To help low back pain, the first goal is elongation of the spine, then movement—twisting, flexion (forward), and extension (back). Building core strength is key in supporting the back (see chapter 6 for practices). Additionally, you can suggest that students use a rolled yoga mat or towel to sit more completely on the sitting bones, even while driving.

A good warm-up for the spine and back is Cat/Cow Pose. Making sure the students' weight is not on their wrists, have them press their fingers and feel a slight lift of their wrists away from the ground as they inhale and let their spine move down between their shoulder blades and the crown of the head, keeping their neck long like a cow's on the front and back, as shown in figure 9.3 (left). On the exhale, have them round up like a mad cat, using the abdominal core to hold for a few breaths as shown in figure 9.3 (right), then move back into Cow Pose. They can lift a leg up with the opposite arm, then curve back and look at each hip, making a "C" shape with the spine. Finally, have them engage the abdominal core, especially on the exhale, using the breath, the *bandhas*, the skeleton, and the muscles.

You can address lengthening the psoas muscles in a variety of poses, especially lunging. Have students begin in a Low Lunge Pose with their back knee on the ground, lowering their hips while isometrically pulling their legs toward each other, with their front heel moving back and their back leg moving forward, without actually going anywhere. Then have the students lower their hips toward the floor and forward, making sure their front heel stays solidly down (they may need to move it forward as they open). They can use blocks under their arms as they rise up. They should tuck their tailbone as they gently peel their torso away from the front thigh as shown in figure 9.4. Their arms can be moved to the side, raised up, or placed on their knee. You may also want to tuck a blanket under their back knee if there is any sensation in it. Have them practice the pose on both sides.

Opening the hip joints also helps ease low back pain, and Pigeon Prep Pose (Eka Pada Raja Kapotasana) is a good way to work. Ask the students to start in Cat/Cow Pose, then bring a knee up to the same-side hand, extending the opposite leg back as shown in figure 9.5. Some may want

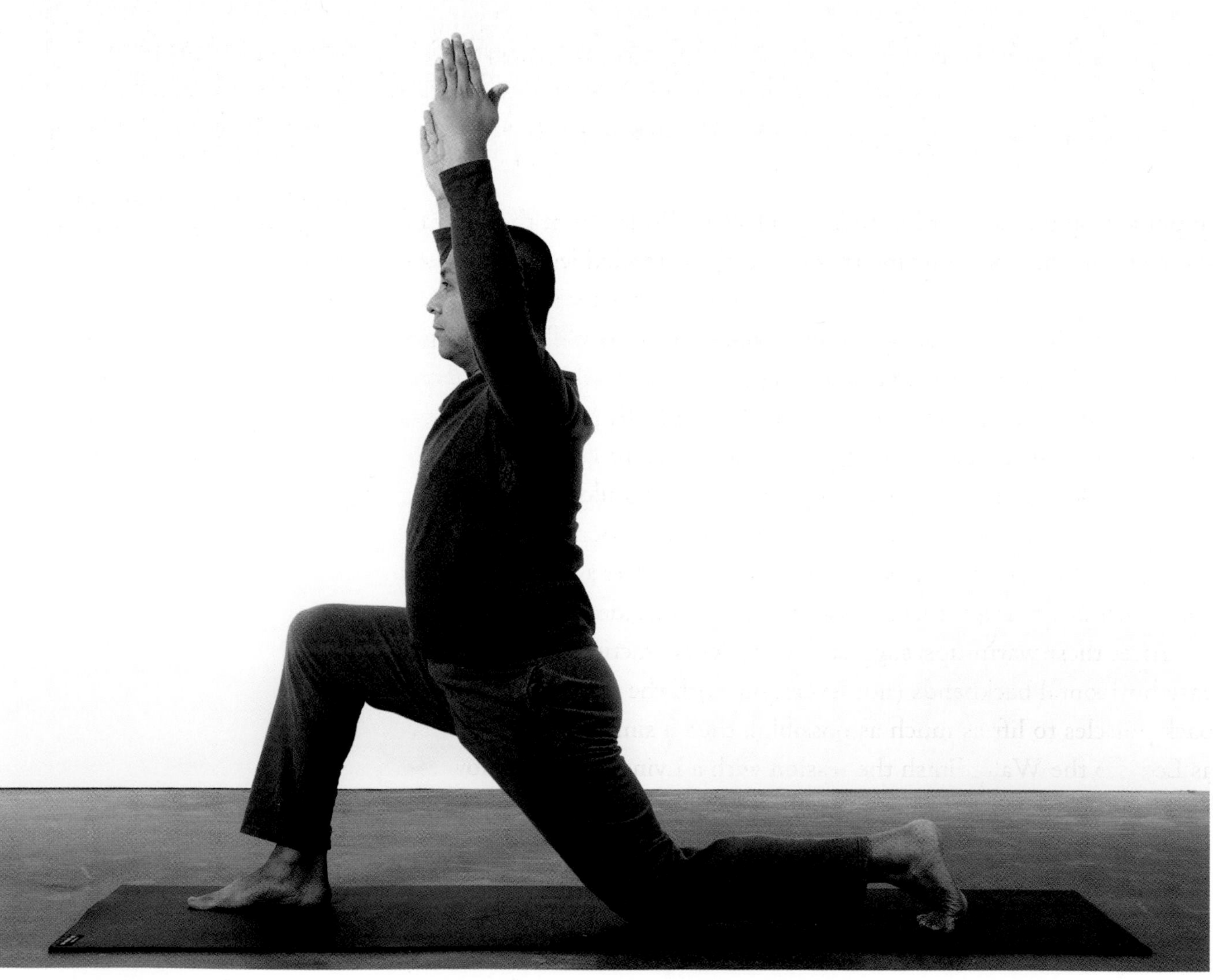

Figure 9.4. Low Lunge Pose for psoas stretch

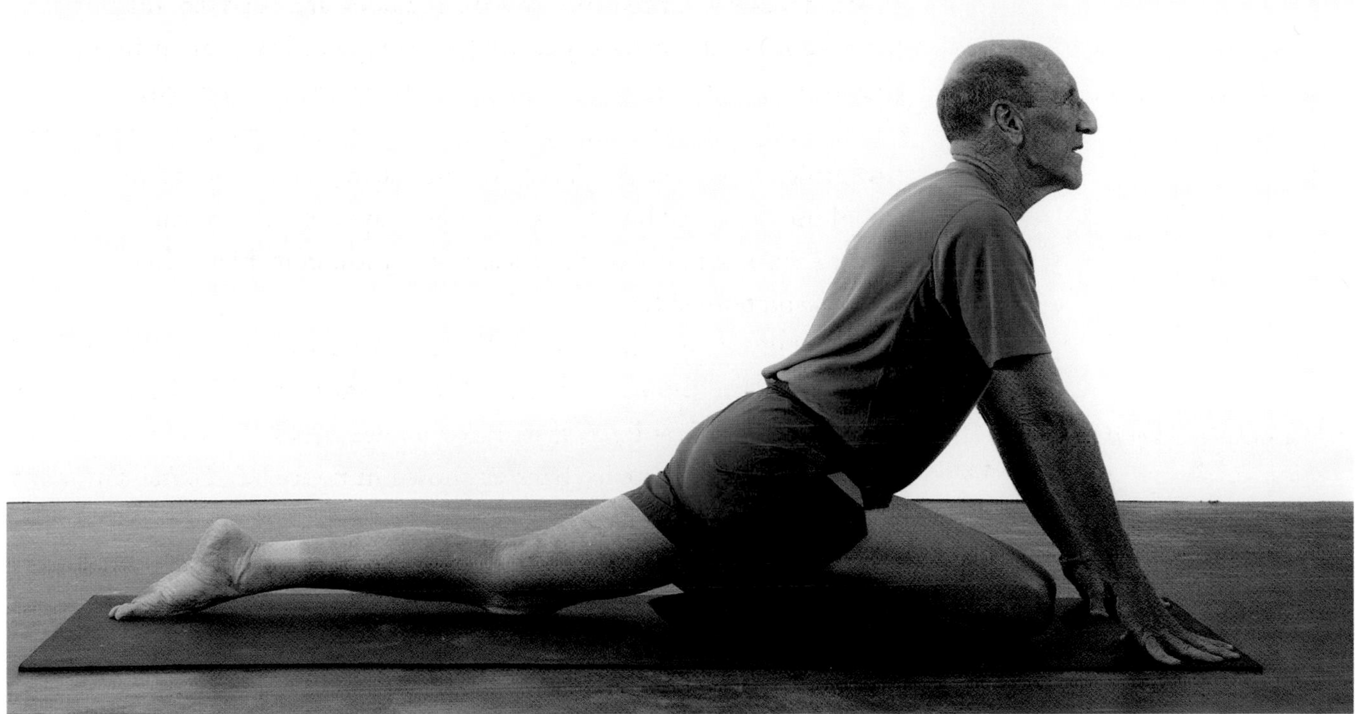

Figure 9.5. Pigeon Prep Pose to open hips, with sandbags for stability

to put a prop under their hip to keep hips equidistant from the front of the mat and the floor, moving them with the extended leg slightly forward and down. Check to make sure students have no knee pain. If there is knee pain, have them bring the foot farther back, as well as putting a knot, made from any available fabric or a scarf, behind the knee. Advise them to breathe deeply in this pose, working with the mind to dive into the sensation rather than avoid it. If the sensation is too intense for them to breathe deeply, they are too low in the pose and should bring their foot back. If there is no sensation, have them bring the foot farther forward. Then have them put their elbows under their shoulders and let their mid-spine melt down. Have them repeat on the second side.

After these warm-ups, suggest that students practice standing poses, easy horizontal backbends (not leveraging with the arms but using the back muscles to lift as much as possible), then a simple inversion, such as Legs up the Wall. Finish the session with a Lying Twist as shown in figure 9.6. Have the students lie on their backs, bring their knees up on an inhale, and let them go to the side on an exhale, extending both arms out to the side, making their body expansive. While inhaling, the spine elongates; while exhaling, the core pulls in and up as the spine twists. Have them repeat on the second side and then do Corpse Pose.

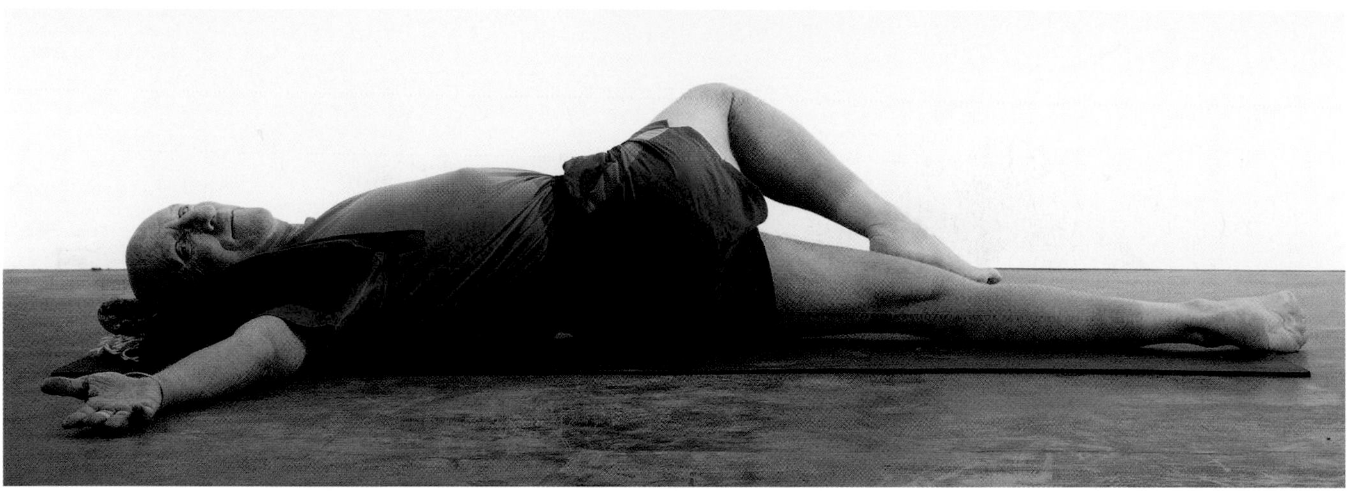

Figure 9.6. Lying Twist Pose to release the spine, with sandbags for stability

Meditation practice, too, can alleviate back pain, and you may recommend a simple one from chapter 5, practicing it with your students. Chanting may also help if they are open to it. Have them start simply, such as by chanting *Aum* nine times, and then sitting and watching, gradually increasing the number to twenty-seven (quarter *mala*) or fifty-four (half *mala*).

One yoga student was benefited significantly when, in addition to practicing poses, he began chanting a Sanskrit mantra 108 times each morning before his established meditation practice. He had come to yoga therapy complaining of low back pain and pain shooting down his right leg, manifesting when he was working as a script supervisor for the movie industry, which required long hours of standing on his feet in very stressful situations in which he had to get stars to use correct words and movements. He had been practicing yoga for many years, and it was clear that his pain was not just physical, as his body was flexible, balanced, and strong—that there was an underlying emotional and spiritual cause. He was given specific poses to practice aimed at opening his hips and lengthening his spine (Cat/Cow, Pigeon Prep, and Downward Facing Dog poses) and the mantra to chant. Thereafter, whenever he felt stressed on the job he mentally chanted the mantra and, in just a few weeks, his back and leg pain were gone.

Shoulder and Neck Pain

When treating shoulder or neck pain, before addressing the shoulders or neck the spine needs to be lengthened and made more flexible. One way to begin—especially for students whose torso and head are slightly forward and rounded and who show tightness in the mid-spine, the thoracic

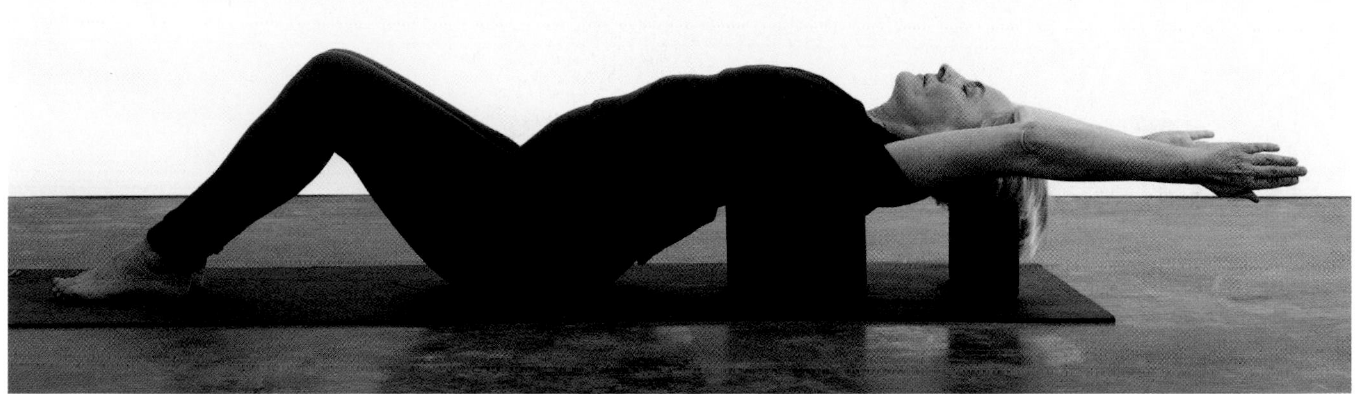

Figure 9.7. Shoulder opening on blocks with arms extended to lengthen spine

spine—is to lift the mid-spine by putting something underneath, such as a sandbag or block as shown in figure 9.7. With conscious breaths, students can feel the front body surrendering around the prop, allowing the thoracic spine to deepen into the body. Once the spine has flexibility, the students can lift their arms straight up, with their shoulders off the back, and then sink them down, feeling the armpits deepen as the head of the upper bone, the humerus bone, moves into the shoulder girdle. Once the humerus bone feels stabilized, they can bend the elbows and roll slightly to the floor a few times, then begin to move the arms back, staying at the minimum edge to avoid injury. The students should breathe deeply, holding the pose as long as the breath moves freely, there is no gripping in the body, such as in the jaws, chest, or legs, and the abdominal core is working to support the opening of the shoulders.

A student named Jenny used this pose successfully to treat shoulder pain. She had suffered from an intense "frozen shoulder" and was in so much pain that sleeping was difficult. She went to a doctor and physical therapist and made some progress but felt ready for more. This pose, along with additional core abdominal work, helped her regain 80 percent mobility in her shoulder in a month and normalcy a few months later. Jenny especially liked the fact that she could practice the pose at home each day and didn't need to rely on medication, making her feel more instrumental in healing.

Knee Pain

The first principle in addressing knee problems in yoga is to be aware of preventative measures. A regular asana practice that builds strength in the muscles around the knees can help protect them from the negative impact of too much pressure, which occurs especially while running, hiking, or playing sports.

Since knees can also be stressed when the outer leg is stronger than the inner leg, it is helpful to build strength around the knees by practicing balancing postures on one leg. Students can begin with the feet aligned correctly, pointing straight forward and building the arches by finding the four continents of connection on the bottom of the foot, with knees pointing straight forward and both hip points equally forward. The students can then practice balancing on one leg in a variety of poses (review balancing poses in chapter 6), eventually moving between poses, as that always takes extra balance and focus. Ensure that the knee remains facing forward, the muscles of the legs lifting strongly, perhaps bending the standing leg to be certain the knee is not hyperextending.

A therapeutic pose to open joints and release compression in the knees, is Hero Pose, Virasana (described in chapter 6), with knots tucked behind each knee. Have students kneel and place knots directly behind

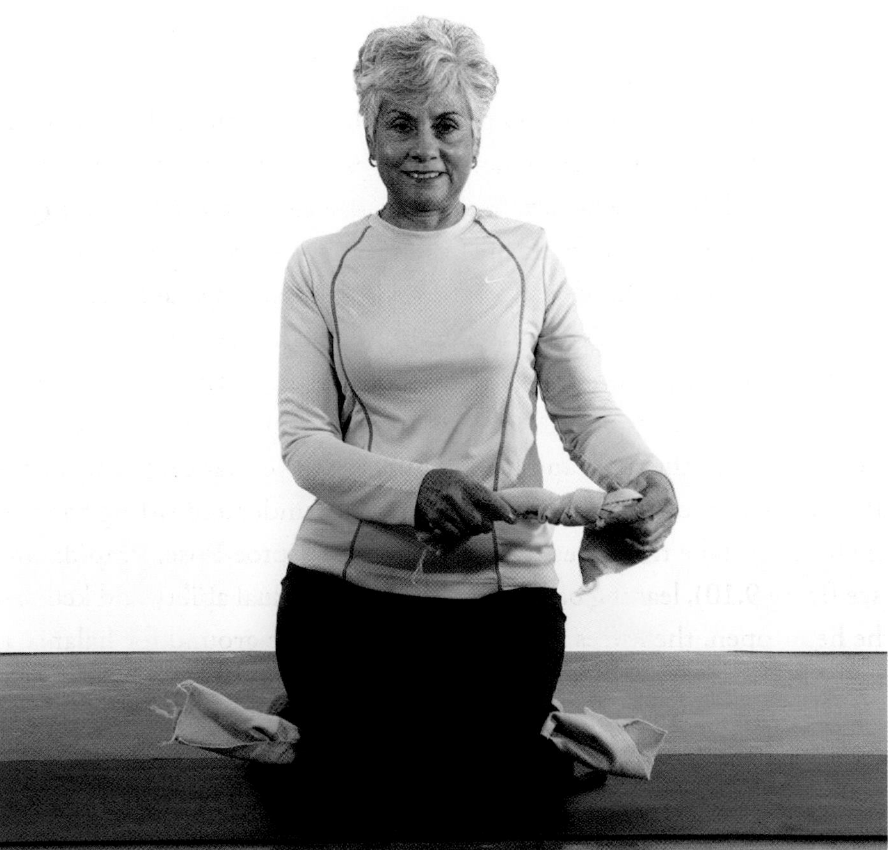

Figure 9.8. Hero Pose with knots to open knees

their knees, then move forward and sit down, probably on a block as shown in figure 9.8. The students can sit in this pose for a few minutes, working with the breath and lengthening the spine while lifting and extending the arms. When they come out of the pose and remove the knots, they should first sit for a few moments in Virasana and assess how their body feels. Then they should come up to their hands and knees, massage the calves, and reach one leg back at a time, tucking the toes and pressing back equally from all five ball mounts—one on the base of each toe—to lengthen the back of the knees. Next they can practice Downward Facing Dog or Standing Forward Fold Pose (figures 6.34 on page 155 and 6.23 on page 145).

One student, Irene, had chronic knee pain for years and felt immediate relief the first time she did Virasana using knots. Afterward, she practiced this at home every day, especially if she felt any discomfort, eventually becoming pain free. She still takes the knots on trips, as sitting in a car for long periods can cause knee pain. Irene's ability to both prevent and treat her pain herself gives her a sense of personal power.

Foot Pain

Foot pain can have a variety of causes, so the student is the best guide regarding therapy. In general, standing poses help align the entire body so that the weight is correctly on the feet. Specifically, you can help students with foot pain by first softening the calf muscles—having them roll a mat behind the knees and sit on it (see figure 9.9), making sure there is no pain, and using a block under the hips if the sensation is too intense. After two to five minutes in this Calves Release Pose, have the students move to Downward Facing Dog Pose and work one foot at a time, bringing the heel toward the floor and lengthening the lower back leg. Then have them work in the other direction, tucking toes under and sitting back on the heels, or take the knees out to the side in Tiptoe Pose, Prapidasana (see figure 9.10), leaning back according to individual ability and keeping the heart open, the knees lifted, and hands on the ground for balance if necessary.

One student came to yoga therapy because of nightly foot pain that interrupted her sleep. Within two weeks of practicing Prapidasana regularly in the morning and at night before bed, she had no more foot pain and could sleep well again.

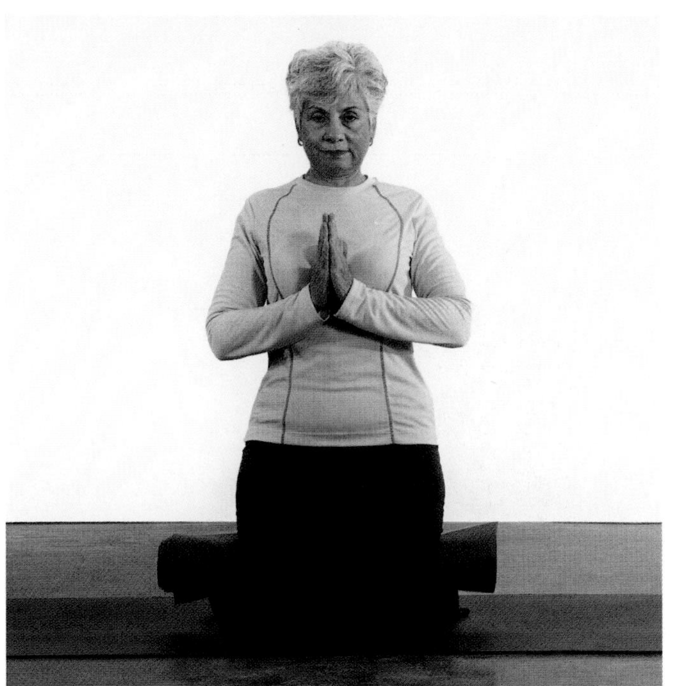

Figure 9.9. Rolled mat behind knees to relax calf muscles and open knees

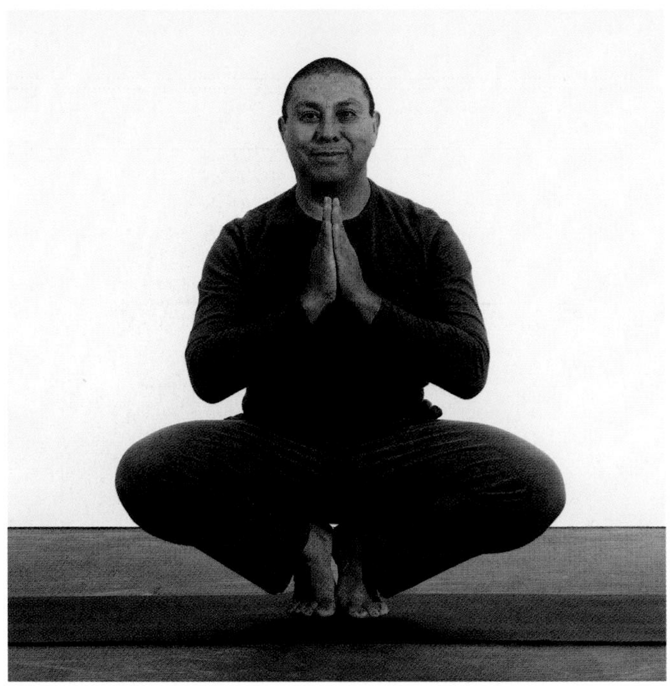

Figure 9.10. Tiptoe Pose—Prapidasana to open feet

Sciatica Pain

Sciatica pain, which emanates from the lower back, above the hip, is thought to be caused by the sciatic nerve, which travels from the lower back through the buttocks and into the leg. This type of pain can be treated by practicing poses that open the spine, especially at the sacrum, open the hips, and lengthen the hamstrings.

A series of Sacrum Release poses can help with a number of problems, as they address tightness and asymmetry in the sacrum.[3] Contractions around the sacrum can interrupt the free flow of *prana* and neurological information to the lower limbs of the body because the spinal cord runs through the spine from the brain and some neurological information from it exits the spinal column through the sacrum, traveling down the legs.

Have students begin the Sacrum Release poses by sitting on the edge of a chair, with sitting bones firmly on the chair. Then have them lean forward, pull the flesh away from their sitting bones, and move side to side. If their knees are below the top of the thighs, put blocks under their feet to stabilize the legs. Have them put their hands on their hips, inhale, lengthen their spine, and lift their sternum to the sky, moving

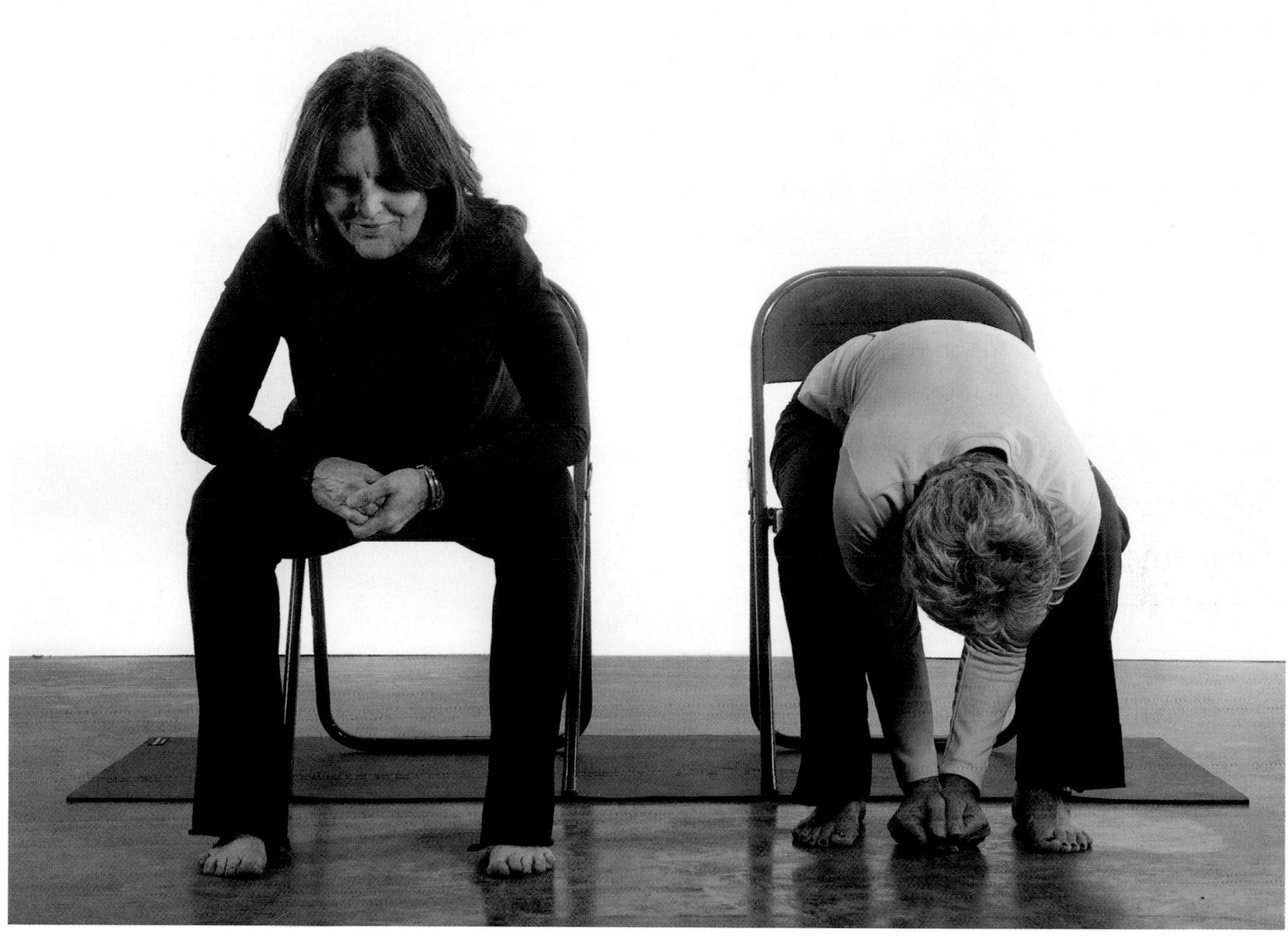

Figure 9.11. Sacrum Release sequence to lengthen spine

the elbows back. Next, have them exhale, round forward, pull their belly back, and let their elbows go forward. This is Cat/Cow Pose on a chair. They should practice this movement for about ten breaths, then come to inhale position and slowly move down until their elbows are on their knees and exhale.

Now have the students inhale and feel their back waist expand, then exhale and press their low back down between their legs (see figure 9.11). Have them stay in this pose, keeping their back long and movement isolated to the low back and sacrum. Then have them let their arms go between their legs, push their feet down with their hands, breathe, and hold for about ten breaths. Next, ask them to inhale and move up so their elbows are on their knees, pause, and lengthen the spine. On the next inhale, have them come up to a vertical position, closing their eyes and feeling the sensation.

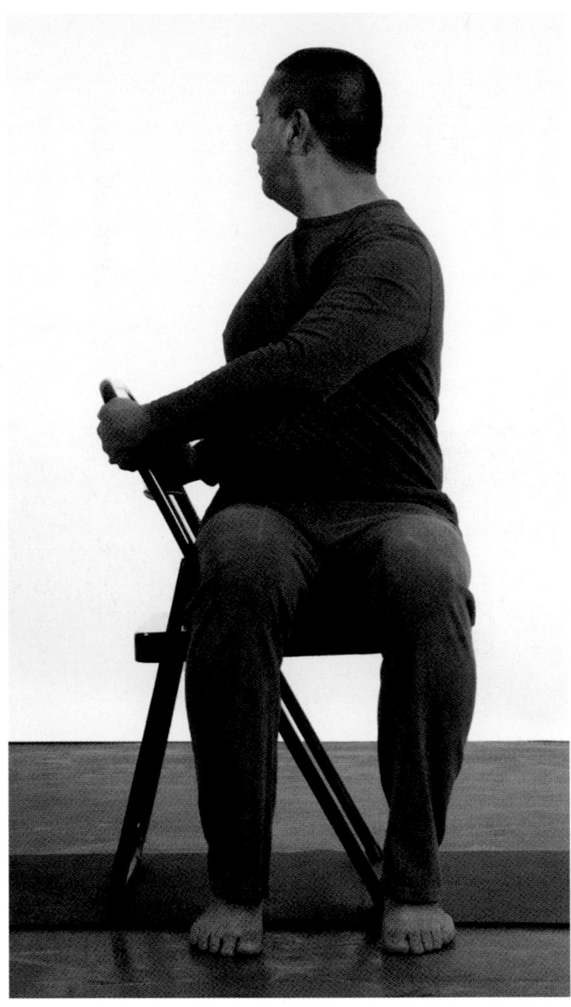

Figure 9.12. Chair Twist to lengthen spine and massage internal organs

Next, have them turn to one side of the chair and, pressing their feet firmly down, inhale and twist toward the back of the chair, putting their arms on the back to gently apply pressure on the exhale to twist, beginning from the belly (see figure 9.12). Have them inhale and elongate the spine, feeling their head reach to the sky, then exhale and twist, beginning with the lowest part of the spine. Have the students put their back hand on their sacrum and move it up and into the body as they inhale, then twist with that length. Have them practice it for about ten breaths, turn, and then practice it on the other side for ten breaths.

To open the hips, have students do the Pigeon Pose and Threading the Needle Pose, which is described as follows. Students begin by lying down with their legs bent, breathing easily, then bringing one knee to their chest and pulling it in as they resist with the other foot, still on the floor, and find the oppositional energy between the leg actions. Then have them put the lifted foot on the opposite thigh and press the knee away without letting their hip lift, holding it down with their hand. Keeping their lifted foot flexed, after some breaths have them raise their leg and thread the needle by putting one hand between their legs and the other on the outside, moving their leg toward their torso, and pressing their knee away with their elbow (see figure 9.13). Have them release after counting ten to fifteen breaths and repeat on the other side.

To lengthen the hamstrings and open the hips, have students do Lying Leg Lift. To begin, have them lie down, bring one leg to their chest, hook their foot with a belt, and slowly straighten the leg, keeping the knee, hip, and ankle in the same plane. Next, with breath, have them bring their leg toward their torso, keeping their hips level (see figure 9.14). After ten breaths, have them turn their foot and leg out and open to the side, keeping the opposite hip down. After ten more breaths, have them lift their leg and cross it over their torso in a Lying Twist for ten breaths, then repeat on the other side.

One student came for a yoga therapy session having suddenly experienced excruciating pain running from his low back down his right leg. He had been hospitalized and seen many specialists, who had diagnosed his condition as sciatica, but other than injecting a numbing medicine into his spine doctors had told him there was no treatment for his pain. Through

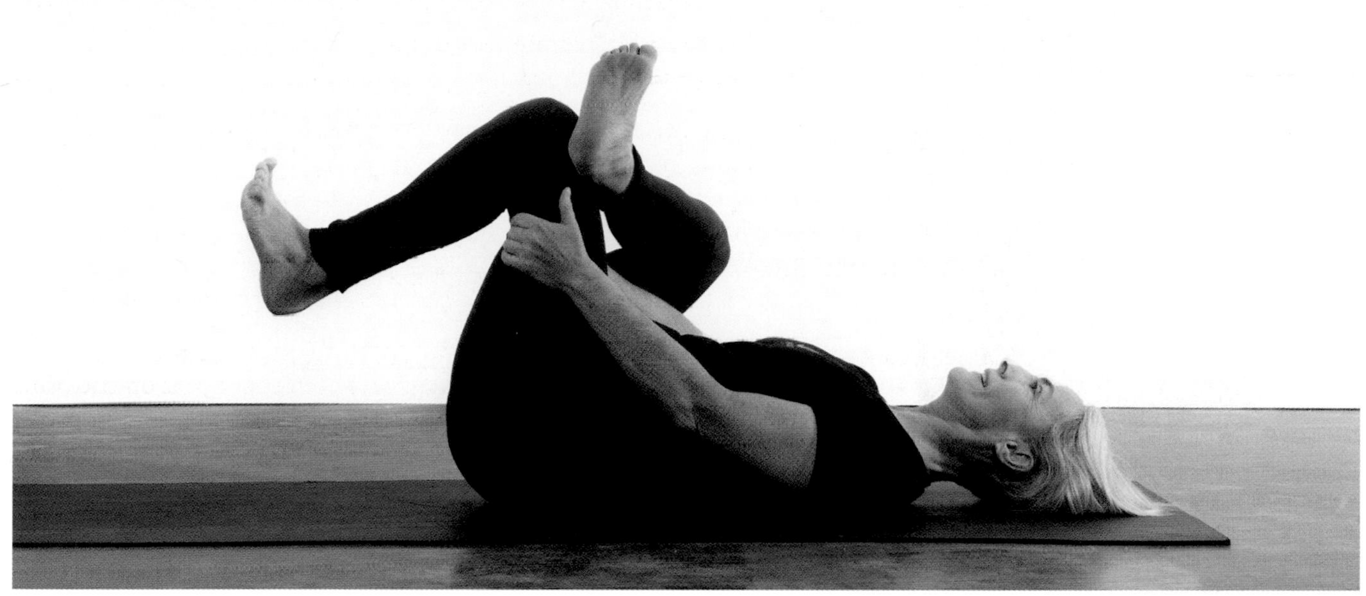

Figure 9.13. Threading the Needle Pose to open hips

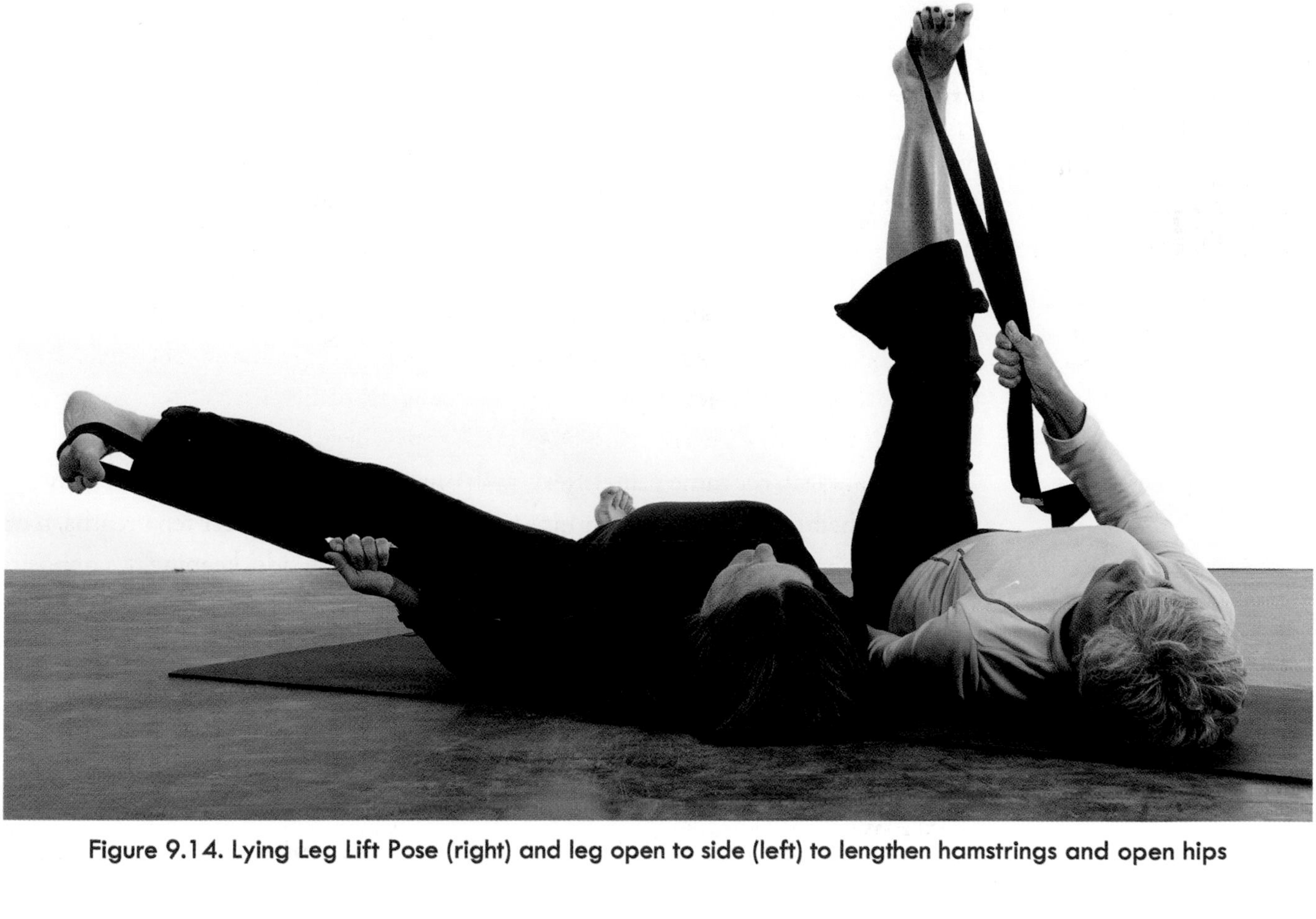

Figure 9.14. Lying Leg Lift Pose (right) and leg open to side (left) to lengthen hamstrings and open hips

regular practice of the poses in this section, however, his condition was relieved. Additionally, to prevent future problems he also changed the way he worked at his computer, standing instead of sitting for at least half of his work time, which was ten to twelve hours a day.

Depression

A regular well-balanced yoga practice helps many students find relief from depression. A yogi named Jean, a psychotherapist who treats people for depression, not only recommends yoga to her clients but says that yoga allows her to shift her own energy so that she can continue to be helpful and compassionate.

An especially excellent elixir for a depression that manifests as feeling lethargic and unmotivated is backbends, such as those described in chapter 6, depending on student ability. For best results, a practice composed largely of backbends should be balanced with standing poses, inversions, seated poses, and twists. If a depression manifests as agitation, however, calming practices are advisable, such as Seated Forward Fold Pose, Child's Pose, or Legs up the Wall Pose.

In addition to the specific forms of yoga therapy discussed in this section, teachers may devise other forms for these and other ailments, depending on the appropriateness of each situation.

YOGA AS A PROFESSION

As yoga comes to inform your life and worldview, you may want to make yoga your profession Today, many opportunities exist for working in the field of yoga, including teaching at hospitals, schools, prisons, in the workplace, and on the Internet. Corporate yoga is a way to work through the Human Resources Department of an organization offering yoga to workers and thus establishing contacts.[4]

To begin your career, you may want to first start volunteering and practice teaching yoga. Then, as you gain experience and expertise, you may wish to freelance, teaching at a number of venues, including perhaps teaching yoga to neighbors and friends in your own home. To prepare for freelance teaching, you should become a Registered Yoga Teacher (RYT) through the Yoga Alliance, a national nonprofit organization that sets minimum educational standards for yoga teachers and maintains a registry of yoga teachers and Registered Yoga Schools (RYS) qualified to offer teacher training. As yoga increasingly interfaces with our health-care system, there will be more need for regulation. The International Association of Yoga Therapists is currently implementing additional regulation, but for teaching yoga and practicing yoga therapy now, registration with the Yoga Alliance establishes a minimum level of professionalism.

As protection, you will want some kind of liability insurance in case a student sues you, even though such lawsuits occur infrequently. If you are teaching at a studio, health spa, or gym, they will have insurance to cover their liability, but you can also be sued personally and you don't want your personal assets at risk. You can purchase insurance from a variety of sources, ranging from the insurance carrier for your house or car to specialty brokers listed on the Yoga Alliance Web site.[5] Also be sure to collect personal information from students and a waiver statement saying they are responsible for their well-being and that you are not a medical professional (see appendix 2).[6] Although students who sign such a waiver statement can still sue you and force you to defend yourself, insurance will cover the costs of most cases that might arise.

After you've been teaching for some years and have a group of dedicated students, you may decide to open your own yoga studio. Running a yoga studio, however, requires significant management, business, and marketing skills, which are different from the skills necessary to teach yoga or apply yoga therapy. Management skills are needed to match teachers to classes, schedule classes, and arrange other events. The management skills I learned while working in corporate America have helped in running my yoga studio.

The numerous business skills required to successfully run a yoga studio include, first, keeping expenses as low as possible, which is critical to making a profit because the current cost of yoga classes is minimal. This involves watching the cost of rent; basic expenses, such as utilities, phone, and supplies; as well as the initial cost of props. It is also essential to keep careful track of all financial data for tax purposes.

Marketing skills are necessary to successfully attract the right kind of teachers and students to your studio. Since as studio owner you can only teach a limited number of classes a week, you will need a group of reliable, talented yoga teachers who, in turn, will draw a sufficient number of students to fill classes. My experience is that what brings students to classes is a teacher who has the ability not only to teach asana but to transmit knowledge about all eight limbs with heart.

To attract good teachers and interested students, it is wise to create a marketing plan. Such a plan does not have to rely heavily on paid media, the cost of which is usually prohibitive. Instead, it can focus primarily on methods of attracting teachers and students by word of mouth. Since yoga is a practice in which students are physically, mentally, and emotionally vulnerable, recommendations from friends concerning the positive energy and safety of a studio can be the most effective way to attract teachers and students. Such recommendations are likely if you make students feel valued by demonstrating your concern for them, learning their names, and remaining aware of any problems they express during practice. You can also attract students by offering incentives, such as a free class to anyone who brings a friend. In addition, free media advertising may be possible if you send press releases to local weeklies, newspapers, radio, TV, and community calendars, especially if you are able to create a news story about yoga with local interest. For example, you might focus on how advantageous it is to become more flexible before summer to avoid injury while engaging in summer vacation activities like biking and hiking.

An increasingly effective means of marketing is the Web, and so it is crucial to have a Web site that conveys the atmosphere of your studio and attracts good students. At a minimum, your site should show the class schedule, fees, location, and teachers, but as you expand you can add other features, such as links and yoga store items. Due to yoga's increasing popularity, not only do local individuals find prospective yoga classes online but travelers often use the Web to find classes at their destinations.

Once you have attracted a sufficient number of students, it is a good idea to invest in software programs to help you administer classes. Most are now Web based, so you can check on how classes are going even if you aren't there. By constantly assessing attendance you can see problems developing before they become critical.

Perhaps the single most important skill you need to maintain a successful yoga studio is the ability to stay alive in your own personal practice, constantly learning by reading and attending classes, paying attention to your students, and working to embody the yogic precepts in the *yamas* and *niyamas*, living and working from the eight limbs of yoga with enthusiasm and joy.

Glossary of Sanskrit Words and Phrases

Adho Mukha Svanasana. Downward Facing Dog Pose.

Adho Mukha Vrksasana. Headstand Pose; literally, Upward Facing Tree Pose.

Ahimsa. Abstention from harming others; nonviolence; love.

Ajna. Command; the sixth chakra, located at the third eye, between and slightly above the eyebrows, and associated with the seed syllable *Aum*, intuition, inner wisdom, and the color indigo.

Anahata. Unstruck; the fourth chakra, or heart chakra, located in the center of the body near the heart and associated with the seed syllable *Yam*, air, the sense of touch, and the color green.

Anandamaya kosha. The bliss body, or fifth—and subtlest—layer of experience, where all things become one, derived from the word *ananda* (bliss).

Anj. To adorn, honor, or celebrate.

Anjali. Offering.

Annamaya kosha. The physical body, or outermost layer of experience, derived from the words *anna* (food), *maya* (full of), and *kosha* (sheath or layer).

Aparigraha. Abstention from greed; awareness of abundance and fulfillment.

Ardha Chandrasana. Half Moon Pose.

Ardha Matshendrasana. Half Fish Twist Pose.

Asana. Pose; to sit.

Ashtanga. The eight-limbed path of yoga described by Patanjali in the Yoga Sutras, derived from the words *ashta* (eight) and *anga* (limbs, or component parts).

Ashtanga vinyasa. A form of yoga that focuses on synchronizing a type of breathing, called *ujjayi* breath, with a progressive series of postures so the body produces intense internal heat and a purifying sweat that detoxifies muscles and organs.

Asteya. Nonstealing; noncovetousness; generosity; honesty.

Atharva Veda. One of the four Vedas, composed around 4000 BCE.

Aum. The most famous seed syllable; associated with the sixth chakra.

Ayurveda. The science of life, derived from the words ayur (life) and veda (knowledge).

Bakasana. Crow Pose.

Bandha. Hold, lock, or tighten; energetic lifts or holds used to implement breathing patterns.

Bhagavad Gita. A foundational text of yoga that constitutes a portion of the *Mahabharata* describing the yoga of action, devotion, and wisdom.

Bhujangasana. Cobra Pose.

Brahmacharya. Moderation; boundaries; balance and protection of creative life forces.

Chakras. Vortices; wheels.

Chaturanga Dandasana. Four Limb Staff Pose.

Chikitsa. The first series in Ashtanga vinyasa yoga, which detoxifies and aligns the body.

Chin mudra. Gesture of consciousness.

Darshans. Six classical schools of Indian philosophy, one of which is yoga.

Devanagari. The main script used to write Sanskrit, written from left to right and containing a distinctive horizontal line linking the tops of the letters; derived from the words *deva* (god, brahman, or celestial) and *nāgarī* (city or sacred script of the city).

Dharana. Focus.

Dharma. A person's purpose or occupation; rules of proper conduct; duty to a higher law; principle or law that orders the universe.

Dhyana. Concentration.

Drishti. Gaze of the eyes.

Eka Pada Raja Kapotasana. Pigeon Prep Pose.

Garuda. The king of birds.

Gunas. The fundamental elements of nature: stability, activity, and lightness.

Harshad. Great joy.

Hatha. Today's most practiced form of yoga, derived from the words *ha* (sun) and *tha* (moon), meaning forceful; the balance of oppositional forces.

Hum. Seed syllable associated with the fifth chakra.

Ida. The female lunar *nadi* opposite *pingala nadi* going about the central *sushumna nadi.*

Isvara-pranidhana. Wholehearted dedication to others in the world; surrender to the Divine.

Jalandhara. Refers to throat and is derived from the words *jala* (net) and *dhara* (carrying or upward pull).

Jalandhara bandha. An energetic hold in the throat, with the sternum lifting up and the chin tucked down.

Janusirsasana. Knee to Head Pose.

Jathara Parivartanasana. Lying Twist Pose.

Jnana mudra. Gesture of knowledge.

Kaivalya. Liberation; happiness.

Kaivalya Pada. Fourth *pada* of the Yoga Sutras, translated as Cultivating Inner Freedom.

Kalyana mitra. An auspicious friend.

Kama Sutra. An ancient text, written between the first and sixth century CE, about how to reach enlightenment through conscious sexual practices, derived from the words *kama* (love) and *sutra* (treatise).

Kapalabhati. Shining skull, derived from the words *kapala* (skull) and *bhati* (shining); a form of breath cultivation.

Karma. Action or deed.

Kirtan. Devotional chanting.

Kitchari. Nourishing and strengthening mixture recommended during Ayurvedic cleansing programs.

Kosha. Sheath, layer.

Kula. Community of the heart.

Kumbhaka. Breath retention, derived from the word *kumbhah* (pot, either full or empty).

Kundalini. The upward flow of masculine and feminine forces from the base of the spine to the crown of the head; coiling like a snake.

Laksmi. Female manifestation of prosperity and abundance.

Lam. Seed syllable associated with the first chakra.

Maha. Big, great, noble.

Maha mantra. A great mantra.

Maha mudra. A gesture sometimes translated as the great psychic attitude.

Mahabharata. One of two great epic stories of ancient India, derived from the words *maha* (big, great) and *bharatas* (descendants of the legendary king Bharata); see also *Ramayana*.

Mahaprana. Cosmic energy.

Maharishi. A great one with the ability to see.

Mandala. Circle; center; completion.

Manipura. Jeweled city; the third chakra, the solar plexus, associated with the seed syllable *Ram*, power to affect the world (physically and psychically), fire, the sense of sight, and the color yellow.

Manomaya kosha. The mental body, or third layer of experience, derived from the word *mano* (mind, intellect, wisdom) and composed of *manas* (the rational mind) and *buddhi* (intellect).

Mantra. A chant with meaning beyond the reach of the mind or protection of the mind, derived from the words *man* (to think) or *manas* (mind) and *tra* (without or protection).

Marmas. Energy intersections in the subtle body, like chakras, except formed by the convergence of fewer energy lines.

Matsyendrasana. Fish Pose.

Maya. Full of.

Mimamsa. School of Indian philosophy providing rules for interpreting the Vedas and for justifying Vedic ritual.

Moksha. Liberation; happiness.

Mudra. A gesture, usually of the hands, that channels energies to energetic pathways, *nadis*, and centers, chakras, to create specific experiences in the body, mind, and spirit; attitude.

Mula. Root.

Mula bandha. An energetic hold used to lock *prana* in the organs of the pelvis.

Muladhara. The first chakra, derived from the words *mula* (root) and *adhara* (supporting), located at the base of the spine and associated with the seed syllable *Lam*, the earth, the color red, the sense of smell, and the feeling of being grounded.

Nadi shodhana. Alternate-nostril breathing, derived from the words *nadi* (channel, or flow) and *shodhana* (purification); the second series in Ashtanga vinyasa yoga, which purifies the nervous system.

Nadis. Energetic pathways throughout the body, forming vortices, or wheels, along the spine; channels, or flows.

Namaste. A salutation meaning, "I bow to you," or "From the still quiet place in me I bow to the quiet still space in you, and when we are both in that place we are one."

Nataraj. Cosmic dancer, derived from the words *nata* (dance) and *raj* (royal); a manifestation of Shiva as Lord of Yoga.

Navasana. Boat Pose.

Niyama. Personal observances; our attitudes toward ourselves; evolution toward harmony.

Nyaya. That which leads the mind to a conclusion; school of Indian philosophy focusing on study of the elements and states of matter.

Pada. Foot; also, part or chapter.

Parivrtta Janusirsasana. Revolved Knee to Head Pose.

Parivrtta Parsvakonasana. Revolved Side Angle Pose.

Parivrtta Trikonasana. Revolved Triangle Pose.

Parivrtta Utkatasan. Revolved Fierce Pose.

Parsva Bakasana. Side Crow Pose.

Parsvakonasana. Side Angle Pose.

Parsvotanasana. Side Stretched Out Pose.

Pascimottanasana. Seated Forward Fold Pose.

Pingala. The male solar *nadi* opposite *ida nadi* going about the central *sushumna nadi.*

Plankasana. Plank Pose.

Prakriti. Matter.

Prana. Life force.

Pranamaya kosha. The energy body, or second layer of experience, derived from the words *prana* (life force), *maya* (full of), and *kosha* (layer or sheath); the layer comprising the expansion of our vital energies.

Pranayama. Breath control.

Prapidasana. Tiptoe Pose.

Prasarita Padottanasana. Pyramid Pose.

Pratyahara. Sense withdrawal.

Purusha. Spirit.

Ram. Seed syllable associated with the third chakra.

Ramayana. One of two great epic stories of ancient India; see also *Mahabharata.*

Rig Veda. Considered the most ancient book in the world, composed around 4000 BCE; the earliest of the four Vedas and place where the word *yoga* first appears.

Sadhana Pada. Second *pada* of the Yoga Sutras, translated as Creating Spiritual Practice.

Sahasrara. Thousand-spoke wheel; the seventh chakra, the crown of the head, visualized as a thousand-petal lotus and the connection between self and the universe.

Salamabasana. Locust Pose.

Salamba Sarvangasana. Shoulderstand Pose.

Sama Veda. One of the four Vedas, composed around 4000 BCE.

Sama vritti. Full complete breathing.

Samadhi. Ecstasy; also bliss, freedom, pure consciousness, enlightenment.

Samadhi Pada. First *pada* of the Yoga Sutras, translated as Merging with Divine Self.

Samatvam. Equanimity.

Samyama. Self-control, derived from the words *sam* ([full/protection] self) and *yama* (control); also perfect discipline and integrated, regulated consciousness.

Sangha. Community of like-minded individuals.

Sankalpa. Intention, determination, purpose.

Sankhya. That which explains the whole; school of Indian philosophy espousing a method for dealing with all levels of manifestation.

Santosha. Contentment; cultivating happiness and peace with self and others; being comfortable with what we have.

Sarvaushadha. A panacea consisting of all herbs; quieting the heat of the body.

Satsang. A gathering of like-minded individuals.

Satya. Truth; right communication; integrity.

Sauca. Purity; cleanliness; simplicity, refinement.

Savasana. Corpse Pose.

Shakti. Creative female energy.

Shambhavi mudra. Focusing on the third eye.

Shanmukti mudra. A hand gesture for withdrawing the senses, derived from the words *shan* (six) and *mukti* (mouth).

Shiva. A major Hindu deity representing death.

Shodana. Purification.

Shrim. A seed syllable.

Sirsasana. Headstand Pose.

So hum. An ancient Sanskrit mantra meditation practice involving silently repeating the words *so* ("I am") and *hum* ("that"), meaning "I am that," or "I am that I am."

Sputa Virasana. Lying Hero Pose.

Sthira bhaga. The third series in Ashtanga vinyasa yoga, which integrates the other practices.

Sukkasana. Happy Pose.

Sushumna nadi. The central channel of the body, derived from the words *sushumna* ("She who is most gracious") and *nadi* (conduit).

Sutra. Thread—as in the medical term suture, a stitch to close a wound; also a style of writing used in many ancient Indian texts.

Svadhishthana. The second chakra, located a few fingers below the navel and above the root chakra, derived from the words *sva* (self) and *adhishthana* (base) and associated with the seed syllable *Vam*, safety, water, the sense of taste (literally or aesthetically), the color orange, and sexual desire.

Svadhyaya. Self-study; study of the Divine through scripture, nature, and introspection.

Swaha. Honoring.

Tadasana. Mountain Pose.

Tantra. That which expands wisdom; book; to weave.

Tapas. Focus; inner fire for self-discipline; passion for the work of yoga; purification.

Trataka. To look; a meditation practice involving gazing at an object.

Uddiyan bandhi. An energetic hold that builds core strength in the body.

Uddiyana. Upward flying.

Ujjayi. Victory; a type of breath control that generates inner heat and leads to an audible hiss.

Upanishad. Inner or mystic teaching; knowledge portion of the Vedas, derived from the words *upa* (near), *ni* (down), and *s(h)ad* (to sit).

Upavista Konasana. Seated Angle Pose.

Urdhva Danurasana. Upward Bow Pose.

Urdhva Hastasana. Upward Facing Arms Pose.

Urdhva Mukha Svanasana. Upward Facing Dog Pose.

Ustrasana. Camel Pose.

Utkatasana. Fierce Pose.

Uttanasana. Standing Forward Fold Pose.

Uttitha Trikonasana. Triangle Pose.

Vaisesika. School of Indian philosophy postulating that all objects in the physical universe are reducible to a finite number of atoms.

Vam. Seed syllable associated with the second chakra.

Vasisthasana. Side Plank Pose.

Veda. Knowledge, derived from the root *vid* (to know).

Vedanta. End of the Vedas, or the cultivation of knowledge; school of Indian philosophy advocating contemplative self-inquiry leading to the realization of one's true nature.

Vibhuti Pada. Third *pada* of the Yoga Sutras, translated as Manifesting Divine Power or On Supernatural Abilities and Gifts.

Vidyas. Wisdom knowers.

Vijnanamaya kosha. The intellectual body, or fourth layer of experience, derived from the words *vi* (intensity for all experiences) and *jnana* (knowledge, intellect, wisdom).

Vinyasa. To place in a special way; flowing sequence with breath.

Viparita Karani. Legs up the Wall Pose.

Virabhradrasana. Warrior Pose.

Virasana. Hero Pose.

Vishuddha. Pure; the fifth chakra, located at the throat and associated with the seed syllable *Hum*, finding your voice (literally as well as creatively), space, the sense of hearing, and the color blue.

Vrkrasana. Tree Pose.

Yajur Veda. One of the four Vedas, composed around 4000 BCE.

Yam. Seed syllable associated with the fourth chakra.

Yama. Abstinences.

Yantra. A specific geometric image, derived from the words *yan* (to support) and *trana* (freedom).

Yoga. Yolk; union.

Yoga-Bhashya. First commentary on the Yoga Sutras, written by Vyasa and translated as Discussion on Yoga.

Appendix One
Table of Yoga Poses

PRACTICE GUIDELINES

TEACHING GUIDELINES

THERAPEUTIC GUIDELINES

Appendix Two
Student Waiver Agreement

This waiver is not intended as a substitute for liability insurance coverage.

I, ____, understand that yoga
(print name)
includes physical movements as well as an opportunity for relaxation, stress reeducation, and relief of muscular tension. As is the case with any physical activity, the risk of injury, even serious or disabling, is always present and cannot be entirely eliminated. If I experience any pain or discomfort, I will listen to my body, adjust the posture, and ask for support from the teacher. I will continue to breathe smoothly.

Yoga is not a substitute for medical attention, examination, diagnosis, or treatment. Yoga is not recommended and is not safe under certain medical conditions. I affirm that I alone am responsible to decide whether to practice yoga. I hereby agree to irrevocably release and waive any claims that I have now or hereafter may have against (name of instructor, studio, and/or center).

____

Signature of student, parent, or guardian

____

Date

Appendix Three
Sample Classes

Gentle Class

- Lying Release Pose
- Three-part yogic breath with *kumbhaka* on inhale only
- Set intention as an offering
- Lying Twist Pose
- Lying Release with Leg Lift Variations
- Cat/Cow Pose
- Moon Salutations—slow, holding each position for five to eight breaths (in Puppy Dog Pose, with knees on floor, instead of Downward Facing Dog Pose)
- Warrior II Pose
- Pyramid Pose with blocks
- Revolved Side Angle Pose with back knee on floor
- Tree Pose
- Hero Pose with props
- Bridge Pose with block
- Camel Pose at wall
- Table Pose using wall or with legs up the wall
- Seated Forward Fold Pose with bent knees
- Lying Twist Pose
- Corpse Pose

Level 1 Class

- Lying Release Pose
- Three-part yogic breath with *kumbhaka* on inhale and exhale
- Set intention as an offering
- Shoulder opening on blocks with arms extended

- Lying Twist Pose
- Cat/Cow Pose
- Cat/Cow Pose with leg lifts
- Mountain Pose
- Standing Forward Fold Pose with props
- Warrior I Pose facing and using wall for stability
- Side Stretched Out Pose facing and using wall for stability
- Warrior II Pose
- Side Angle Pose
- Revolved Side Angle Pose
- Half Moon Pose using wall and props
- Handless Cobra Pose
- Camel Pose at the wall
- Downward Facing Dog Pose
- Table Pose using wall or with legs up the wall
- Tiptoe Pose
- Half Fish Twist Pose
- Seated Forward Fold Pose
- Lying Twist Pose
- Corpse Pose

Mixed Level Class

- Comfortable seated posture
- Set intention as an offering
- *Ujjayi* breath practice
- Cat/Cow Pose
- Mountain Pose
- Upward Facing Arms Pose
- Fierce Pose
- Standing Forward Fold Pose

- Warrior I Pose with arms behind back, fingers interlaced
- Torso folded forward on front or inside thigh
- Plank or Four Limb Staff Pose
- Cobra or Upward Facing Dog Pose
- Downward Facing Dog Pose
- Side Plank Pose and leg variations
- Warrior II Pose, Side Angle Pose, Triangle Pose
- Revolved Triangle Pose
- Pyramid Pose with arm variations
- Half Moon Pose flowing to Warrior III Pose
- Hero Pose and Reclined Hero Pose
- Full Wheel Backbend Pose (or Bridge Pose)
- Headstand or Legs up the Wall Pose
- Knee to Head Pose
- Revolved Knee to Head Pose
- Boat Pose
- Seated Forward Fold Pose
- Lying Twist Pose
- Corpse Pose

Flow Class

- Comfortable seated posture
- Set intention as an offering
- *Ujjayi* breath practice
- Cat/Cow Pose
- Sun Salutations with variations—holding for eight breaths with each pose, two rounds:
    - Mountain Pose, Upward Facing Arms Pose, Standing Forward Fold Pose, Warrior I Pose, Side Stretched Out Pose, Plank or Four Limb Staff Pose, Cobra Pose, Downward Facing Dog Pose. Repeat on the second side.

- Sun Salutations with variations—holding for eight breaths with each pose, two rounds:
    - Mountain Pose, Upward Facing Arms Pose, Fierce Pose, Warrior II Pose, Triangle Pose, Plank or Four Limb Staff Pose, Cobra Pose, Downward Facing Dog Pose. Repeat on the second side.
- Plank or Four Limb Staff Pose flowing to Cobra Pose flowing to Downward Facing Dog Pose, with a vinyasa between each one
- Side Plank Pose
- Pyramid Pose with arm variations
- Revolved Fierce Pose
- Warrior III Pose flowing to Tree Pose flowing to Pigeon Prep Pose
- Full Wheel Backbend Pose (or Bridge Pose) with leg lifts
- Handstand or Supine Bound Angle Pose
- Handstand variations, moving away from the wall
- Half Fish Twist Pose
- Crow Pose flowing to Side Crow Pose
- Seated Angle Pose flowing to Boat Pose, with legs apart then together
- Seated Forward Fold Pose
- Corpse Pose

Notes

Preface

1. Vyaas Houston, *The Yoga Sutra Workbook: The Certainty of Freedom* (Warwick, NY: American Sanskrit Institute, 1995), I.1.
2. Mahatma Gandhi, http://www.brainyquote.com/quotes/quotes/m/mohandasga131253.html.

Introduction

1. All dates regarding ancient texts in India are disputed; this date was routinely quoted as 1100–1700 BCE until archaeological evidence indicated an earlier date, for example.
2. Phil Catalfo, http://www.yogajournal.com/lifestyle/283.
3. International Sivananda Yoga *Vedanta* Centers, http://www.sivananda.org/ ttc/schedule.html.
4. Mukunda Stiles, *Yoga Sutras of Patanjali* (Boston: Red Wheel/Weiser, 2002), 25.
5. Ibid.
6. http://www.allspiritfitness.com/library/features/aa120400a.shtml.
7. Bill Harper, http://www.yogajournal.com/advertise/press_releases/10.
8. *Pema Chödrön and Alice Walker in Conversation: On the Meaning of Suffering and the Mystery of Joy*, Audio CD, Sounds True (1 Oct. 2005).
9. *The Principal Upanishads: The Essential Philosophical Foundation of Hinduism*, trans. Alan Jacobs (London, England: Watkins Publishing, 2007), 5.

Chapter 1. A Panoramic View of History and Ideas

1. Max Muller, http://www.dlshq.org/religions/vedas.htm.
2. Ravindra Raj Singh, *Death, Contemplation and Schopenhauer* (Farnham Surrey, England: Ashgate Publishing, 2007), 61.
3. Sogyal Rinpoche, *The Tibetan Book of Living and Dying* (San Francisco: HarperCollins, 1994).
4. "There are currently 16.5 million people who practice yoga [in the United States]," said Lynn Lehmkuhl, an editor at *Yoga Journal*. "And since 2002 that's been literally an increase of 43 percent, which is phenomenal." http://abcnews. go.com/GMA/Health/story?id=615557&page.

5. David Frawley, *Gods, Sages and Kings: Vedic Secrets of Ancient Civilization* (New Delhi, India: Motilal Banarsidass Publishers, 1993), 210.
6. Jacobs, trans., *The Principal Upanishads*, 5–6.
7. Stephen Mitchell, *Bhagavad Gita: A New Translation* (New York: Three Rivers Press, 2000), 68.
8. Sri Swami Satchidananda, *The Yoga Sutras of Patanjali* (Buckingham, VA: Integral Yoga Publications, 1978), 231–32.
9. Jaideva Singh, *Siva Sutras: The Yoga of Supreme Identity* (Delhi, India: Narendra Prakash Jain for Motilal, 1979), 58–59.
10. Rod Stryker, http://www.parayoga.com/, od@parayoga.com.
11. Swami Vishnu-devananda, *Hatha Yoga Pradipika* (New York: OM Lotus Publishing, 1987), 22.
12. Ibid., 128.
13. Ibid., 119.
14. Betheyla (circa Spring 2004).
15. Stiles, *Yoga Sutras of Patanjali*, 24–25 (see intro., n. 4).
16. Krishna Das, http://www.krishnadas.com/chanting.cfm.
17. Yoga student (name withheld for privacy purposes).
18. Yoga student Claudia Reiter (24 October 2005).
19. B.K.S. Iyengar, *Light on Yoga* (New York: Schocken Books, 1966), 41.
20. Patricia Walden, excerpted from "Genius in Action," http://www.yoga.com/www/patriciawalden/Reflections.html (October 2008); originally appeared on www.iynaus.org.
21. http://www.vermontwoman.com/articles/0206/yoga.shtml.
22. Pattabhi Jois, *Yoga Mala* (New York: Eddie Stern/Patanjali Yoga Shala, 1999), 42.
23. T.K.V. Desikachar, *The Heart of Yoga: Developing a Personal Practice* (Rochester, VT: Inner Traditions, 1995), xxvi.
24. Vanda Scaravelli, *Awakening the Spine: The Stress-Free Yoga That Works with the Body to Restore Health, Vitality, and Energy* (New York: Harper Collins, 1991), 28.
25. Much of this material about Indra Devi is from http://www.allspiritfitness.com/library/IndraDevi.shtml.
26. Paraphrased from a workshop at Upaya Zen Center in Santa Fe, New Mexico (July 2006).

Chapter 2. The Foundational Texts of Yoga

1. Web resources for the Yoga Sutras include: http://hrih.hypermart.net/patanjali/library/, http://www.sacredtexts.com/ hin/yogasutr

.htm, http://www.swamij.com/yoga-sutras.htm, http://www.daily readings.com/sutras_1.htm, and http://www.patanjalisutras.com/.

2. Stiles, *Yoga Sutras of Patanjali*, 11–12.
3. David MacKenzie, yoga teacher (23 April 2008).
4. Houston, *The Yoga Sutra Workbook*, I.1 (see pref., n. 1).
5. First seen on a bumper sticker from Northern Sun, http://www.northernsun.com/n/s/5434.html.
6. Barbara Miller, *Yoga Discipline of Freedom* (New York: Bantam, 1998), 29.
7. Stiles, *Yoga Sutras of Patanjali*, 2.
8. Jois, *Yoga Mala*, 16 (see ch. 1, n. 21).
9. T.K.V. Desikachar, *Reflections on Yoga Sutras of Patanjali* (Chennai, India: Krishnamacharya Yoga Mandiram, 1987), 19.
10. Chip Hartranft, *The Yoga-Sutra of Patanjali: A New Translation with Commentary* (Boston: Shambhala Publications, 2003), 2.
11. B.K.S. Iyenger, *Light on the Yoga Sutras of Patanjali* (London, England: Thorsons, 1993), 50.
12. Stiles, *Yoga Sutras of Patanjali*, 5.
13. Desikachar, *Reflections on Yoga Sutras of Patanjali*, 129.
14. Christopher Isherwood and Swami Prabhavananda, *How to Know God: The Yoga Aphorisms of Patanjali* (Hollywood, CA: *Vedanta* Press, 1953), 141–143.
15. Desikachar, *The Heart of Yoga*, 174–176.
16. Stiles, *Yoga Sutras of Patanjali*, 23–24.
17. Nischala Joy Devi, *The Secret Power of Yoga* (New York: Three Rivers Press, 2007), 163–164.
18. Lynne Twist, *The Soul of Money: Reclaiming Our Inner Resources* (New York: W. W. Norton, 2003), 74–77.
19. Desikachar, *Reflections on Yoga Sutras of Patanjali*, 64.
20. Mitchell, *Bhagavad Gita*, 62.
21. Ibid., 66.
22. Ibid., 62.
23. *The Bhagavad Gita*, Juan Mascaró, trans. (London, England: Penguin Books, 1962), 17.
24. Mitchell, *Bhagavad Gita*, 68.
25. Ibid., 78.
26. Ibid., 55.
27. Edward Waldo Emerson and Waldo Emerson Forbes, eds., *Journals of Ralph Waldo Emerson* (Boston: Houghton-Mifflin, 1909–1914), vol. 7: 241–42, 511; http://www/*vedanta*-newyork.org/articles/bhagavad_gita_5.htm.

28. *Journals of Ralph Waldo Emerson*, ibid.
29. Mahatma Gandhi, http://hinduism.about.com/library/weekly/extra/ bl-gitacomments.htm.
30. Ram Dass, *Paths to God: Living the Bhagavad Gita* (New York: Harmony Books, 2004), 52.

Chapter 3. Vibration As Tool

1. Mark Wheeler, "Signal Discovery?" *Smithsonian Magazine* (March 2004): http://www.smithsonianmag.com/science-nature/Signal_Discovery. html?c=y&page=1,
2. Jacobs, trans., *The Principal Upanishads*, 45–46.
3. Stiles, *Yoga Sutras of Patanjali*, 8–9, I.27–28.
4. http://www.psyking.net/id36.htm.
5. Thomas Ashley-Farrand, *Healing Mantras* (New York: Random House, 1999), 36–61.

Part II. On the Mat

1. Desikachar, *The Heart of Yoga*, 181.

Chapter 4. Breath, Bandhas, and Mudras: The Subtle Realm

1. Dr. David Anderson, a scientist who heads research on behavior and hypertension at the National Institute on Aging at the National Institutes of Health, believes the way we breathe may hold a key to how the body regulates blood pressure and that it has less to do with relaxation than with breaking down the salt we eat. Currently, he is attempting to prove his premise, which could shed new light on the relationship between hypertension, stress, and diet. See http://www.foxnews.com/story/0,2933,206454,00.html.
2. http://www.clevelandclinic.org/health/health-info/docs/2900/2963.asp?index=10684.
3. Stiles, *Yoga Sutras of Patanjali*, 30, II. 52–53.
4. Scaravelli, *Awakening the Spine*, 28 (see ch. 1, n. 23).
5. Animated anatomical depiction of swallowing, http://www.linkstudio.info/images/portfolio/medani/Swallow.swf.
6. Satchidananda, *Yoga Sutras of Patanjali*, 57.
7. Swami Niranjanananda Saraswati, *Prana Pranayama Prana Vidya* (Bihar, India: Yoga Publications Trust, 2002), 1.
8. Jill Bolte Taylor, http://www.ted.com/index.php/talks/view/id/229.
9. Sarahjoy Marsh, personal correspondence (2 Jan 2008).

10. Some experts say up to 50 percent of women who have had more than one child will eventually develop a prolapse; http://www.bbc.co.uk/health/womens_ health/issues_pelvicprolapse.shtml.
11. Vishnu-devananda, *Hatha Yoga Pradipika*, 128.
12. Ibid., 133.
13. Swami Svatmarama, *Hatha Yoga Pradipika* (New York: Om Lotus Publishing, 1987), 105.
14. Gertrud Hirschi, *Mudras: Yoga for the Hands* (San Francisco: Red Wheel/Weiser, 2000), 60, 150.
15. Gratitude produces more serotonin and melatonin than any other emotional state. These neurotransmitters are responsible for states of happiness and peace.
16. Swami Muktibodhananda, *Hatha Yoga Pradipika* (Bihar, India: Yoga Publications Trust, 1985), 294–97.

Chapter 5. Meditation for Beauty and Bliss

1. Stiles, *Yoga Sutras of Patanjali*, 30.
2. Ibid., 31–32.
3. See http://www.dhamma.org/ for more information.

Chapter 6. Poses for Freedom

1. Vishnu-devananda, *Hatha Yoga Pradipika*, 17.
2. American philosopher Joseph Campbell, http://www.yogajournal.com/lifestyle/1318?print=1.
3. Swami Poornaseva, "Sowing the Seeds of Change," *Australian Yoga Life* 21, p. 6.
4. To learn more about anatomy and physiology in relation to yoga, see the bibliography.
5. Women's Sports Foundation, "Her Life Depends on It: Sport, Physical Activity and the Health and Well-Being of American Girls" (May 2004) is the most comprehensive compilation of research to date about the impact of physical activity on the physical, psychological, and social health of girls. The report points to physical activity and sport as solutions for many serious health and social problems faced by girls, including obesity, heart disease, substance abuse, teen pregnancy, and depression—which account for much of the more than $1 trillion spent on health care for treating these issues. See http://www.womens colleges.org/news/depends-onit.htm.
6. Stiles, *Yoga Sutras of Patanjali*, 46.
7. http://www.sivananda.org/teachings/asana/exercise.html.

8. Sris Chandra Vasu, *Gherand Samhita: A Treatise on Hatha Yoga* (London, England: Theosophical Publishing House, 1895), 25–26.
9. Swami Sivananda Radha, *Hatha Yoga: The Hidden Language, Symbols, Secrets, and Metaphors* (Montreal, Canada: Timeless Books, 2006), 57.
10. Vanda Scaravelli's backbends and inspiring discussions of life can be viewed in the documentary video *Vanda Scaravelli on Yoga*, http://www.yoga. net.au/benefits2.
11. Vishnu-devananda, *Hatha Yoga Pradipika*, 137.
12. Inversions often help reduce high blood pressure but should be done cautiously and with the consent of a physician. Research concerning yoga and hypertension can be found on the Web site PubMed, a service of the United States National Laboratory of Medicine, part of the National Institutes of Health.
13. Iyengar, *Light on Yoga*, 190.
14. Leslie Kaminoff, *Yoga Anatomy* (Champagne, IL: Human Kinetics, 2007), 88.

Chapter 7. Yoga in Everyday Life

1. There is an engaging and informative discussion of the *Kama Sutra* by Wendy Doniger on a six-CD set entitled *Erotic Spirituality and the Kama Sutra* (Boulder, CO: Sounds True, 2003).
2. Georg Feuerstein, *Tantra: The Path of Ecstasy* (Boston: Shambhala Publications, 1998), 242 and Sudhir Kakar, *Kamasutra* (Philadelphia, PA: Running Press, 2003), 77–98.
3. Thomas Moore, "Sex (American Style)," *Mother Jones* (Sept/Oct 1997), http://motherjones.com/politics/1997/09/sex-american-style.
4. To learn more about NVC, including training sessions domestically and internationally, visit www.cnvc.org.
5. *The Upanishads*, trans. Max Müller; http://www.sacred-texts.com/hin/sbe15/sbe15035.htm.
6. Ayurvedic Institute, Albuquerque, NM, offers books, online resources.
7. Mohandas Gandhi, *Anasaktiyoga: The Gospel of Selfless Action: The Gita According to Gandhi* (Ahmedabad, India: Navajivan Publishing House, 1946), 131.

Chapter 8. Teaching Yoga

1. Scaravelli, *Awakening the Spine*, 46.
2. Indra Devi, *Yoga Unveiled*. A DVD (2004), disc 1.

3. For a state-by-state teacher training program list, including Kripalu, White Lotus, Anusara, and Iyengar styles of yoga, visit http://www.yogajournal.com/directory/.
4. Yoga Alliance, a nonprofit, tax-exempt organization, maintains a national Yoga Teachers' Registry to recognize and promote teachers with training that meet their standards.
5. http://yogaalliance.org/Conduct.html.
6. http://www.yogajournal.com/for_teachers/mentor_experts.

Chapter 9. Yoga Therapy Training and Yoga As a Profession

1. Well-known yoga therapy training centers include Integrative Yoga Therapy (IYT), Phoenix Rising Yoga Therapy, Mukunda's Yoga Therapy Center, American Viniyoga Institute, Samata Yoga Center, Yoga Biomedical Trust, and the Yoga Therapy and Training Center.
2. http://www.iayt.org/; choose Professional Resources.
3. The sequence was adopted and modified from teachings of Rama Birch, the founder and creator of Svaroopa Master Yoga.
4. http://www.corporateyoga.org/.
5. http://yogaalliance.org/Insurance.html.

Bibliography

BOOKS AND ARTICLES

Alcamo, Edward I. *Anatomy Coloring Workbook*. New York: Random House, 1997.

Ashley-Farrand, Thomas. *Healing Mantras: Using Sound Affirmations for Personal Power, Creativity, and Healing*. New York: Random House, 1999.

Bachman, Nicolai. *The Language of Yoga: Complete A to Y Guide to Asana Names, Sanskrit Terms, and Chants*. Louisville, CO: Sounds True, 2005.

Bouanchaud, Bernard. *The Essence of Yoga: Reflections on the Yoga Sutras of Patanjali*. Portland, OR: Rudra Press, 1997.

Buddhananda, Swami. *Moola Bandha: The Master Key*. Bihar, India: Yoga Publications Trust, 1996.

Carroll, Cain, and Lori Kimata, ND. *Partner Yoga: Making Contact for Physical, Emotional, and Spiritual Growth*. Emmaus, PA: Rodale Books, 2000.

Catalfo, Phil. http://www.yogajournal.com/lifestyle/283.

Chödrön, Pema. *When Things Fall Apart: Heart Advice for Difficult Times*. Boston: Shambhala Publications, 2000.

Clarke, Michaela, and Sally Griffyn. *Ashtanga Yoga for Women: Invigorating Mind, Body, and Spirit with Power Yoga*. Berkeley, CA: Ulysses Press, 2003.

Coulter, H. David, and Timothy McCall. *Anatomy of Hatha Yoga: A Manual for Students, Teachers, and Practitioners*. Honesdale, PA: Body and Breath, 2001.

Das, Krishna. http://www.krishnadas.com/chanting.cfm.

Dass, Ram. *Paths to God: Living the Bhagavad Gita*. New York: Harmony Books, 2004.

Desikachar, Kausthub. *The Yoga of the Yogi: The Legacy of T Krishnamacharya*. Chennai, India: Krishnamacharya Yoga Mandiram, 2005.

Desikachar, T.K.V. *The Heart of Yoga: Developing a Personal Practice.* Rochester, VT: Inner Traditions, 1995.

_______. *Reflections on Yoga Sutras of Patanjali.* Chennai, India: Krishnamacharya Yoga Mandiram, 1987.

Devi, Indra. *Yoga for Americans: A Complete Six Weeks' Course for Home Practice.* Englewood Cliffs, NJ: Prentice Hall, 1969.

Devi, Nischala Joy. *The Secret Power of Yoga: A Woman's Guide to the Heart and Spirit of the Yoga Sutras.* New York: Three Rivers Press, 2007.

Devi, Nischala, Dean Ornish, MD, and Shaye Areheart. *The Healing Path of Yoga: Time-Honored Wisdom and Scientifically Proven Methods That Alleviate Stress, Open Your Heart, and Enrich Your Life.* New York: Three Rivers Press, 2000.

Emerson, Edward Waldo, and Waldo Emerson Forbes, eds. *Journals of Ralph Waldo Emerson.* Boston: Houghton-Mifflin, 1909–1914.

Feuerstein, Georg. *The Shambhala Encyclopedia of Yoga.* Boston: Shambhala Publications, 1997.

_______. *Tantra: The Path of Ecstasy.* Boston: Shambhala Publications, 1998.

Frawley, David. *Gods, Sages and Kings: Vedic Secrets of Ancient Civilization.* New Delhi, India: Motilal Banarsidass Publishers, 1993.

_______. *Yoga and Ayurveda: Self-Healing and Self-Realization.* Twin Lakes, WI: Lotus Press, 1999.

Gandhi, Mahatma. http://hinduism.about.com/library/weekly/extra/bl-gitacomments.htm.

_______. http://www.brainyquote.com/quote/m/ mohandasga131253.html.

Gandhi, Mohandas. *Anasaktiyoga: The Gospel of Selfless Action: The Gita According to Gandhi.* Ahmedabad, India: Navajivan Publishing House, 1946.

Gannon, Sharon, and David Life. *Jivamukti Yoga: Practices for Liberating Body and Soul.* New York: Random House, 2002.

Hafiz. *The Gift.* New York: Penguin, 1999.

Hartranft, Chip. *The Yoga-Sutra of Patanjali: A New Translation with Commentary*. Boston: Shambhala Publications, 2003.

Hirschi, Gertrud. *Mudras: Yoga for the Hands*. San Francisco: Red Wheel/Weiser, 2000.

Houston, Vyass. *The Yoga Sutra Workbook: The Certainty of Freedom*. Warwick, NY: American Sanskrit Institute, 1995.

Isherwood, Christopher, and Swami Prabhavananda. *How to Know God: The Yoga Aphorisms of Patanjali*. Hollywood, CA: *Vedanta* Press, 1953.

Iyengar, B.K.S. *Light on Yoga*. New York: Schocken Books, 1966.

_______. *Light on the Yoga Sutras of Patanjali*. London, England: Harper Collins 1993.

_______. *Yoga: The Path to Holistic Health*. New York: Dorling Kindersley: 2001.

Iyengar, B.K.S., and Yehudi Menuhin. *Light on Pranayama: The Yogic Art of Breathing*. New York: Crossroad Publishing, 1999.

Jacobs, Alan, trans. *The Principal Upanishads: The Essential Philosophical Foundation of Hinduism*. London, England: Watkins Publishing, 2007.

Jois, Pattabhi, *Yoga Mala*. New York: Eddie Stern/Patanjali Yoga Shala, 1999.

Juhan, Deane. *Job's Body: A Handbook for Bodywork*. Barrytown, NY: Barrytown, Ltd., 1998.

Kabat-Zinn, Jon. *Wherever You Go There You Are: Mindfulness Meditation in Everyday Life*. New York: Hyperion, 1994.

Kaminoff, Leslie. *Yoga Anatomy*. Champaign, IL: Human Kinetics, 2007.

Kirk, Martin, Brooke Boon, and Daniel DiTuro. *Hatha Yoga Illustrated: For Greater Strength, Flexibility, and Focus*. Champaign, IL: Human Kinetics, 2004.

Kraftsow, Gary. *Yoga for Wellness: Healing with the Timeless Teachings of Viniyoga*. New York: Penguin, 1999.

Lasater, Judith. *Relax and Renew: Restful Yoga for Stressful Times*. Berkeley, CA: Rodmell Press, 1995.

Little, Tias. *Sthira Sukham Asanam: Handbook for Yoga Postures*. Santa Fe, NM: Yogasource, 2003.

Long, Ray. *The Key Muscles of Hatha Yoga*. Plattsburgh, NY: Bandha Yoga Publications, 2005.

Mascaró, Juan, trans. *The Bhagavad Gita*. London, England: Penguin Books, 1962.

_______, trans. *The Upanishads*. New York: Penguin, 1965.

McCall, Timothy. *Yoga As Medicine: The Yogic Prescription for Health and Healing*. New York: Random House, 2007.

Mehta, Silva, Mira, and Shyam. Yoga: *The Iyengar Way*. New York: Dorling Kindersley, 1990.

Mesko, Sabrina. *Healing Mudras: Yoga for Your Hands*. New York: Ballantine, 2000.

Miller, Barbara Stoler. *The Bhagavad-Gita: Krishna's Counsel in Time of War*. New York: Bantam Books, 1986.

_______. *Yoga Discipline of Freedom: The Yoga Sutra Attributed to Patanjali*. New York: Bantam Books, 1998.

Mitchell, Stephen. *Bhagavad Gita: A New Translation*. New York: Three Rivers Press, 2000.

Mittra, Dharma. *Asanas: 608 Yoga Poses*. Novato, CA: New World Library, 2003.

Muktibodhananda, Swami. *Hatha Yoga Pradipika*. Bihar, India: Yoga Publications Trust, 1985.

Müller, Max, trans. *The Upanishads*. http://www.sacred-texts.com/hin/sbe15/sbe15035.htm.

Myers, Esther. *Yoga and You: Energizing and Relaxing Yoga for New and Experienced Students*. Boston: Shambhala Publications, 1996.

Myers, Esther, and Lynn Wylie. *The Ground, the Breath, and the Spine*. Toronto, Ontario, Canada: Esther Myers, 1992.

Netter, Frank H. *Atlas of Human Anatomy*. Teterboro, NJ: Icon Learning Systems, 2003.

Pappas, Stephanie. *Yoga Posture Adjustments and Assisting*. Victoria, BC: Trafford Publishing, 2006.

Poornaseva, Swami. "Sowing the Seeds of Change," *Australian Yoga Life* 21, 6.

Radha, Swami Sivananda. *Hatha Yoga: The Hidden Language, Symbols, Secrets, and Metaphors*. Montreal, Canada: Timeless Books, 2006.

Radhakrishnan, Sarvepalli. *Indian Philosophy*. Princeton, NJ: Princeton University Press, 1989.

Roach, Geshe Michael, and Christie McNally. *The Essential Yoga Sutra: Ancient Wisdom for Your Yoga*. New York: Three Leaves Press, 2005.

_______. *How Yoga Works*. Pompton Plains, NJ: Diamond Cutter Press, 2004.

Rosen, Richard. *The Yoga of Breath: A Step-by-Step Guide to Pranayama*. Boston: Shambhala Publications, 2002.

Rosenberg, Marshall. *Nonviolent Communication: A Language of Life*. Encinitas, CA: Puddle Dancer Press, 2003.

Ross, Steve. *Happy Yoga: 7 Reasons Why There's Nothing to Worry About*. New York: HarperCollins, 2003.

Salzberg, Sharon. *Lovingkindness: The Revolutionary Art of Happiness*. Boston: Shambhala Publications, 2002.

Saraswati, Swami Niranjanananda. *Prana Pranayama Prana Vidya*. Bihar, India: Yoga Publications Trust, 2002.

_______. *Yoga Nidra*. Bihar, India: Yoga Publications Trust, 2005.

Saraswati, Swami Satyananda. *Asana Pranayama Mudra Bandha*. Bihar, India: Bihar School of Yoga, 1999.

_______. *Kundalini Tantra*. Bihar, India: Bihar School of Yoga, 1984.

_______. *Yoga Darshan*. Bihar, India: Yoga Publications Trust, 1993.

Sargeant, Winthrop. *The Bhagavad Gita*. Albany: State University of New York Press, 1994.

Satchidananda, Sri Swami. *The Yoga Sutras of Patanjali*. Buckingham, VA: Integral Yoga Publications, 1978.

Scaravelli, Vanda. *Awakening the Spine: The Stress-Free Yoga That Works with the Body to Restore Health, Vitality, and Energy*. New York: HarperCollins, 1991.

Schiffmann, Erich. *Yoga: The Spirit and Practice of Moving into Stillness*. New York: Pocket Books, 1996.

Shantananda, Swawi. *The Splendor of Recognition*. South Fallsburg, NY: SYDA Foundation, 2003.

Singh, Jaideva. *Siva Sutras: The Yoga of Supreme Identity*. Delhi, India: Narendra Prakash Jain for Motilal, 1979.

Singh, Ravindra Raj. *Death, Contemplation and Schopenhauer*. Farnham Surrey, England: Ashgate Publishing, 2007.

Sogyal, Rinpoche. *The Tibetan Book of Living and Dying*. San Francisco: HarperCollins, 1994.

Sparrowe, Linda, Patricia Walden, and Judith Hanson Lasater. *The Woman's Book of Yoga and Health: A Lifelong Guide to Wellness*. Boston: Shambhala Publications, 2002.

Stiles, Mukunda. *Structural Yoga Therapy*. Boston, MA: Weiser Books, 2000.

_______. *Yoga Sutras of Patanjali*. Newburyport, MA: Weiser Books, 2002.

Stryker, Rod. http://www.parayoga.com.

Svatmarama, Swami. *Hatha Yoga Pradipika*. New York: Om Lotus Publishing, 1987.

Svoboda, Robert E. *Ayurveda for Women*. Newton Abbot, Devon, England: David and Charles, 1999.

_______. *Prakruti*. Albuquerque, NM: Geocom, 1989.

Swenson, David. *Ashtanga Yoga: The Practice Manual*. Houston, TX: Ashtanga Yoga Productions, 1999.

Tolle, Eckhart. *A New Earth: Awakening to Your Life's Purpose*. New York: Penguin Group, 2005.

Twist, Lynne. *The Soul of Money: Reclaiming the Wealth of Our Inner Resources*. New York: W.W. Norton, 2003.

Vasu, Sris Chandra. *The Gheranda Samhita: A Treatise on Hatha Yoga*. London, England: Theosophical Publishing House, 1895.

Vishnu-devananda, Swami. *Hatha Yoga Pradipika*. New York: OM Lotus Publishing, 1997.

Yee, Rodney. *Moving Toward Balance: 8 Weeks of Yoga with Rodney Yee*. Emmaus, PA: Rodale, 2004.

DVDS AND CDS

Aburdene, Patricia. *Megatrends 2010*. Boulder, CO: Sounds True DVD, 2007.

Chasse, Betsy, Mark Vicente, and William Arntz. *What the Bleep Do We Know!?* Beverly Hills, CA: Captured Light and Lord of the Wind Films DVD, 2004.

Chödrön, Pema. *Pema Chödrön and Alice Walker in Conversation: On the Meaning of Suffering and the Mystery of Joy*. Boulder, CO: Sounds True Audio CD, 2005.

Chopra, Deepak. *Sacred Verses, Healing Sounds: The Bhagavad Gita, vols I and II*. Novato, CA: New World Library/Amber-Allen Publishing CD, 1994.

Devi, Indra. *Yoga Unveiled: The Evolution and Essence of a Spiritual Tradition*. Directed by Gina and Mukesh Desai. Canada: Gita Desai, DVD, 2004.

Doniger, Wendy. *Erotic Spirituality and the Kama Sutra*. Boulder, CO: Sounds True 6-CD set, 2003.

Grilley, Paul. *Anatomy for Yoga*. San Francisco: *Pranayama* Inc. DVD, 2003.

Myers, Esther. *Vanda Scaravelli on Yoga*. Toronto, Ontario, Canada: Esther Myers DVD and video, 1991.

Rosenberg, Marshall. *Nonviolent Communication with Marshall Rosenberg*. Peace Talks Radio.

Image Credits

PHOTOGRAPHS

Grateful acknowledgment is made for permission to reprint the following:

Dedication page: Betheyla, *Ed Zadlo.*

Figure 1.2: Pashupati seal drawing, *Jodi Call-Swedberg.*

Figure 1.3: Map of India, *Stasys Eidiejus/BigStockPhoto.com.*

Figure 1.8 Kundalini energy channels, *Chakras: Energy Centers of Transformation by Harish Johari, Peter Weltevrede (artist), Inner Traditions/Bear & Co., www.InnerTraditions.com.*

Figure 1.9: Swami Vivekananda, *Advaita Ashrama.*

Figure 1.10: Krishnamacharya, *Indra Devi Foundation, Buenos Aires, Argentina, www.fid.org.ar.*

Figure 1.11: Iyengar and Scaravelli, *Rossella Baroncini.*

Figure 1.12: Krishna Das, *Dan Steinberg.*

Figure 1.13: Richard Rudis, *James Daley Photographs.*

Figure 1.14: Indra Devi (Mataji), *Indra Devi Foundation, Buenos Aires, Argentina, www.fid.org.ar.*

Figure 2.1: Patanjali drawing, *Jodi Call-Swedberg.*

Figure 3.1 Chakra petals with Sanskrit letters, *Chakras: Energy Centers of Transformation by Harish Johari, Peter Weltevrede (artist), Inner Traditions/Bear & Co., www.InnerTraditions.com.*

Figure 4.5: Diaphragm, *Andrea Danti/BigStockPhoto.com.*

Figure 5.8: Mandala for meditation, *Desiree Walstra/BigStockPhoto.com.*

Figure 6.2: Bones of the Body and Spine, *The Key Muscles of Hatha Yoga by Ray Long, MD, Chris Macivor (illustrator), Bandha Yoga, 3rd edition.*

Figure 6.3: Sitting bones, ibid.

Figure 6.4: Hip joint, ibid.

Figure 6.5: External rotators of hips, ibid.

Figure 6.6: Psoas muscle group, ibid.

Figure 6.7: Quadricep muscles, ibid.

Figure 6.8: Hamstring muscles, ibid.

Figure 6.9: Abdominal muscles, ibid.

Figure 6.44: Vanda Scaravelli in Backbend Pose, *Rob Howard.*

Figure 6.58: Seated twisting anatomy, *The Key Muscles of Hatha Yoga by Ray Long, MD, Chris Macivor (illustrator), Bandha Yoga, 3rd edition.*

Figure 7.1: Temple at Konark Orissa, *Jeremy Richards/BigStockPhoto.com.*

Figure 7.8: Needs Mandala, inspired by the work of Marshall Rosenberg, PhD (developer of *Nonviolent Communication*), and Chilean economist Manfred Max-Neef, PhD. Copyright © 2005 PeaceWorks, Jim and Jori Manske (radicalcompassion.com), CNVC Certified Trainers in *Nonviolent Communication* (cnvc.org).

Figure 9.2: Psoas muscle group, *The Key Muscles of Hatha Yoga by Ray Long, MD, Chris Macivor (illustrator), Bandha Yoga, 3rd edition.*

Author photograph on page 312 copyright © Muki Pictures, LLC.

All other photographs and renderings are from the author's studio collection.

ILLUSTRATIONS

Figure 1.1: Historical Timeline of Yogic Philosophies, Texts, and Key Figures, *conceived by Meta Chaya Hirschl, rendered by Felicia Montoya.*

Figures 2.2, 2.3, 2.4, 4.1, 5.1, 5.3, 5.4, 5.5: Ashtanga map and series, *Angela Werneke.*

Figure 3.3: Aum, *Cypresse Emery.*

Figure 3.6: The five koshas, *Felicia Montoya.*

Figure 5.10: Ashtanga Primary Series, *Jodi Call-Swedberg.*

Figure 6.64: Sun Salutations, *Jodi Call-Swedberg.*

Figure 6.65: Moon Salutations, *Jodi Call-Swedberg.*

Figure 8.1: Golden Rule of Teaching, *Felicia Montoya.*

In Gratitude . . .

My first bow of gratitude is for the practice of yoga, which supports me in ways that continually astound me, and for the guidance I receive from meditation.

A special thank you to my agent, Gareth Esersky, for finding Matthew Lore, of The Experiment, who shares my enthusiasm for spreading the vision of yoga through this second edition.

The first edition owes much to Ellen Kleiner, editor and muse; Angela Werneke, designer; Felicia Montoya, graphic stylist of the charts and timeline; and Tina Larkin, photographer. Deep bows and gratitude to Gary Cordova, who created the Sanskrit Devanagari names for the poses with aplomb despite adversity. Special thanks to Nicolai Bachman, MA, for his wise consultation on dates and details of history, philosophy, and Sanskrit. And thanks to Ray Long, MD, for the generous permission to use his anatomy illustrations.

Thanks also to the models—Cypresse Emery, Wyatt Heard, Dharmashakti McBride, Felice Garcia, Irene Kersting, Jenny DeBouzek, Kelly Coogan, Leah Roberts, Lisa Keck, and Ross Perkal—for showing up with patience and good humor in sometimes hard conditions, or as Wyatt said, under circumstances that "would require combat pay in peacetime."

Thanks as well to the artists Cypresse Emery and Jodi Call-Swedberg, who gave their creative efforts with yogic devotion.

Thanks, too, to Albuquerque's Rio Grande Botanic Garden, for providing the backdrop for the mudra photos, and to Maryann Torrez and Toni Martorelli, for their vision of yoga at the Japanese Garden Pond.

In addition, I want to express abundant gratitude for all the ways my family, friends, and yoga community have supported me and this project: to my daughters, Shona and Bella, who cheered me on and kept me going when the boulder seemed to do nothing but roll back down on me; to my parents, Pat Browne and Harry Hamel Hirschl, for their enduring love and now friendship; to Amy Anixter Scott for her friendship and encouragement; to Charlene and David Schroeder, who were there when the teaching light struck, and for their beautiful space for YogaNow; to my family of yogis at YogaNow, especially Heidi Heard, who single-handedly filled my Gentle yoga classes; and to all students everywhere whom I've had the honor to teach and who have also taught me. There is no doubt that, for me, it does take a village to write a book.

Finally, I bow deeply, with great respect, to the teachers who have come before me, including my teachers, and to beings everywhere. May we all be happy, free, know liberation from pain, and come together in union, in yoga, to help one another thrive on this sacred place we call Mother Earth.

INDEX

Page numbers in *italics* indicate photographs or drawings.
Page numbers followed by "n" refer to the Notes.

C

D

E

F

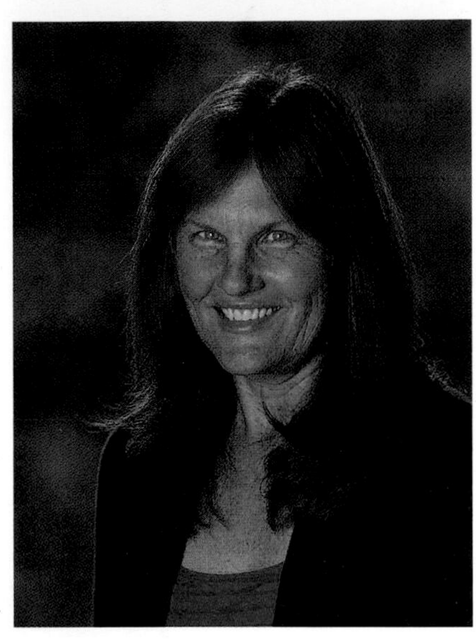

About the Author

Meta Chaya Hirschl's path to yoga was circuitous, and ultimately powered by her passion for vitality of body and mind. She began her professional career in the food industry, supervising the production of beer for Miller Brewing Company, graham cracker pie shells for Nestle in Milwaukee, and soda for Pepsi in Brooklyn. Meta earned an MBA at New York University to support her transition to another field, then worked at Arthur Anderson & Co. installing large systems for IBM, NJ Dept. of Labor, NYNEX, and ConEd. After moving to Indiana, she taught systems at Purdue University.

After having her first child in 1987, Meta developed severe asthma and was stunned by the prospect of a lifetime of drugs and curtailed activities. For the next twenty years, she challenged that fate. Yoga was her vehicle to a full and vibrant life.

Meta's yoga quest included seven teacher-training programs from a wide variety of teachers and styles. Always a voracious reader, she drew and continues to draw knowledge and inspiration from the ancient texts of yoga, particularly the Bhagavad Gita, the Yoga Sutras, and the Radiant Sutras. She studies Sanskrit and chants and meditates daily. By meditating for eleven hours daily at a ten-day Vipassana retreat, she honed her skills and deepened her understanding of quieting within.

In 2001, Meta opened a yoga studio in Albuquerque. She has since developed a nationally certified teacher-training program that is the basis of this book. Her vision for *Vital Yoga* is to elevate understanding of all that yoga offers—which includes both learning body and mind poses on the mat and working with the body and mind out in the real world.

Meta's new focus is the huge population suffering from asthma. She hopes to embody the message that the radiant health she enjoys thanks to the holistic approach of yoga is available to other asthmatics as well. With her renewed vigor, Meta has hiked down and up the Grand Canyon five times, and has also completed the Big Sur marathon. Meta is now in training for another outdoor adventure, and she hits the trail with her beloved dog, Dharma, whenever she can.